T0313805

Tethered Cord Syndrome in Children and Adults

Second Edition

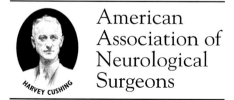

American Association of Neurological Surgeons

and the American Association of Neurosurgeons

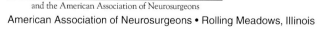

American Association of Neurosurgeons • Rolling Meadows, Illinois

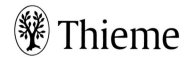

Tethered Cord Syndrome in Children and Adults

Second Edition

Shokei Yamada, MD, PhD, FACS
Professor and Chairman Emeritus
Department of Neurosurgery
Loma Linda University School of Medicine
Loma Linda, California

Visiting Professor
Department of Neurosurgery
University of Mississippi Medical Center
Jackson, Mississippi

Consultant
Department of Neurosurgery
Arrowhead Regional Medical Center
Colton, California

Consultant
Department of Neurosurgery
Kaiser Permanente Medical Center
Fontana, California

Thieme
New York • Stuttgart

American Association of Neurosurgeons
Rolling Meadows, Illinois

Thieme Medical Publishers, Inc.
333 Seventh Ave.
New York, NY 10001

American Association of Neurosurgeons (AANS)*
5550 Meadowbrook Drive
Rolling Meadows, Illinois 60008-3852

*The abbreviation AANS refers to both the American Association of Neurological Surgeons and the American Association of Neurosurgeons.

Editorial Director: Michael Wachinger
Executive Editor: Kay D. Conerly
Editorial Assistant: Lauren Henry
International Production Manager: Andreas Schabert
Production Editor: Print Matters, Inc.
Vice President, International Marketing and Sales: Cornelia Schulze
Chief Financial Officer: James W. Mitos
President: Brian D. Scanlan
Compositor: Thomson
Printer: Everbest Printing Company Ltd.

Library of Congress Cataloging-in-Publication Data

Tethered cord syndrome in children and adults / [edited by] Shokei Yamada. — 2nd ed.
    p. ; cm.
  Rev. ed. of: Tethered cord syndrome / edited by Shokei Yamada. c1996.
  Includes bibliographical references and index.
  ISBN 978-1-60406-241-0 (alk. paper)
  1. Spinal cord—Abnormalities. I. Yamada, Shokei. II. Tethered cord syndrome.
  [DNLM: 1. Neural Tube Defects. WL 101 T347 2009]
  RD768.T435 2009
  617.5'6—dc22
                          2009022008

Important note: Medical knowledge is ever-changing. As new research and clinical experience broaden our knowledge, changes in treatment and drug therapy may be required. The authors and editors of the material herein have consulted sources believed to be reliable in their efforts to provide information that is complete and in accord with the standards accepted at the time of publication. However, in view of the possibility of human error by the authors, editors, or publisher of the work herein or changes in medical knowledge, neither the authors, editors, or publisher, nor any other party who has been involved in the preparation of this work, warrants that the information contained herein is in every respect accurate or complete, and they are not responsible for any errors or omissions or for the results obtained from use of such information. Readers are encouraged to confirm the information contained herein with other sources. For example, readers are advised to check the product information sheet included in the package of each drug they plan to administer to be certain that the information contained in this publication is accurate and that changes have not been made in the recommended dose or in the contraindications for administration. This recommendation is of particular importance in connection with new or infrequently used drugs.

Some of the product names, patents, and registered designs referred to in this book are in fact registered trademarks or proprietary names even though specific reference to this fact is not always made in the text. Therefore, the appearance of a name without designation as proprietary is not to be construed as a representation by the publisher that it is in the public domain.

The material presented in this publication by the AANS is for educational purposes only. The material is not intended to represent the only, nor necessarily the best, method or procedure appropriate for the medical or socioeconomic situations discussed, but rather it is intended to present an approach, view, statement, or opinion of the faculty, which may be helpful to others who face similar situations.

Neither the content, the use of a specific product in conjunction therewith, nor the exhibition of any materials by any parties coincident with this publication, should be construed as indicating endorsement or approval of the views presented, the products used, or the materials exhibited by the AANS, or its Committees, Commissions, or Affiliates.

Printed in China

5 4 3 2 1

ISBN 978-1-60406-241-0

To my dearest wife, Rachel for her support and patience, and my children Vivian, Cheryl, and Brian for their understanding

Contents

Continuing Medical Education Credit Information and Objectives

■ Objectives

Upon completion of this activity, the learner should be able to:

1. Discuss and describe the embryology and pathophysiology necessary to diagnose and treat tethered cord syndrome.
2. Discuss the anatomic and functional diagnosis of tethered cord syndrome using both neurologic examinations and imaging procedures.
3. Discuss and evaluate the various medical and surgical treatments of tethered cord syndrome.

■ Accreditation

This activity has been planned and implemented in accordance with the Essentials and Standards of the Accreditation Council for Continuing Medical Education through the American Association of Neurological Surgeons (AANS*). The AANS is accredited by the Accreditation Council for Continuing Medical Education to provide continuing medical education for physicians.

■ Credit

The AANS designates this educational activity for a maximum of 15 *AMA PRA Category 1 credits*™. Physicians should only claim those hours of credit commensurate with the extent of their participation in the activity.

The Home Study Examination is online on the AANS Web site at: http://www.aans.org/education/books/tetheredcord.asp

Estimated time to complete this activity varies by learner, and activity equaled up to 15 Category 1 credits of CME.

■ Release/Termination Dates

Original Release Date: January 12, 2010
The CME termination date is: January 12, 2013

The acronym AANS refers to both the American Association of Neurological Surgeons and the American Association of Neurosurgeons.

Continuing Medical Education Disclosure

The AANS controls the content and production of this CME activity and attempts to ensure the presentation of balanced, objective information. In accordance with the Standards for Commercial Support established by the Accreditation Council for Continuing Medical Education, authors (and the significant others of those mentioned) are asked to disclose any relationship they or their co-authors have with commercial companies that may be related to the content of their chapter.

Authors (and the significant others of those mentioned) who have disclosed a relationship* with commercial companies whose products may have a relevance to their chapter are listed below.

Author Name	Disclosure	Type of Relationship
J. Paul Jacobson	Genelux	Shareholder
David S. Knierim	Company LDR visit to factory in France 2008	other financial support
George T. Mandybur	Medtronic Corp.	Industry Grant Support

The following authors have disclosed that they do not have a relationship with commercial companies whose products may have a relevance to their chapter(s):

Author Name:

Austin R. T. Colohan	Bermans Iskandar	W. Jerry Oakes	John Walsh
Mark S. Dias	Antoine Khoury	Dachling Pang	Daniel J. Won
Anthony J. DiPatri	Daniel K. Kido	Sharad Rajpal	Brian Yamada
James Drake	Samir Lapsiwala	Gideon D. Richards	Shokei Yamada
Robin L. Gilmore	Sun Ik Lee	Elias B. Rizk	Shoko Yamada
Nalin Gupta	Russell R. Lonser	Herbert Ruckle	Vivian A. Yamada
Roger Hadley	David McLone	Sanford Schneider	Alexander Zouros
David B. Hinshaw	Kenji Muro	Javed Siddiqi	
Jason L. Hwang	Marvin D. Nelson	R. Shane Tubbs	

*Relationship refers to receipt of royalties, consultantship, funding by research grant, receiving honoraria for educational services elsewhere, or any other relationship to a commercial company that provides sufficient reason for disclosure.

Foreword to the First Edition

There are many kinds of textbooks written today but nearly all of them are more technical and less interesting than they should be, and few of them are written to provide a clear and understandable approach to the problem under discussion.

A good textbook should grip the reader in much the same way as a well-crafted adventure story and should appeal to many levels of expertise. One should feel the urge to continue reading beyond the initial area of interest, even though one's comprehension is being stretched to the limit and the new thoughts are sometimes difficult to integrate.

Since my first experience with the operative repair of a lumbar myelomeningocele some 45 years ago, I have had an intense interest in the complex ramifications of developmental anomalies of the central nervous system. Here at last in Professor Yamada's book are the answers to some of these intriguing puzzles.

The chapters on embryology and physiology are brilliant in their clarification of the abnormalities of structure and function, while those on radiology and clinical studies are current not only procedurally but also in theory. I hope that the chapter entitled "Tethered Cord Syndrome in Adults" will demonstrate to "adult" neurosurgeons, urologists, and orthopedists that the tethered cord is not confined to the arena of interest of the pediatric subsections of their specialties!

This is not just a book for neurosurgeons and neurologists. It will be a source of information for senior medical students, residents, internists, and other health care providers.

All chapters are eminently readable, stand alone, and avoid the use of technical jargon. This is unusual and most welcome in these days of information flood.

I recommend most strongly *Tethered Cord Syndrome* to all those who have an interest in or even a passing involvement with the patient with problems of the central nervous system and, in particular, spinal cord dysfunction.

I enjoyed every chapter.

E. Bruce Hendrick, MD, FRCS(C)
Emeritus Professor
Department of Neurology
Hospital for Sick Children
Toronto, Ontario, Canada

Foreword to the Second Edition

One might wonder just when the word *tether* made its way into the medical lexicon and what the implications of this label were. Some would be familiar with its application to animals and a tether limiting their ability to roam within the radius allowed. By contrast, radius fixation is moot when the term is applied to the consequences of multiple forms of intrinsic intradural spinal column developmental pathology. The feature of this form of tethering inhibits "the ascent of the intrathecal nervous tissue within the vertebral canal during growth."[1] Several years passed following this alert before there began an effort to explain the disturbed anatomy of the tethered spinal cord. In 1981, the editor of this text became the leading academic of this disorder, a devotion that remains with him to this day.[2]

The various applications of "tether" were incorporated first into the multiple and intriguing patterns of "closed" spinal dysraphism (e.g., diastematomyelia, lipomyelomeningocele, the benign dermoid and epidermoid tumors, and the whimsically labeled "fatty filum"). Children's neurosurgeons also began regretting their earlier repairs of open neural tube defects in newborn infants. As time passed, many noted that the intradural landscape was cluttered with adhesions that were "anchoring the cord" and that such could only have resulted from operative technique. These architectural features became apparent to clinicians coincident with the emergence of magnetic resonance imaging technology.

The second edition of this book brings forth source information with respect to folate supplementation and the reduction of neural tube defects, modern imaging features of the dysraphic spine, the accomplishments of intrauterine myelomeningocele repair, and appropriately for the continuum through to adulthood the features of the tethered cord as well as urological management that even in its mildest forms is a given in every aging patient. This book is directed at those with career paths identical to its authors but also to those in the fields of rehabilitation medicine and physio- and occupational therapy, as well as to frontline pediatricians and others who take care of an aging population.

Robin P. Humphreys, MD
University of Toronto
Toronto, Ontario, Canada

---

[1] James CCM, Lassman LP. Spinal Dysraphism. Spina Bifida Occulta. London, Butterworths; 1972:83.

[2] Yamada S, Zinke D, Saunders D. Pathophysiology of "tethered cord syndrome." J Neurosurg 1981;54:494–503.

Preface

In the first edition (1996), the editor expressed his gratitude for the acceptance of tethered cord syndrome (TCS) as a standard of medical practice. This acceptance followed many decades of skepticism that viewed the expression *tethered cord* as limited to visual impressions without scientific background or merit. Today's practice of neurosurgery and the associated research that will lead to even better neurosurgerical practice in the future is indebted to the many clinicians and scientists who defined TCS as a clinical syndrome and brought understanding to the pathophysiology, diagnosis, and treatment of this syndrome. The excellent contributions of the many clinicians and investigators in that edition and in this updated second edition underscore the importance for health care professionals to know the signs and symptoms of TCS and of treatment options and prognoses.

The first edition, published by AANS (1996), emphasized that accurate diagnosis and proper treatment of TCS requires understanding TCS pathophysiology and its links with TCS symptomatology. Responses were such that the book was sold out within a few years. This second edition was prompted by such acceptance of the first edition and also by the facts that (1) many patients with disabling TCS symptomatology are still unaware of such a syndrome, (2) the range of knowledge about TCS among medical professionals continues to be variable, and (3) there are still multiple interpretations of TCS among neurosurgeons and related specialists.

Goals of this edition were to weave its 21 chapters among themes in a manner that provides new information and answers to questions that have developed since the first edition. The first of these themes is the essential background necessary for understanding TCS, its diagnosis, and treatment. Chapter 2 (embryology) explains with beautiful illustrations the complexities of central nervous system growth and the clinical problems found in spinal cord patients when there are deviations from normal spinal development. Chapter 3 (pathophysiology) reviews basic understandings of TCS and distinguishes this syndrome from that which occurs in patient with similar symptomatology when there is visual cord tethering.

The second theme is TCS diagnosis, which is complex given that TCS requires a functional diagnosis in a manner similar to epilepsy. This is because TCS is not strictly anatomical, which would allow it to be regarded in the same manner as spinal cord tumors.

Within this broad topic, Chapter 4 describes key techniques for neurologically examining TCS patients, whereas Chapters 5 and 6 summarize imaging procedures that are essential to demonstrate anomalies in the spinal canal and to assist in accurately diagnosing this syndrome. These chapters emphasize the importance of carefully evaluating the locus of anomalies by magnetic resonance imaging (MRI) or ultrasonography when categorizing TCS in the manner described in Chapter 1. Chapters 7 and 8 center on the urological aspects of TCS, which may include incontinence with or without motor and sensory dysfunction. These chapters report that a goal of TCS treatment should be early correction of urinary dysfunction and prevention of irreversible incontinence. Chapter 10 discusses neurological lesions of cervical TCS that can be localized either cephalic or caudal to the tethering site, whereas Chapter 9 relates TCS to pediatric patients, revisiting the original "tethered spinal cord" by Hoffman et al and updating new development.

Adult TCS was expanded to include late teenage patients whose follow-up is often lost in the gap between pediatric and adult neurosurgeons. Chapter 15 summarizes findings in TCS patients without neural spinal dysraphism. These patients are often referred to neurosurgeons because they suffer disabling back and leg pain for many months or years without definite diagnosis. The diagnosis in this age group requires physicians' familiarity with the specific symptomatology and imaging features, and an understanding of the pathophysiology of TCS. In contrast, Chapter 16 describes occult TCS, which includes patients with lipomyelomeningoceles and those with cord elongation and filum thickening. Also within this theme is Chapter 11, which considers surgical treatment of a variety of lipomyelomeningoceles. Related as well are Chapter 12, which describes epidermoid or dermoid to be related to TCS, and Chapters 17 and 18, which review diagnostic-related findings in the caudal end of the spinal cord, the diameter of the terminal filum. These two chapters support the inelastic nature of the filum to be the mechanical cause of TCS as a functional disorder.

The third theme relates to TCS treatment, including surgery for myelomeningoceles and lipomyelomeningoceles (cf. Chapters 11, 13, and 16). Chapter 13 describes in utero surgical attempts to prevent progressive and permanent neurological deficit that might develop during gestation. Chapter 14 details results of folate administration in pregnant women for prevention of myelomeningoceles. Chapters 19 and 20 detail progress in neurophysiological testing (preoperative and postoperative somatosensory or motor evoked potential recording) for enhancing TCS diagnosis, and intraoperative recording of lumbosacral cord or sacral nerve root stimulation to protect the nerve elements.

■ Acknowledgments

At this opportunity, I would like to acknowledge my remarkable mentor and longtime associate, Dr. George Austin, an outstanding neurosurgeon and scientist who became the first professor and chairman of neurosurgery at Loma Linda University School of Medicine. Dr. Austin encouraged my scientific studies of tethered cord syndrome, and it was under his aegis that I studied and conducted research on spinal cord physiology and surgery. I am also grateful for the authoritative and friendly cooperation of professors Bruce Hendrick, Harold Hoffman, and Robin Humphreys, and the continuing support of their colleagues. I am also indebted to Dr. Myron Rosenthal, professor of neurology and physiology and vice provost for human subject research at the University of Miami, for our many critical discussions on this topic and for his collaborative support in studies of experimental spinal cord tethering.

I am pleased also to express my appreciation for the contributions and support of professors E. Harry Botterell, Charles H. Tator, Michael G. Fehlings (Toronto, Ontario), Joseph P. Evans, Sean F. Mullan (Chicago, Illinois), Julian R. Youmans, Phanor L. Perot (Charleston, South Carolina), Francis Jobsis, George Somjen (Durham, North Carolina), Joseph LaManna (Cleveland, Ohio), Reiji Natori, and Toshio Sakai (Tokyo, Japan). My gratitude extends to Dr. Richard Start (Brantford, Ontario), Dr. and Mrs. Henry Sugiyama (Toronto, Ontario), and Dr. Alice Felten (Chicago, Illinois) for their encouragement during my neurosurgical training.

I further wish to express my special admiration and gratitude to the contributors for their accomplishments, which made this publication possible. For the past year, the editor has received the special assistance of two dedicated neurosurgeons who provided the momentum to the book completion. Professor Mark Linskey (Irvine, California), the chair of the AANS Publication Committee, gained the cooperation of Dr. Bermans Iskandar (Madison, Wisconsin). Dr. Iskandar shared communications with the editor in persuading authors to complete their chapters promptly. It was with his consistent, selfless, and conscientious assistance that the book was completed within one year of his involvement. In addition, perfect understanding of the principle of the tethered cord syndrome was most valuable for this new edition.

I appreciate my late brothers Drs. Shotoku and Shotetsu Yamada for the constant encouragement and financial support for my research, and my parents Dr. Shoan and Mrs. Toki Yamada for directing my life in my young days.

I thank the editorial staff—Kay Conerly, Lauren Henry, and Ivy Ip—for their consistent communication throughout the publication process; and Richard Rothschild for his clear and capable responses to the editor with appropriate discussions during the editing of proofs, which made the process very effective. I value the initial impetus with which Professor Daniel L. Barrow and Ms. Joanne Needham promoted the first edition of *Tethered Cord Syndrome*. Further I thank Professor James Rutka for bridging the AANS and Thieme Medical Publishers for the second edition. Finally, I acknowledge President Brian Scanlan's insight into this publication, and Dr. Javed Siddiqi's coordinating between the editor and the Thieme president.

Contributors

Editor

Shokei Yamada, MD, PhD, FACS
Professor and Chairman Emeritus
Department of Neurosurgery
Loma Linda University School of Medicine
Loma Linda, California

Visiting Professor
Department of Neurosurgery
University of Mississippi Medical Center
Jackson, Mississippi

Consultant
Department of Neurosurgery
Arrowhead Regional Medical Center
Colton, California

Consultant
Department of Neurosurgery
Kaiser Permanente Medical Center
Fontana, California

Contributors

Austin R. T. Colohan, MD, FACS
Professor and Chairman
Department of Neurosurgery
Loma Linda University School of Medicine
Loma Linda University Medical Center
Loma Linda, California

Mark S. Dias, MD, FAAP
Professor and Vice-Chair of Clinical
    Neurosurgery
Director of Pediatric Neurosurgery
Department of Neurosurgery
Penn State Milton S. Hershey
    Medical Center
Hershey, Pennsylvania

Arthur J. DiPatri Jr., MD
Assistant Professor
Department of Neurological Surgery
Northwestern University Feinberg School
    of Medicine
Attending Neurosurgeon
Division of Pediatric Neurosurgery
Children's Memorial Hospital
Chicago, Illinois

**James M. Drake BSE, MBBCh, MSc,
    FRCS(C), FACS**
Professor
Department of Neurosurgery
University of Toronto
Neurosurgeon
Division of Surgery
The Hospital for Sick Children
Toronto, Ontario, Canada

Robin L. Gilmore, MD
Professor Emeritus
Department of Neurology
University of Florida College of Medicine
Gainesville, Florida

Nalin Gupta, MD, PhD
Associate Professor
Department of Neurological Surgery
University of California San Francisco
San Francisco, California

H. Roger Hadley, MD
Dean and Professor
Department of Urology
Loma Linda University School of Medicine
Loma Linda, California

David B. Hinshaw Jr., MD
Professor and Chairman
Department of Radiology
Head
Magnetic Resonance Science Division
Loma Linda University School of Medicine
Loma Linda, California

Harold J. Hoffman, MD, BSc(Med), FRCS(C), FACS†
Emeritus Faculty
Department of Neurology
The Hospital for Sick Children
Toronto, Ontario Canada

Robin P. Humphreys, MD, FRCSC, FACS, FAAP
Emeritus Faculty
Department of Neurology
The Hospital for Sick Children
Toronto, Ontario Canada

Jason Hwang, MD
Attending Staff
Department of Radiology
Loma Linda University Medical Center
Loma Linda, California

Bermans J. Iskandar, MD
Associate Professor
Department of Neurological Surgery
    and Pediatrics
University of Wisconsin School of Medicine
    and Public Health
University of Wisconsin Hospital and Clinics
American Family Children's Hospital
Madison, Wisconsin

J. Paul Jacobson, M.D.
Assistant Professor and Program Director
Department of Radiology
Loma Linda University School of Medicine
Loma Linda University Medical Center
Loma Linda, California

Antoine E. Khoury, MD, FRCS(C), FAAP
Professor and Head
Department of Urology
University of Toronto
The Hospital for Sick Children
Toronto, Ontario, Canada

Daniel K. Kido, MD, FACR
Professor
Department of Radiology
Head of Division of Neuroradiology
Loma Linda University School of Medicine
Loma Linda University Medical Center
Loma Linda, California

David S. Knierim, MD, FACS
Department of Neurosurgery
University of California San Francisco
Attending Staff
Children's Hospital Central California
Madera, California

Samir B. Lapsiwala, M.D.
Department of Neurosurgery
The Cleveland Clinic
Cleveland, Ohio

---

†Deceased

Sun Ik Lee, MD
Resident
Tulane University Medical Center
New Orleans, Louisiana

Russell R. Lonser, MD, FACS
Chair
Surgical Neurology Branch
National Institutes of Health
Clinical Center at the National Institutes of Health
Bethesda, Maryland

George T. Mandybur, MD, FACS
Associate Professor
Director of Stereotactic
  and Functional Neurosurgery
Department of Neurosurgery
University of Cincinnati College of Medicine
The Neuroscience Institute/Mayfield Clinic
Cincinnati, Ohio

David G. McLone, MD, PhD, FACS
Professor
Division of Pediatric Neurosurgery
Attending Neurosurgeon
Department of Neurological Surgery
Children's Memorial Hospital
Northwestern University Feinberg School
  of Medicine
Chicago, Illinois

Kenji Muro, MD
Assistant Professor
Department of Neurological Surgery
Northwestern University Feinberg School
  of Medicine
Chicago, Illinois

Marvin D. Nelson Jr., MD, MBA
Professor
Department of Radiology
University of Southern California Keck School
  of Medicine
Chairman
Childrens Hospital Los Angeles
Los Angeles, California

W. Jerry Oakes, MD
Professor
Department of Surgery
Division of Neurosurgery
University of Alabama at Birmingham
Children's Hospital
Birmingham, Alabama

Dachling Pang, MD, FRCS(C), FRCS(Eng), FACS
Professor of Pediatric Neurosurgery
Department of Neurological Surgery
University of California Davis School of Medicine
Sacramento, California
Chief of Pediatric Neurosurgery
Regional Department of Pediatric Neurosurgery
Kaiser Permanente Medical Center
Oakland, California

Sharad Rajpal, MD
Chief Resident
Department of Neurological Surgery
University of Wisconsin School of Medicine
  and Public Health
University of Wisconsin Hospital and Clinics
Madison, Wisconsin

Gideon D. Richards, MD
Resident
Department of Urology
Loma Linda University Medical Center
Loma Linda, California

Elias B. Rizk, MD
Neurosurgical Resident
Department of Neurosurgery
Penn State Hershey Milton S. Hershey
  Medical Center
Hershey, Pennsylvania

Herbert C. Ruckle, MD, FACS
Professor and Chairman
Department of Urology
Loma Linda University School of Medicine
Loma Linda, California

Sanford Schneider, MD
Former Chief of Division of Neurology
University of Oklahoma College of Medicine
Oklahoma City, Oklahoma

Javed Siddiqi, MD, DPhil, FRCS(C), FACS
Chairman and Residency Program Director
Department of Neurosurgery
Arrowhead Regional Medical Center
Colton, California

R. Shane Tubbs, MS, PAC, PhD
Associate Professor
Department of Surgery
Division of Neurosurgery
University of Alabama at Birmingham
Division of Pediatric Neurosurgery
Children's Hospital
Birmingham, Alabama

John Walsh, MD, PhD
Professor
Department of Neurosurgery
Director of Pediatric Neurosurgery
Tulane University School of Medicine
New Orleans, Louisiana

Daniel J. Won, MD, FACS, FAAP
Attending Neurosurgeon
Department of Neurosurgery
Chief of Pediatric Neurosurgery
Kaiser Permanente Medical Center
Fontana, California

Brian S. Yamada, MD, FACS
Attending Staff
Capital Region Urological Surgeons
Residency Program Staff
Medical College of Albany
St. Peters Hospital
Albany, New York

Cheryl T. Yamada, BA
Research Assistant
Department of Communication Studies
Chapman University
Orange, California

Shokei Yamada, MD, PhD, FACS
Emeritus Professor
Department of Surgery
Loma Linda University School of Medicine
Loma Linda, California

Shoko M. Yamada, MD, DMSci
Associate Professor
Department of Neurosurgery
Teikyo University Chiba Medical Center
Anesaki, Ichihara, Chiba-ken Japan

Vivian A. Yamada, BS, DPsy
Associate Director for Clinical Services
Counseling Center
University of Central Florida
Orlando, Florida

Alexander Zouros, MD FRCS(C)
Assistant Professor
Department of Neurosurgery
Loma Linda University School of Medicine
Loma Linda University Medical Center
Loma Linda, California

1 Introduction to Tethered Cord Syndrome

Shokei Yamada

The word *tether* means to restrain, an example of which is an animal held to the maximal range of motion by a rope. This definition leads to the connotation "the harder the pull on the rope, the tenser the rope." Applying the word *tethered* to the lumbosacral spinal cord, one visualizes an unnatural, unmitigated, abnormal constraint that aptly applies to the medical condition called tethered cord syndrome (TCS). However, there has been much uncertainty about this syndrome and its diagnosis and treatment because clinicians and scientists did not agree with the usage of this term and because perceptions were based on visual rather than on scientific evidence (F. Anderson, personal communication, 1984). Interestingly, there is no word that has the same definition and connotation as English *tether* in any other language. The delay in recognizing this syndrome may be due in part to this linguistic difference.

There is now agreement that TCS is a functional disorder caused by stretching of the spinal cord with its caudal end fastened by an inelastic structure.[1] The disorder is made worse as spinal cord tension increases with such influences as rapid growth in children, or forceful spinal flexion and extension.

■ Historical Background of Tethered Cord Syndrome

The concept of TCS evolved slowly but with increasing interest among clinicians and pathologists. A suggestion that stretching of the spinal cord could induce a disorder came from a case with myelomeningocele in 1910.[2] Other articles followed on disorders such as a sacral lipoma,[3,4] and occult spinal dysraphism[5]; however, the expression *tethered cord* was avoided in such writings, which appeared to have linked the characteristic neurological deficits to "lipoma infiltration or congenital neuronal dysgenesis." Although Garceau and others attributed the neurological deficits to the traction effect that a tight filum[6,7] or myelomeningocele (MMC)[8] exerted on the spinal cord, none of these articles were published in neurosurgical journals.

In 1940, Lichtenstein, an authoritative neuropathologist, was first to propose that tethering of the spinal cord may cause paraplegia and herniation of the brain stem and cerebellum through the foramen magnum.[9] However, his hypothesis was not accepted, particularly for the development of Chiari malformation.[10-12] Although surgeons noticed neurological improvements in their patients after what is currently called untethering of the spinal cord, two questions remained unanswered. First, if tethering-induced symptoms exist, what part of the nervous system is affected? And second, what is the pathophysiological basis for any reversible lesion?

In 1976 Hoffman et al adopted the term *tethered spinal cord* in a report on 31 patients presenting with incontinence and motor and sensory deficits in the lower limbs. These symptoms subsided after sectioning of a thickened filum terminale,[13] which indicated that the neurological lesion was in the lumbosacral cord. In 1981, Yamada et al demonstrated impairments of oxidative metabolism in the lumbosacral cord before surgery and recovery from the impairments after surgery in patients who had the same clinical presentations as those described by Hoffman et al.[13] Simultaneously, electrophysiological impairments and recoveries were recorded before and after cord untethering, respectively.[1,14]

McLone [moderator] and a panel reviewed such pathophysiological and clinical information during a debate titled "Is the TCS Fact or Fiction?" One conclusion was that tethered spinal cord is a clinical entity based on scientific evidence.[15] Since then, the term *TCS* has increasingly appeared in the neurosurgical literature.[16–20]

■ Current Understanding of Tethered Cord Syndrome

Expanding the stretch-induced disorder from tethered spinal cord to TCS, Yamada et al included patients with neural spinal dysraphism located in the caudal end of the spinal cord, such as MMCs and lipomyelomeningoceles (LMMCs).[1] This definition engendered misinterpretations and questions despite the fact that these patients presented with the same symptomatology and oxidative metabolic impairment and postoperative metabolic and neurological improvement as those of tethered spinal cord of Hoffman et al.[13]

Two questions evolved: (1) How could the theory of TCS pathophysiology explain the downhill course in some MMC patients after repeated surgical repairs?[21] and (2) Why are surgical results of TCS patients so variable?[22]

Answers to these questions may be derived from a better definition of the differences between TCS and the expressions *cord tethering* or *tethered cord* and from studies of TCS pathophysiology. Analyzing these questions, it became apparent that they are missing the fact that TCS is the manifestation of a stretch-induced lesion above the inelastic structure that exerts traction force to the spinal cord. In contrast, MMCs and LMMCs that are located dorsal to the spinal cord can cause neurological deficits by local compression or ischemia, or as a part of neuronal dysgenesis. It is clear that the lumbosacral neurological symptomatology in these patients is not caused by caudal traction effects and is not considered TCS.[23]

At the request of Professor Sergio DiRocco to clarify the diagnosis of TCS (DiRocco S, personal communication, 2006), the editor felt it necessary to categorize such expressions as *cord tethering* and *tethered cord*, which are derived only from visuals. Based on the pathophysiological analysis on caudal spinal cord anomalies, Yamada and Won divided these into three categories based on experience with individual clinical cases.[24]

Category 1 represents patients with true TCS who exhibited neurological signs and symptoms due to anchoring structures restricting the spinal cord movement at its caudal end. They include an inelastic filum terminale, caudal lipoma or LMMC, or sacral MMC.[25]

Category 2 includes patients whose signs and symptoms resemble those of true TCS; however, signs and symptoms are associated with large MMCs, extensive dorsal or transitional LMMCs (see Chapter 11), and postoperative MMCs with extensive fibrous adhesions (category 2A). These structures cause local compression or ischemia to the spinal cord resulting in neurological deficits. In some cases the deficits are related to neuronal dysgenesis. These patients do not belong to true TCS. Only when a part of the signs and symptoms is indicative of a lesion above the anomalies is partial TCS an appropriate diagnosis (category 2B).

Category 3 patients typically present with thoracolumbar MMC and exhibit total paraplegia and urinary and bowel incontinence due to the lack of functional neurons in the lumbosacral region of the cord.

Surgical results differ depending on the patient's category. After surgical untethering, category 1 patients can expect excellent outcome with pain relief and neurological improvement. Category 2B patients also have good outcome with similar symptomatic improvement. Category 2A patients have good pain relief with deficits stabilized but no neurological improvement. Category 3 patients have no predictable neurological improvement. No surgical treatment is indicated for category 3 patients. There is no hope for reversing incontinence in patients who have been performing intermittent catheterization for more than a few years.

There are special case reports other than the ordinary untethering surgery. One is a report of relief of severe back and leg pain after cord transection was performed on patients with severe adhesive arachnoiditis around the caudal spinal cord and cauda equina.[26] When the neurological signs indicate a neurological lesion above the transection, the diagnosis of TCS can be appropriate. Another report indicated reversal of TCS symptomatology by lumbar corpectomy in patients with magnetic resonance imaging (MRI) evidence of severe arachnoiditis. This method relieved spinal cord tension by shortening the length of the vertebral column.[27] These atypical treatments will further stimulate the advancement of TCS studies.

Other chapters included in this book cover the pathophysiology of TCS (Chapter 3), embryological analysis of TCS (Chapter 2), neurological examination (Chapter 4), imaging studies of TCS (Chapters 5 and 6), pediatric tethered spinal cord (Chapter 9), adult TCS (Chapters 15 and 16), cervical tethered spinal cord (Chapter 10), TCS associated with MMCs and LMMCs (Chapter 11), folate studies in families of neural spinal dysraphism (Chapter 12), in utero repair of myelomeningocele (Chapter 13), TCS associated with dermoid (Chapter 14), urological aspects of TCS (Chapters 7 and 8), intraoperative stimulation studies on sacral cord and roots (Chapter 19), anomaly of the lumbosacral cord (Chapter 17), spinal cord length and filum thickness (Chapter 18), electrophysiology with somatosensory evoked potentials (SSEPs) for TCS evaluation (Chapter 20), and conservative and operative treatment (Chapter 21). Each chapter follows the principle of TCS with expertise and endeavors by proper diagnosis and treatment to improve the care of TCS patients to help them achieve their full potential capacities.

Topics regarding TCS discussed in this book include the following:

- Correlation of pathophysiology to clinical manifestation of TCS
- Signs and symptoms of TCS to the spinal cord level of neurological lesions
- Distal motor and sensory lesions in lower limbs
- Patchy motor and sensory lesions in TCS patients
- Incontinence becoming irreversible earlier than motor and sensory dysfunction
- Hypoactive deep tendon reflex (DTR) seen in TCS patients
- Mechanism of later development of TCS in adult and late teenagers
- Difference in neurological improvement after what appeared to be complete untethering procedures
- Surgical indications and surgical techniques for TCS patients
- Essential parts of surgical procedures for untethering
- Complications to be anticipated
- Rationale for surgical treatment and alternative treatment

The editor recommends that neurosurgeons identify the three categories in patients who present with so-called cord tethering: the true TCS (category 1), relative TCS (category 2B), and non-TCS patients with symptoms similar to TCS. By following the categorization of cord tethering, neurosurgeons can correctly envisage the surgical outcome for the patients in each group. They will be able to convince referring physicians as well as patients and families of their ability to properly diagnose and treat adult TCS patients and to handle those who show similar symptomatology but belong to categories 2A and 3.

References

1. Yamada S, Zinke DE, Sanders D. Pathophysiology of "tethered cord syndrome." J Neurosurg 1981;54: 494–503
2. Fuchs A. Über Beziehungen der Enuresis Nocturna zu Rudimentarformen der Spina Bifida Occulta (Myelodysplasie). Wien Med Wochenschr 1910;80: 1569–1573
3. Bassett RC. The neurologic deficit associated with lipomas of the cauda equina. Ann Surg 1950;131: 109–116, illust
4. Rogers HM, Long DM, Chou SN, French LA. Lipomas of the spinal cord and cauda equina. J Neurosurg 1971;34:349–354
5. James CCM, Lassman LP. Spinal dysraphism: the diagnosis and treatment of progressive lesions in spina bifida occulta. J Bone Joint Surg Br 1962;44B:828–840
6. Garceau GJ. The filum terminale syndrome (the cord-traction syndrome). J Bone Joint Surg Am 1953;35-A: 711–716
7. McKenzie KG, Dewar FP. Scoliosis with paraplegia. J Bone Joint Surg Am 1949;31B:162–174
8. Hoffmann GT, Hooks CA, Jackson IJ, Thompson IM. Urinary incontinence in myelomeningoceles due to a tethered spinal cord and its surgical treatment. Surg Gynecol Obstet 1956;103:618–624
9. Lichtenstein BW. "Spinal dysraphism": spina bifida and myelodysplasia. Arch Neurol Psychiatry 1940; 44:792–809
10. Barry A, Patten BM, Stewart BH. Possible factors in the development of the Arnold-Chiari malformation. J Neurosurg 1957;14:285–301
11. Barson AJ. The vertebral level of termination of the spinal cord during normal and abnormal development. J Anat 1970;106(Pt 3):489–497
12. Gardner WJ, Smith JL, Padget DH. The relationship of Arnold-Chiari and Dandy-Walker malformations. J Neurosurg 1972;36:481–486
13. Hoffman HJ, Hendrick EB, Humphreys RP. The tethered spinal cord: its protean manifestations, diagnosis and surgical correction. Childs Brain 1976;2:145–155
14. Gilmore RL, Walsh J. The clinical neurophysiology of tethered cord syndrome and other dysraphic syndromes. In: Yamada S, ed. Tethered Cord Syndrome. Park Ridge, IL: American Association of Neurological Surgeons; 1996:167–182
15. McLone DG, Reigel DH, Pang D, Mickle JP. Tethered Cord: Fact or Fiction. TCS Seminar at: Annual Meeting of the American Association of Neurological Surgeons: 1987; Dallas, TX
16. Pang D, Wilberger JE Jr. Tethered cord syndrome in adults. J Neurosurg 1982;57:32–47
17. McLone DG, Naidich TP. The tethered spinal cord. In: McLaurin RL, Schut I, Venes JL, Epstein F, eds. Pediatric Neurosurgery. 2nd ed. Philadelphia: WB Saunders; 1989:76–96
18. Reigel DH. Spina bifida. In: McLaurin RL, Venes JL, Schut L, Epstein F, eds. Pediatric Neurosurgery. 2nd ed. Philadelphia: WB Saunders; 1989:35–52
19. Pang D. Tethered cord syndrome. In: Hoffman HJ, ed. Advances in Neurosurgery, vol 1, no 1. Philadelphia: Hanley & Belfus; 1986:45–79
20. Harwood-Nash D. Neuroradiology A: computed tomography. In: Holtzman RNN, Stein BM, eds. The Tethered Spinal Cord. New York: Thieme-Stratton; 1985:41–46
21. Yamada S, Won DJ, Yamada SM. Pathophysiology of tethered cord syndrome: correlation with symptomatology. Neurosurg Focus 2004;16:E6
22. Lee GYF, Paradiso G, Tator CH, Gentili F, Massicotte EM, Fehlings MG. Surgical management of tethered cord syndrome in adults: indications, techniques, and long-term outcomes in 60 patients. J Neurosurg Spine 2006;4:123–131
23. Yamada S, Colohan ART, Won DJ. Neurosurgical Forum, The Letter To The Editor. J Neurosurg, In press
24. Yamada S, Won DJ. What is the true tethered cord syndrome? Childs Nerv Syst 2007;23:371–375
25. Yamada S, Won DJ, Pezeshkpour G, et al. Pathophysiology of tethered cord syndrome and similar complex disorders. Neurosurg Focus 2007;23:1–10
26. Blount JP, Tubbs RS, Wellons JC III, Acakpo-Satchivi L, Bauer DB, Oakes WJ. Spinal cord transection for definitive untethering of repetitive tethered cord. Neurosurg Focus 2007;23:1–4
27. Grande AW, Maher PC, Morgan CJ, et al. Vertebral column subtraction osteotomy for recurrent tethered cord syndrome in adults: a cadaveric study. J Neurosurg Spine 2006;4:478–484

2 Normal Spinal Cord Development and the Embryogenesis of Spinal Cord Tethering Malformations

Mark S. Dias and Elias B. Rizk

Understanding normal and abnormal embryology of the nervous system is vital for the neurosurgeon treating patients with dysraphic malformations, and not just as an academic exercise. Such understanding not only allows an appreciation for how (and when) these malformations might arise during embryogenesis, it also improves the surgeon's understanding of the anatomical relationships between the malformation and spinal cord during repair and/or tethered cord release. This chapter briefly reviews several of the earlier embryological events in the formation of the spinal cord, as well as the various ways in which development might go awry. The chapter provides a detailed review of the principles underlying normal early neural development and applies these principles to the embryogenesis of dysraphic malformations.

■ Normal Early Human Neural Development

Blastogenesis

During the first 4 days after fertilization postovulatory day (POD) 1 to 4, the human embryo undergoes approximately five cell divisions to form a mass of ~32 cells (the blastocyst), which surrounds a central cavity (the blastocystic cavity). The blastocyst contains an eccentrically located inner cell mass (ICM), the embryonic cell proper, and a thinner surrounding ring of cells,

the trophoblast (**Fig. 2.1**). By POD 4, the ICM develops two distinct layers: cells on the dorsal surface, adjacent to the trophoblast, form the epiblast, whereas cells on the ventral surface, adjacent to the blastocystic cavity, form the hypoblast.[1]

By POD 7 to 12 two additional cavities develop (**Fig. 2.1**): the *amnionic cavity* appears between the epiblast and the overlying trophoblast cells, while the *umbilical vesicle* (or *yolk sac*) appears below the hypoblast. The epiblast is therefore adjacent to the amnionic cavity, and the hypoblast is adjacent to the umbilical vesicle. By POD 13, the hypoblast thickens cranially; this portion of the hypoblast is the prochordal plate. The prochordal plate will eventually give rise to the cephalic mesenchyme and to portions of the foregut.[1]

Gastrulation and Formation of Germ Layers

During the second embryonic week *gastrulation* transforms the embryo from a two-layered structure containing epiblast and hypoblast into a three-layered structure containing ectoderm, mesoderm, and endoderm. A midline structure, the primitive streak, first develops at the caudal end of the blastocyst at POD 13 and elongates cranially over the next 3 days. It reaches its full length by POD 16 and then begins to regress back toward the caudal pole of the embryo. The primitive streak is contiguous cranially with the *primitive knot*, or *Hensen node*;

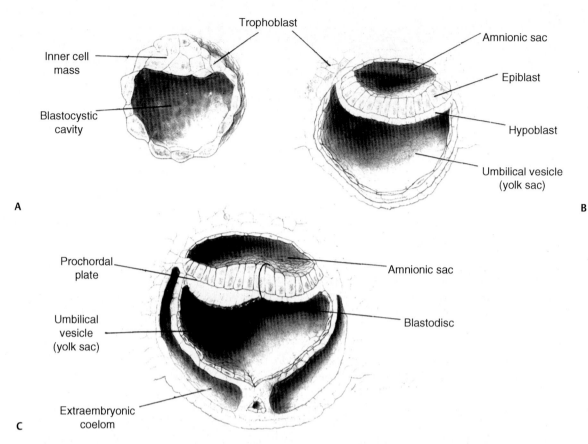

Fig. 2.1 Development of the blastocyst; midsagittal illustrations. **(A)** Continued proliferation of cells produces a sphere containing a blastocystic cavity surrounded by an eccentrically located inner cell mass and a surrounding ring of trophoblast cells. **(B)** The inner cell mass develops further into a two-layered structure, the blastodisc, containing the epiblast adjacent to the amnionic cavity and the hypoblast adjacent to the yolk sac. **(C)** With further development, the blastodisc thickens cranially to form the prochordal plate.

in the middle of Hensen node is a small indentation, the *primitive pit*. Along the length of the primitive streak is located a midline trough, the *primitive groove*, which is contiguous cranially with the primitive pit.[1]

During gastrulation, cells in the epiblast migrate medially toward the primitive streak and invaginate through the primitive groove (**Fig. 2.2A**). The initial wave of cells displaces the hypoblast cells laterally and forms the definitive *endoderm*, whereas the next wave migrates between the epiblast and endoderm to form *mesoderm*. Cells remaining in the epiblast will spread out to replace those that have

migrated through the primitive streak and will form the ectoderm (*neuroectoderm* and *cutaneous* ectoderm).

During primitive streak regression, prospective notochordal cells located in the Hensen node at the cranial end of the primitive streak (**Fig. 2.2B**) invaginate through the primitive pit to form the midline notochordal process between the epiblast and hypoblast[1,2]; as gastrulation proceeds, the notochord is eventually sandwiched between the endoderm ventrally and the neuroectoderm dorsally. The notochord, together with the paraxial mesoderm, will form the vertebral column.

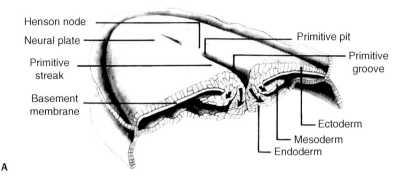

A

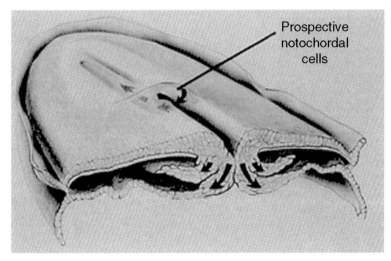

B

Fig. 2.2 Normal human gastrulation. **(A)** Prospective endodermal and mesodermal cells of the epiblast migrate toward the primitive streak and ingress (*arrows*) through the primitive groove to become the definitive endoderm and mesoderm. **(B)** Prospective notochordal cells in the cranial margin of the Hensen node will ingress through the primitive pit during primitive streak regression to become the notochordal process.

Intercalation and Excalation of the Notochordal Process

In primate embryos,[3,4] the developing notochord undergoes a peculiar series of morphogenetic events between POD 17 and 25. The notochordal process initially consists of a median cord of cells radially arranged about a central lumen; the central lumen (or notochordal canal) is continuous dorsally with the amnionic cavity through the primitive pit (**Fig. 2.3A**).

The notochordal process continues to elongate between POD 17 and 19 and reaches its full length by POD 19 to 21. It is initially rod shaped and lies between the neuroectoderm and the endoderm; however, between POD 18 and 20 it fuses, or *intercalates*, with the underlying endoderm to form the *notochordal plate* (**Fig. 2.3B**), bringing the notochordal canal into communication with the yolk sac. The most caudal portion of the notochordal canal is the primitive neurenteric canal, which is continuous both with the amnion through the primitive pit and with the yolk sac as a result of intercalation; this communication is called the *neurenteric canal*.[4]

The neurenteric canal remains open until POD 21 to 23 at which time the notochordal plate folds dorsoventrally and separates (or

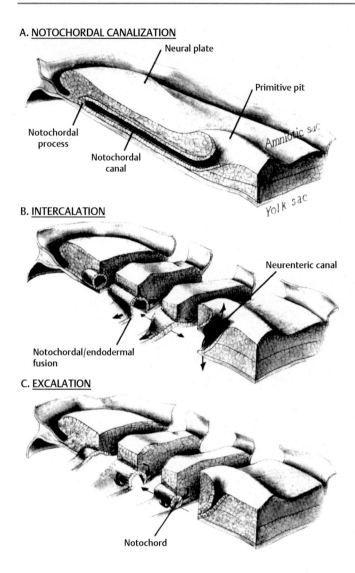

A. NOTOCHORDAL CANALIZATION

Neural plate

Primitive pit

Notochordal process

Notochordal canal

Amniotic sac

Yolk sac

B. INTERCALATION

Neurenteric canal

Notochordal/endodermal fusion

C. EXCALATION

Notochord

Fig. 2.3 Formation of the notochord. **(A)** The notochordal process contains a central lumen (the notochordal canal), which is continuous with the amnionic cavity through the primitive pit. **(B)** During intercalation, the canalized notochordal process fuses with the underlying endoderm; the communication of the amnion with the yolk sac forms the primitive neurenteric canal. **(C)** During excalation, the notochord rolls up and separates from the endoderm to become the definitive notochord; the primitive neurenteric canal becomes obliterated.

excalates) from the endoderm; by POD 23 to 25 the notochordal process has completely separated once again from the underlying endoderm (**Fig. 2.3C**). Thereafter, the *true notochord* exists as a solid rod of notochordal cells.[4]

Formation of the Neural Tube: Primary Neurulation

Primary neurulation involves the shaping of the neuroectoderm to form the neural plate, and bending of the neural plate to form the neural tube (**Fig. 2.4**). The neural plate is evident by POD 17 to 19, with the neural groove forming a midline crease immediately above the notochord. By POD 19 to 21, the neural groove has deepened considerably and neural folds are developing laterally.[1] The neural folds converge toward the midline and meet to form a closed neural tube between POD 21 and 23. Closure of the neural tube is accompanied by separation of neural from cutaneous ectoderm (called *dysjunction*). Neural crest cells arise from the neural tube at the junction between the neural

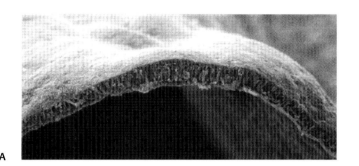

A

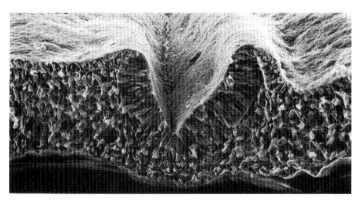

B

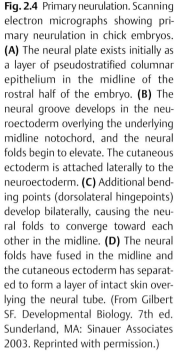

Fig. 2.4 Primary neurulation. Scanning electron micrographs showing primary neurulation in chick embryos. **(A)** The neural plate exists initially as a layer of pseudostratified columnar epithelium in the midline of the rostral half of the embryo. **(B)** The neural groove develops in the neuroectoderm overlying the underlying midline notochord, and the neural folds begin to elevate. The cutaneous ectoderm is attached laterally to the neuroectoderm. **(C)** Additional bending points (dorsolateral hingepoints) develop bilaterally, causing the neural folds to converge toward each other in the midline. **(D)** The neural folds have fused in the midline and the cutaneous ectoderm has separated to form a layer of intact skin overlying the neural tube. (From Gilbert SF. Developmental Biology. 7th ed. Sunderland, MA: Sinauer Associates 2003. Reprinted with permission.)

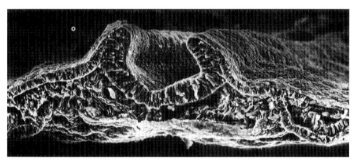

C

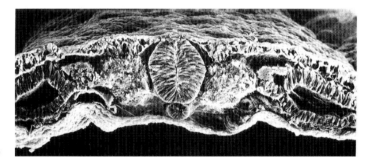

D

folds and adjacent surface ectoderm, and differentiate into several different cell types, including the pharyngeal arches, the meninx (pia and arachnoid), the cranial and spinal Schwann cells and melanocytes, the cranial ganglia, and the dorsal root ganglia and roots. Neural tube closure takes place over 4 to 6 days and may occur simultaneously at several initiation sites along

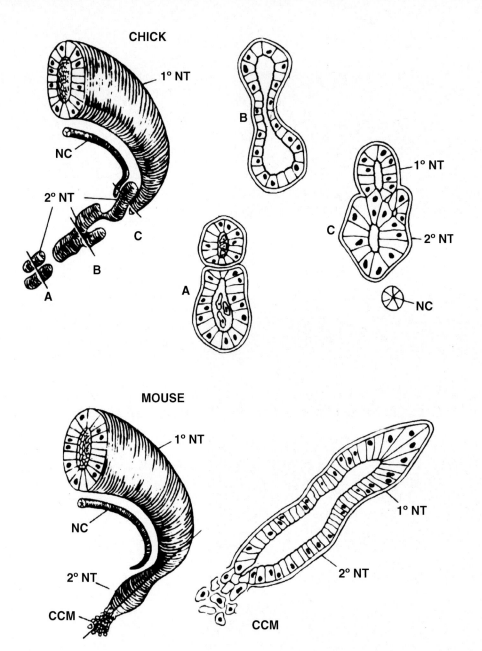

Fig. 2.5 Secondary neurulation. Upper illustration depicts secondary neurulation in avian embryos. **(A)** The medullary cord consists of multiple luminae, each surrounded by an outer layer of tightly packed, radially oriented cells and containing an inner group of more loosely packed cells. **(B)** Adjacent cords coalesce to form larger aggregates; simultaneously, the inner cells are lost. Eventually a single structure is formed, having a single lumen that is *not* yet in direct communication with the lumen formed by primary neurulation. **(C)** Later, the neural tube (NT) formed by secondary neurulation (2° NT) fuses with that formed from primary neurulation (1° NT); at this point, the luminae of the two neural tubes communicate directly. NC, notochord. Lower illustration depicts secondary neurulation in mouse embryos. A medullary rosette is composed of cells radially arranged about an empty central lumen. The lumen is always in communication with the central canal formed by primary neurulation. Growth of the secondary neural tube occurs by additional cavitation of the secondary lumen, and by recruiting additional cells from the caudal cell mass (CCM). (From McLone DG, Dias MS. Normal and abnormal embryology of the nervous system. In: Cheek WR, ed, Pediatric Neurosurgery, Surgery of the Developing Nervous System. 3rd ed. Philadelphia: WB Saunders; 1994:3–39. Reprinted with permission.)

the craniocaudal neural axis.[5–8] The last portions to close are the anterior neuropore at the level of the commissural plate (closing during POD 23 to 25), and the caudal neuropore at the level of the *second sacral spinal cord segment* (closing during POD 25 to 27).[9,10] *All neural tissue cranial to the second sacral segment is therefore derived from primary neurulation.*

Formation of the Caudal Conus Medullaris and Filum Terminale: Secondary Neurulation

The caudal neural tube (including the tip of the conus medullaris [CM] caudal to the second sacral segment, as well as the filum terminale) arises by *secondary* neurulation from the caudal cell mass or end bud (the remnants of the Hensen node and primitive streak) at the caudal pole of the embryo (**Fig. 2.5**). Secondary neurulation is species specific—for example, in chick embryos secondary neurulation involves the formation and subsequent coalescence of multiple independent tubules into a caudal neural tube that eventually fuses with the primary neural tube in an area called the *overlap zone.*[11] In contrast, secondary neurulation in mouse embryos involves the progressive extension of the primary neural tube through the addition of cells onto its caudal end.[12] It is unclear whether humans more closely resemble a mouse or a chicken.

Ascent of the Conus Medullaris

Ascent of the CM is a process whereby the conus changes position with respect to the surrounding vertebral column, appearing to rise or ascend over time such that spinal cord segments come to lie opposite more cranial vertebral segments, and the spinal nerves take a progressively more caudal course as they travel from their origins on the spinal cord to their respective neural foraminae (and forming the cauda equina). Ascent begins on POD 42 and continues throughout embryogenesis and perhaps even into the postnatal period. Ascent occurs through two mechanisms. The first, occurring between POD 42 and 54, is an ill-defined process referred to as

retrogressive differentiation, during which the caudal neural tube becomes thinner, develops a rudimentary marginal and no mantle zone, and looks "less well developed." Beyond POD 54, retrogressive differentiation has ceased, and all further ascent occurs because the spinal cord is elongating more slowly than the surrounding vertebral column. The rate of ascent is steeper between gestational weeks 12 and 20 and slows thereafter until term. According to Barson, the CM at birth lies opposite the L2/3 disk space and ascends to its final level opposite the L1/2 disk space by 2 months postnatal.[13] However, several subsequent radiographic studies have demonstrated that the conus already lies opposite the L1/2 disk space at term.[14,15] In a recent study of 100 children undergoing whole spine magnetic resonance imaging (MRI) scans (to evaluate for leptomeningeal seeding from tumors), the *average* level of the normal CM was opposite the inferior third of the L1 vertebral body, the *mode* was opposite the L1/2 disk space, and the *lowest normal level* (95% confidence limits) was opposite the middle third of the second lumbar vertebral segment.[16] Therefore, *any CM that is positioned caudal to the midbody of the second lumbar segment should be considered radiographically tethered.*

■ Abnormal Human Early Neural Development

The following is a classification of central nervous system (CNS) malformations according to their reputed embryogenetic mechanism(s), keeping in mind that few of these have been validated experimentally (**Table 2.1**).

Failure of Neural Tube Closure: Myelomeningocele, Anencephaly

Myelomeningocele (MMC) and anencephaly represent a simple localized failure of a portion of the neural tube to close, yielding an open or exposed malformation on the dorsum of the child. Because MMC and anencephaly reflect a failure of neural tube closure they are, *by definition,*

Table 2.1 Embryologic Classification of Dysraphic Spinal Malformations

Disordered midline axial integration during gastrulation
- Split cord malformations
- Combined spina bifida
- Neurenteric cysts
- Some myelomeningoceles
- Some cervical myelomeningoceles
- Hemimyelomeningoceles
- Some examples of caudal agenesis and Klippel-Feil
- Complex dysraphic malformations

Localized failure of neurulation
- Myelomeningocele
- Anencephaly

Premature ectodermal dysjunction
- Lipomyelomeningoceles

Incomplete ectodermal dysjunction
- Dermal sinus tracts, dermoid/epidermoid tumors
- Meningocele manqué?
- Meningocele?

Disordered formation of the caudal cell mass or secondary neurulation
- Terminal spinal lipomas
- Fatty filum terminale
- Myelocystoceles

Postneurulation disorders (not discussed)
- Encephaloceles
- Chiari II malformation

open malformations still attached circumferentially to the surrounding cutaneous ectoderm (skin). The pathogenesis of MMC and anencephaly involves both genetic and environmental factors; attention has focused largely on the contributions of folate. Folate antagonists can cause neural tube defects (NTDs) both experimentally and clinically, and periconceptional folate supplementation has been shown to reduce NTDs by as much as 80%.[17–19] Further studies have begun to elucidate the importance of folate within the "methylation cycle" and the conversion of homocysteine to methionine.

The genesis of cervical and upper thoracic MMC likely involves a different embryonic mechanism.[20,21] Whereas lumbosacral MMCs are open, have a larger fascial defect, and are commonly associated with a complete loss of sensorimotor function below the level of the malformation, cervicothoracic lesions are usually closed, have a limited fascial defect, and are associated with little or no loss of sensorimotor function below the malformation. Approximately 50% of cervicothoracic malformations are associated with split cord malformations (see below). These more cranial lesions have been hypothesized to arise through a limited failure of the final stages of neural tube closure, through myelocystocele formation[21,22] (see below), or through an abnormality of gastrulation.[23]

Anomalies Resulting from Incomplete Dysjunction: Dermal Sinus Tracts, Meningoceles Manqué, and Meningoceles

Several malformations—dermal sinus tracts, meningoceles manqué, and perhaps even true meningoceles—may represent disorders of dysjunction in which a persistent tract of tissue, variably containing epidermal or dermal elements, fibrous tissue, and/or peripheral nerve elements (nerve roots and/or ganglion cells) extends a variable length from the dorsum of the spinal cord toward the skin.[24] Dermal sinus tracts (DSTs) incorporate a tract of cutaneous ectoderm (with or without fibrous tissue) that extends from the dorsal midline skin to the neural tube. Approximately 60% of dermal sinuses incorporate a dermoid or epidermoid tumor; conversely, 30% of dermoid and epidermoid tumors occur in association with DSTs.[25,26] The proposed embryogenesis involves faulty separation of neuroectoderm from cutaneous ectoderm at the time of dysjunction,[27] most frequently involving the posterior neuropore (**Fig. 2.6**). Accordingly (and importantly from a surgical perspective), the intradural tract usually ends on the *dorsum* of the CM at the level of the second sacral segment, *cranial* to the tip of the CM and *separate* from the origin of the filum terminale.

Meningocele manqué ("failed" meningocele) was a term originally used by James and

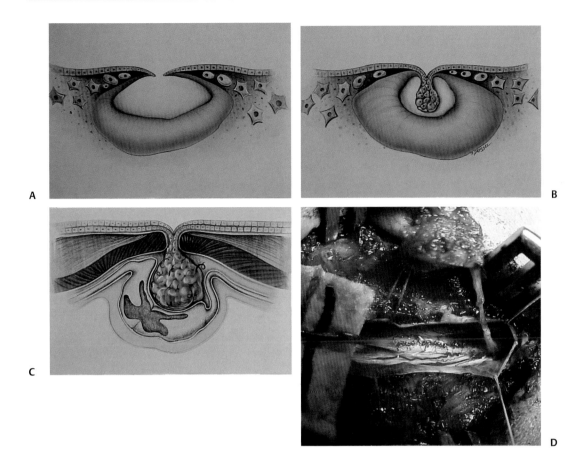

Fig. 2.6 Reputed embryogenesis of dermal sinus tracts. **(A)** During early neurulation, the neural folds have elevated and approach each other in the midline, still connected to the adjacent cutaneous ectoderm. **(B)** A failure of dysjunction of the neuroectoderm from surface ectoderm drags a small tract of cutaneous ectoderm down beneath the skin surface, in association with the neural tube. **(C)** The tract of epidermal cells produces a dermal sinus tract. An accumulating nest of cutaneous ectodermal and mesodermal cells adjacent to the spinal cord produces a dermoid tumor variably containing epidermal and dermal elements, adnexal structures, and hair. **(D)** Operative photograph showing the DST traveling from the skin to the dorsum of the conus medullaris, terminating cephalad to the filum terminale.

Lassman to describe a malformation characterized by a small scarified lesion (sometimes referred to as a "cigarette burn") on the skin, having an underlying fibrous tract (and, in their original description, aberrant nerve roots) that extends a variable distance from the spinal cord to the skin.[28] Although originally described as atretic or abortive meningoceles, these malformations likely represent another example of disordered dysjunction in which the cutaneous ectoderm, rather than being displaced toward the spinal cord, instead incorporates fibrous tissue and/or neural crest cells that are drawn up toward the surface ectoderm. Approximately half have been described in association with split cord malformations[28] and may represent a secondary effect of disordered gastrulation.[23]

Finally, the senior author has seen examples of true meningoceles in which close inspection revealed a tract of fibrous tissue extending between the dorsum of the spinal cord and the

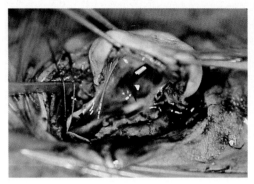

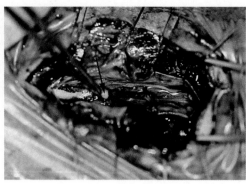

Fig. 2.7 Meningocele. **(A)** The meningocele sac has been cut to expose the contents of the sac. A fibrous band (*arrow*) projects dorsally from the spinal cord (*arrowhead*) to the inner surface of the meningocele sac. **(B)** The cut fibrous band (*arrow*) arises from the dorsum of the conus medullaris, cranial to the tip of the conus and the filum terminale (*arrowhead*).

inner surface of the sac. Notably, these fibrous tracts originate in exactly the same place as DSTs—along the dorsum of the spinal cord just cranial to the tip of the CM and separate from the origin of the filum terminale (**Fig. 2.7**). Meningoceles may therefore represent yet another example of a failure of proper dysjunction.

Anomalies Resulting from Premature Dysjunction: Lipomyelomeningocele (Spinal Lipoma)

Lipomyelomeningoceles most frequently arise in the lumbosacral spinal cord, CM, and filum terminale. Lipomas arising cranial to S2 are thought to represent premature dysjunction of neural from cutaneous ectoderm, allowing mesenchymal cells access to the central canal of the neural tube where they differentiate into fat (**Fig. 2.8**).[29,30] From an anatomical standpoint, the neural crest cells arising from the lateral edges of the neural folds embryologically (and giving rise to the dorsal roots at the dorsal root entry zones) lie ventrolateral to the fatty stalk—an important surgical landmark.

Lipomas involving the terminal CM (below S2), as well as those involving the filum terminale, must arise instead from a disorder of secondary neurulation, although the exact mechanism is not clear.

Anomalies Resulting from Disorders of Gastrulation: Split Cord Malformations

Split cord malformations (SCMs),[31] formerly referred to as diastematomyelia and diplomyelia, involve a partial duplication of the spinal cord over a portion of its length. Two types have been identified and differ in terms of (1) whether they involve a single or dual dural sheath and (2) the nature of the intervening connective tissue elements between the split cords. In a type I SCM two hemicords, each within its own dural sheath, are separated by a midline extradural bony or cartilagenous septum. In a type II SCM both hemicords are contained within a *common* dural sheath often separated by *intradural* fibrous bands of tissue, analogous to the extradural bony or cartilaginous septi of the type I malformations. Both types have dorsal and, less frequently, ventral anomalous (and nonfunctional) paramedian nerve roots that extend from the medial surfaces of one or both hemicords to the intervening mesenchymal tissue[31,32] as well as anomalous blood vessels. SCMs occur as an isolated malformation or in the setting of a variety of other dysraphic malformations—including up to 40% of MMCs, 50% of cervicothoracic MMCs, combined spina bifida (the split notochord syndrome), neurenteric cysts, and other

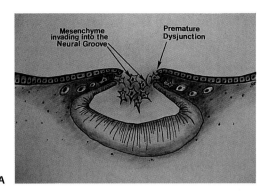

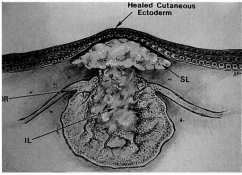

A   B

Fig. 2.8 Reputed embryogenesis of spinal lipomas. **(A)** Premature dysjunction of neuroectoderm from cutaneous ectoderm allows adjacent mesenchyme access to the central canal of the neural tube, where they are induced to form fibrofatty tissue. The cutaneous ectoderm remains intact overlying the malformation. **(B)** The lipoma extends both into the subcutaneous tissues (SLs) and the intramedullary portion of the spinal cord (IL). Dorsal roots (DR) and dorsal root ganglia derived from neural crest cells at the lateral aspects of the neural folds are located immediately ventrolateral to the fibrofatty stalk. (From Pang D. Tethered cord syndrome. In: Neurosurgery: State of the Art Reviews. Vol 1. Philadelphia: Hanley and Belfus; 1986:45–79. Reprinted with permission.)

"complex dysraphic malformations."[23] The midline tissue between the two hemicords may contain normal tissues derived from any of the three germ cell layers, as well as abnormal tissues such as Wilm tumor and suggests an abnormality that arises during gastrulation when these tissues were first being formed (**Fig. 2.9**).[23]

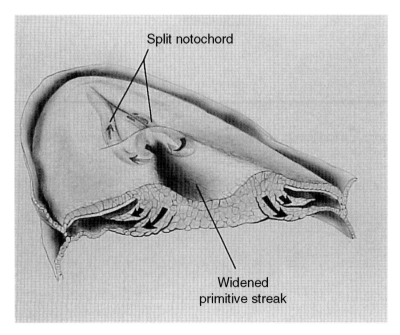

Fig. 2.9 Reputed embryogenesis of split cord malformations (SCM) as a result of disordered midline axial integration during gastrulation. The notochord is split along a portion of its length, perhaps due to a deficiency of midline basement membrane underlying the ectoderm. The overlying neural plate undergoes primary neurulation over a wider area, resulting in the formation of an SCM.

Anomalies Resulting from Disorders of Caudal Cell Mass or Secondary Neurulation: Thickened Filum Terminale, Myelocystocele, Currarino Triad

Thickening of the filum terminale likely arises from an abnormality of secondary neurulation or of retrogressive differentiation, giving rise to the "fatty filum" or "filar lipoma." When extensive, the filar lipoma would be referred to as a terminal lipoma.[33] The underlying mechanism(s) that give rise to these malformations can only be speculated.

Myelocystoceles are rare occult dysraphic lesions characterized by a dilated central spinal cord canal to form a glial or ependyma-lined terminal cyst[34,35] surrounded by an even larger dilated and ectatic dural sleeve. Most arise from the caudal end of the spinal cord and are referred to as terminal myelocystoceles. These malformations are tethered both by the terminal cord attachments to the dural sac as well as by an associated terminal or transitional lipoma. These malformations are covered by full-thickness skin (differentiating them from NTDs) and are erroneously referred to by some as closed myelomeningoceles (which of course they cannot be given that the MMC is, by definition, an open lesion). The embryogenesis is unknown but likely involves some abnormality of the caudal cell mass because they are frequently associated with abnormalities of the cloaca, including cloacal and bladder exstrophy and anorectal malformations, structures also derived from the caudal cell mass. As discussed earlier, the rare cervicothoracic MMCs are referred to by some as myelocystoceles[21,22]; the embryogenesis of these more cranial spinal malformations is also unknown.

A final malformation that may fall into this category is the Currarino triad of hemisacral agenesis, anorectal malformations, and anterior sacral mass (typically either a presacral teratoma or anterior sacral meningocele).[36] The embryogenesis of the Currarino triad was suggested in a recent case report of a child with a Currarino triad having a caudal SCM, the end of one hemicord projecting through the ventral dura and contiguous with a presacral teratoma. The association of a Currarino triad with a caudal SCM suggested that a Currarino triad may represent a disorder of the caudal cell mass during late gastrulation involving inadequate dorsoventral separation of the caudal cell mass into a dorsal neural component and a ventral cloacal component.[37]

Anomalies Resulting from Failure of Caudal Neuraxial Development: Caudal Agenesis

Caudal agenesis (CA) is characterized by a partial or complete absence of a variable number of lumbar and/or sacral vertebrae, as well as the corresponding segments of the caudal neural tube. The distal spinal cord is absent, the terminal spinal cord ending in a dysplastic glial nodule.[38–40] Whereas motor deficits usually correspond to the level of the agenesis, sensory sparing is characteristic. There is an uncommon association of CA with MMC, SCMs, and visceral and limb anomalies such as cloacal or bladder exstrophy.[40–45] The embryogenetic mechanism likely involves a failure of the caudal cell mass to form caudal structures; the increased incidence among offspring of diabetic mothers and production of CA by administration of experimental maternal ketone bodies suggests an underlying abnormality of carbohydrate metabolism. CA may be associated with other malformations of the caudal neuraxis that may cause spinal cord tethering.[46]

■ Conclusion

A thorough understanding of normal embryology provides a solid background for the accurate diagnosis and rational treatment of children with tethering malformations. Although several embryogenetic theories have been put forth to explain the origin of these malformations, none is proven and most are purely speculative. It is

hoped that further research will test the plausi-
bility of these theories and perhaps better elucidate the underlying molecular basis for these
malformations. Even if the theories are ultimately
proven wrong, having a basic understanding of
the anatomy and embryology of these malformations places the neurosurgeon in a better
position to surgically correct them.

References

1. O'Rahilly R, Muller F, Streeter GL. Developmental
Stages in Human Embryos: Including a Revision of
Streeter's "Horizons" and a Survey of the Carnegie
Collection. Washington, DC: Carnegie Institution of
Washington; 1987

2. Nicolet G. Avian gastrulation. Adv Morphog 1971;
9:231–262

3. Hendrickx AG. Description of stages IX, X, and XI. In:
Hendrickx AG, ed. Embryology of the Baboon.
London: University of Chicago Press; 1971:69–85

4. O'Rahilly R, Müller F. Developmental Stages in
Human Embryos. Washington: Carnegie Institution
of Washington; 1987

5. Golden JA, Chernoff GF. Intermittent pattern of neural tube closure in two strains of mice. Teratology
1993;47:73–80

6. Golden JA, Chernoff GF. Multiple sites of anterior
neural tube closure in humans: evidence from anterior neural tube defects (anencephaly). Pediatrics
1995;95:506–510

7. Müller F, O'Rahilly R. The first appearance of the neural tube and optic primordium in the human embryo
at stage 10. Anat Embryol (Berl) 1985;172:157–169

8. Van Allen MI, Kalousek DK, Chernoff GF, et al.
Evidence for multi-site closure of the neural tube in
humans. Am J Med Genet 1993;47:723–743

9. Müller F, O'Rahilly R. The development of the human
brain and the closure of the rostral neuropore at
stage 11. Anat Embryol (Berl) 1986;175:205–222

10. Müller F, O'Rahilly R. The development of the human
brain, the closure of the caudal neuropore, and the
beginning of secondary neurulation at stage 12. Anat
Embryol (Berl) 1987;176:413–430

11. Schoenwolf GC, Delongo J. Ultrastructure of secondary neurulation in the chick embryo. Am J Anat 1980;
158:43–63

12. Schoenwolf GC. Histological and ultrastructural
studies of secondary neurulation in mouse embryos.
Am J Anat 1984;169:361–376

13. Barson AJ. The vertebral level of termination of the
spinal cord during normal and abnormal development. J Anat 1970;106(Pt 3):489–497

14. Jit I, Charnalia VM. The vertebral level of termination
of the spinal cord during normal and abnormal
development. J Anat Soc India 1959;8:93–102

15. Wolf S, Schneble F, Tröger J. The conus medullaris:
time of ascendence to normal level. Pediatr Radiol
1992;22:590–592

16. Kessler H, Dias MS, Kalapos P. The normal position of
the conus medullaris in children: a whole-spine MRI
study. Neurosurg Focus 2007;23:1–5

17. Berry RJ, Li Z, Erickson JD, et al; Collaborative Project
for Neural Tube Defect Prevention. Prevention of
neural-tube defects with folic acid in China.
China–U.S. N Engl J Med 1999;341:1485–1490

18. Czeizel AE, Dudás I. Prevention of the first occurrence
of neural-tube defects by periconceptional vitamin
supplementation. N Engl J Med 1992;327:1832–1835

19. MRC Vitamin Study Research Group. Prevention of
neural tube defects: results of the Medical Research
Council Vitamin Study. Lancet 1991;338:131–137

20. Pang D, Dias MS. Cervical myelomeningoceles.
Neurosurgery 1993;33:363–372, discussion 372–373

21. Steinbok P. Dysraphic lesions of the cervical spinal
cord. Neurosurg Clin N Am 1995;6:367–376

22. Steinbok P, Cochrane DD. The nature of congenital
posterior cervical or cervicothoracic midline cutaneous mass lesions: report of eight cases. J Neurosurg
1991;75:206–212

23. Dias MS, Walker ML. The embryogenesis of complex
dysraphic malformations: a disorder of gastrulation?
Pediatr Neurosurg 1992;18:229–253

24. Rajpal S, Salamat MS, Tubbs RS, Kelly DR, Oakes WJ,
Iskandar BJ. Tethering tracts in spina bifida occulta:
revisiting an established nomenclature. J Neurosurg
Spine 2007;7:315–322

25. Boldrey EB, Elvidge AR. Dermoid cysts of the vertebral canal. Ann Surg 1939;110:273–284

26. Guidetti B, Gagliardi FM. Epidermoid and dermoid
cysts: clinical evaluation and late surgical results.
J Neurosurg 1977;47:12–18

27. Walker AE, Bucy PC. Congenital dermal sinuses; a
source of spinal meningeal infection and subdural
abscesses. Brain 1934;57:401–421

28. James CCM, Lassman LP. Spinal Dysraphism: Spina Bifida Occulta. London: Butterworths; 1972

29. McLone DG, Naidich TP. Spinal dysraphism: experimental and clinical. In: Holtzman RN, Stein BM, eds. The Tethered Spinal Cord. New York: Thieme-Stratton; 1985:14–28

30. Naidich TP, McLone DG, Mutluer S. A new understanding of dorsal dysraphism with lipoma (lipomyeloschisis): radiologic evaluation and surgical correction. AJR Am J Roentgenol 1983;140:1065–1078

31. Pang D, Dias MS, Ahab-Barmada M. Split cord malformation, I: A unified theory of embryogenesis for double spinal cord malformations. Neurosurgery 1992;31s:451–480

32. Pang D. Split cord malformation, II: Clinical syndrome. Neurosurgery 1992;31:481–500

33. Chapman PH. Congenital intraspinal lipomas: anatomic considerations and surgical treatment. Childs Brain 1982;9:37–47

34. McLone DG, Naidich TP. Terminal myelocystocele. Neurosurgery 1985;16:36–43

35. Peacock WJ, Murovic JA. Magnetic resonance imaging in myelocystoceles: report of two cases. J Neurosurg 1989;70:804–807

36. Currarino G, Coln D, Votteler T. Triad of anorectal, sacral, and presacral anomalies. AJR Am J Roentgenol 1981;137:395–398

37. Dias MS, Azizkhan RG. A novel embryogenetic mechanism for Currarino's triad: inadequate dorsoventral separation of the caudal eminence from hindgut endoderm. Pediatr Neurosurg 1998; 28:223–229

38. Frantz CH, Aitken GT. Complete absence of the lumbar spine and sacrum. J Bone Joint Surg Am 1967;49: 1531–1540

39. Price DL, Dooling EC, Richardson EP Jr. Caudal dysplasia (caudal regression syndrome). Arch Neurol 1970;23:212–220

40. Rusnak SL, Driscoll SG. Congenital spinal anomalies in infants of diabetic mothers. Pediatrics 1965;35: 989–995

41. Blumel J, Evans EB, Eggers GWN. Partial and complete agenesis or malformation of the sacrum with associated anomalies; etiologic and clinical study with special reference to heredity; a preliminary report. J Bone Joint Surg Am 1959;41-A:497–518

42. Ignelzi RJ, Lehman RA. Lumbosacral agenesis: management and embryological implications. J Neurol Neurosurg Psychiatry 1974;37:1273–1276

43. Renshaw TS. Sacral agenesis. J Bone Joint Surg Am 1978;60:373–383

44. Sarnat HB, Case ME, Graviss R. Sacral agenesis: neurologic and neuropathologic features. Neurology 1976; 26:1124–1129

45. Stewart SF. Absence of sacrum with report of a case, and a review of the literature. Arch Surg 1924;9: 647–652

46. Pang D. Sacral agenesis and caudal spinal cord malformations. Neurosurgery 1993;32:755–778, discussion 778–779

3 Pathophysiology of Tethered Cord Syndrome

Shokei Yamada, Russell R. Lonser, Daniel J. Won, and Brian S. Yamada

Tethered cord syndrome (TCS) is a stretch-induced functional disorder of the spinal cord with its caudal portion anchored by an inelastic structure. This chapter clarifies the reversible lesions that occur in the cord segments above any of the inelastic structures. In 1957 Hoffman et al localized the reversible lesion in the lumbosacral cord continuous to a thick filum and adopted the term "Tethered Spinal Cord."[1] In 1981, Yamada et al demonstrated impaired oxidative metabolism in the lumbosacral cord of patients with the same presentation and confirmed parallel metabolic and neurological improvement after untethering surgery.[2] All the early signs were completely reversed by sectioning or resectioning of the inelastic filum.

The concept of tethering-caused lesion originated from the surgical experience of various authors.[2–29] However, such expressions as *cord tethering* and *tethered cord* encountered an earlier criticism by many neurosurgeons, for example, Frank Anderson (personal communication, 1985), as only descriptive and of nonscientific significance.[28] To avoid controversies that could originate from unclear terminology Yamada and Won provided three pathophysiological categories.[28] (1) true TCS, associated with an inelastic filum with or without cord elongation or filum thickening, caudal lipomyelomeningoceles (LMMCs) and sacral myelomeningoceles (MMCs), (2) a combination of the lesion above the cord fixation (TCS) and additional local lesion related to

MMCs, or dorsal and large transitional LMMCs, (3) patients without typical signs and symptoms of TCS despite their anatomical appearance of cord tethering: first, those with complete paraplegia and incontinence, associated with MMC, or occasionally with large dorsal or transitional LMMC, indicating that no functional lumbosacral neurons exist; and second, asymptomatic patients with an elongated cord and a thick filum. This chapter concentrates on the pathophysiology of true TCS.

Five basic questions have provided a focus for research on TCS and for clinical advances that have improved diagnosis and treatment. (1) What does tethering do to the spinal cord? (2) What is the mechanism of tethering-induced dysfunction? (3) Is tethering-induced dysfunction reversible? (4) Is the symptomatology of TCS reversible? (5) Are TCS lesions located in the gray matter or the white matter? (6) What is the role of cord elongation and thickening for TCS?

■ What Does Tethering Do to the Spinal Cord?

Although the spinal cord substance is very soft, interlacing fibers of neurons, glia, and vasculature, supported by the pia mater, prevent separation between these structures under the stress of distortion. In addition, the dentate ligaments and the dura mater in the cervical and thoracic cord levels resist cephalad or caudad traction exerted to the spinal cord.[30,31] When the traction force is applied at the caudal end of the spinal cord as seen in the patient whose spine is growing rapidly[32] in the presence of an inelastic filum, no protection by the dentate ligaments and dura mater is available. Instead, viscoelasticity of the filum terminale prevents the cellular components of the cord from dysfunction and disruption. Thus the minor stretching of the spinal cord that occurs during normal movements[33,34] is within the limits of tolerance,[2] and normal lumbosacral cord function is maintained. Despite this protection, however, there are conditions in which further tension increases within the spinal cord and reaches a level sufficient to excessively stretch the cord. If the cord is stretched to moderate levels, functional changes may occur. If the stretching is more severe, lasting derangements in cord function may result.

Insights into the causes and effects of excessive cord stretching have been derived from cat models of tethered spinal cord.[34] Such experimental studies have provided useful information for spinal cord extensibility and the degree

of stretching that can be tolerated. As reviewed in the following sections, studies in such models have resulted in a definition of the physiological and anatomical consequences of stretching the spinal cord, and the mechanisms of dysfunction produced by spinal cord tethering.[2]

Extensibility of the Spinal Cord and Filum Terminale

Typical among studies of TCS in animal models were those in which tension was increased evenly (isotonically) in the various cord segments of cats by ligating the filum terminale and pulling the spinal cord and filum caudad in weight[35] (**Figs. 3.1, 3.2**). Results of increasing cord traction in this manner included the following[2,35]:

1. The extensibility of division 1 (consisting of a half filum and a half coccygeal cord) was like that of a rubber band, forming a linear relationship with the traction weight (**Fig. 3.3A**). The filum worked as a buffer against overstretching the spinal cord.

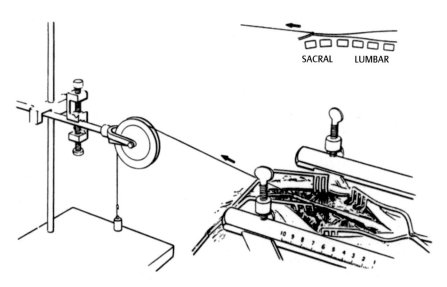

SACRAL   LUMBAR

Fig. 3.1 Animal model of tethered spinal cord: The lumbosacrococcygeal cord was exposed through laminectomy. A ligature was placed around the filum terminale and then threaded over a pulley; various weights were attached to the other end. (From Yamada S, Zinke DE, Sanders DC. Pathophysiology of "tethered cord syndrome." J Neurosurg 1981;54: 494–503. Reprinted with permission.)

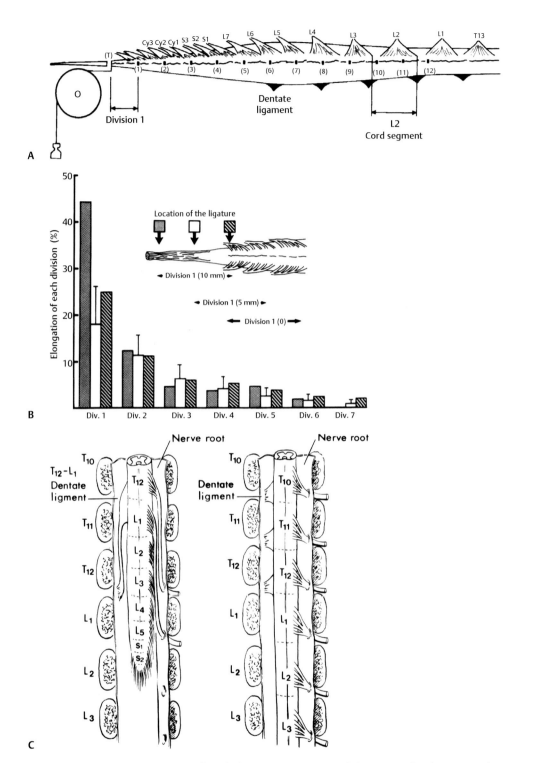

Fig. 3.2 **(A)** The lumbosacrococcygeal cord of cats was divided into 12 divisions of equal length (10 mm). The elongation of each division was measured during traction with various weights during 1 g to 10 g traction. **(B)** The ligature was placed at the caudal end of the spinal cord, 5 mm below, or 10 mm below. The graph shows the percentage of elongation of each segment during 5 g traction. The elongation varied depending on the location of the ligature. **(C)** In humans, the lowest pair of dentate ligaments is attached between the T12 and L1 cord segments, regardless of the length of the spinal cord. (**[A]** Reproduced from Tani et al[49] with permission.)

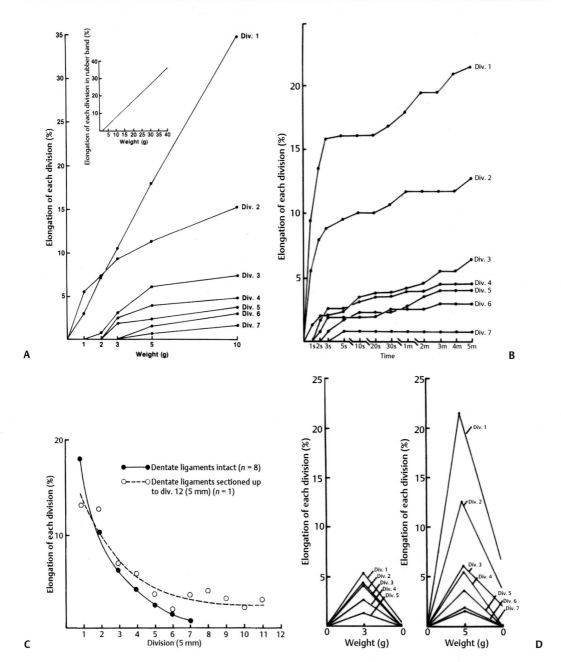

Fig. 3.3 Graphs showing the results in animal models of tethered spinal cord with a ligature placed at 5 mm below the caudal end of the cord. **(A)** The percentage of elongation of each cord division in cats. The percentage of elongation of division 1 (that includes a half filum and a half coccygeal cord) may be compared with that of a rubber band (insert). **(B)** The sequential elongation rate (rapidity of elongation) of each division during 5 g traction; s, seconds; m, minutes. **(C)** The percentage of elongation of each division during 5 g traction with the dentate ligaments intact and sectioned up to division 12 (traction was applied 5 mm below the attachment of the lowest coccygeal nerve). **(D)** The percentage of elongation of each division during 3 g traction (left) and 5 g traction (right) with a ligature placed at the caudal end of the spinal cord. Measurements were taken 5 minutes after the start of traction and 5 minutes after the release of traction.

2. The more caudal the spinal cord segment, the greater was its extensibility, but the percentage of elongation reached a plateau as the weight producing the traction increased (**Fig. 3.3B**).
3. Traction produced no elongation of the spinal cord segments above the lowest dentate ligament attachments to the spinal cord (**Fig. 3.3C**).
4. After release of low-grade (3 g) traction, each cord segment returned to its original length, but after release of high-grade (5 g) traction, the lower cord segments remained slightly elongated (5 minutes or longer) (**Fig. 3.3D**).
5. When the extension of the filum itself (with the ligature placed 10 mm below the caudal end of the cord) was measured, its extensibility was greater than that of the rubber band, signifying its much higher viscoelasticity than the latter (**Fig. 3.4A**).
6. The lower segments stretched faster and more than the higher segments, partly due to the smaller volume in the former

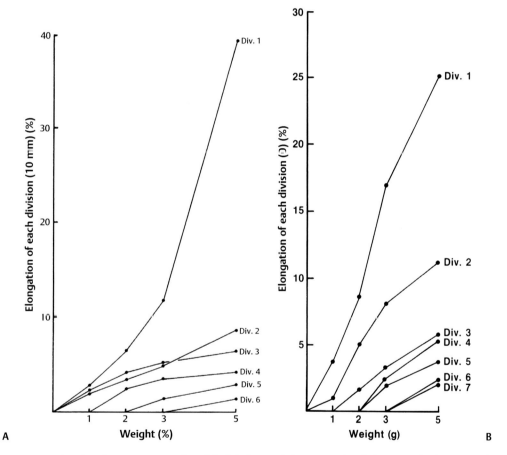

Fig. 3.4 Results of cord traction in animal models. **(A)** The percentage of elongation of each division (with a ligature placed 10 mm below the caudal end of the spinal cord) is shown in relation to weight increases. The elongation rate of the filum itself makes a steeper rise after the first linear increase beyond 3 g traction, indicating its viscoelasticity is greater than that of the rubber band. **(B)** The percentage of elongation of each division with a ligature at the caudal end of the spinal cord is shown. The lowest segment of the spinal cord (division 1) elongates 25%, suggesting that the human tethered spinal cord, anchored by the inelastic filum, elongates similarly. Note: the same segment that corresponds to division 2 in **(A)** elongates only 9% by the protection of the viscoelastic filum.

than the latter, partly to the presence of viscosity in the entire cord. When the ligature was placed at the caudal end of the spinal cord, the lowest cord segment elongated much more than when the filum was tractioned. However, the elongation rate did not form as a steep line as that of the filum, and the higher segments stretched more than they did with filum traction (**Fig. 3.4B**). These findings suggest that the human tethered spinal cord would be affected by the excessive tension, proportionate to the impairment of metabolic and electro-physiological derangement that occurs in similarly stretched conditions, as described later.

7. These studies confirm that isotonic traction of the spinal cord results in different degrees of elongation of various cord segments. The viscoelasticity of the filum terminale is much greater than that of any cord segments and therefore protects the spinal cord from over-stretching (**Fig. 3.5**).

■ What Is the Mechanism of Tethering-Induced Dysfunction?

If the untethering procedure can reverse the symptoms of TCS, tethering may produce electrophysiological dysfunction in the spinal cord that may not be necessarily accompanied by irreversible histopathology. As shown in the following sections, much effort has therefore been directed toward defining the physiological consequences of TCS.

Spinal Cord Evoked Potentials

As usual in elucidating the pathophysiology of disease entities, studies to define the mechanisms of TCS have focused on animal models of this syndrome. An expected result from evidence linking TCS to electrical dysfunction was that, in cats, depression of electrical activity did accompany severe traction.[36,37] For example, stimulation of the S2 and S3 roots produced shifts in interneuron potentials in the corresponding cord

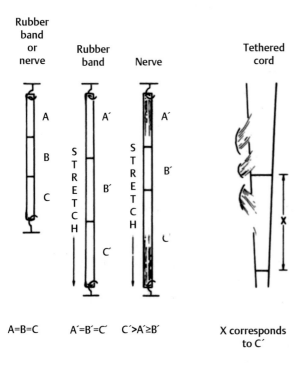

Fig. 3.5 A rubber band and a bundle of cat sciatic nerve fibers were divided into three sections of equal length by markers. Elongation of each section was equal in the rubber band but varied in the nerve fibers, with the greatest elongation in the lower third and the shortest in the middle. Later, the middle section of the nerve fibers gradually elongates as other sections contract. The changes in length are partly due to viscosity and partly to probable contractility of the nerve fibers, similar to those of the spinal cord. (From Yamada S, Knierim D, Yonekura M, et al. Tethered cord syndrome. J Am Paraplegia Soc 1983;6: 58–61. Reprinted with permission.)

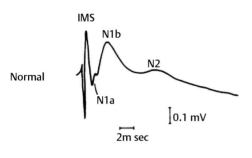

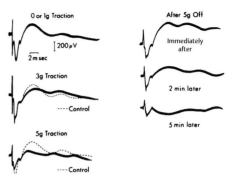

Fig. 3.6 **(A)** Evoked potential recordings at the L7–S1 cord segments in response to stimulation of the corresponding nerve roots. The intramedullary spike (IMS) is the first negative sharp wave, derived from the posterior column. The N1a, the second small negative potential, is derived from the afferent terminal. The N1b and N2 are interneuron potentials.[43] **(B)** Recordings from the S2–3 segments show low potentials and delayed latency, more marked during 5 g traction than during 3 g traction. (From Yamada S, Zinke DE, Sanders DC. Pathophysiology of "tethered cord syndrome." J Neurosurg 1981;54:494–503. Reprinted with permission.)

segments that were diminished during 3 g traction. These evoked potentials recovered after traction was released. In contrast, interneuron potentials were depressed almost to unrecognizable levels during 5 g traction, and recovery after traction release was only to ~50% of control (**Fig. 3.6**). A significant finding also was that after the partial recovery of interneuron potentials following release of (5 g) traction, these potentials again nearly disappeared. This disappearance occurred coincidentally to the secondary changes in oxidative metabolism described below, suggesting a link between these activities.

Redox Shifts of Cytochrome a,a₃

A hypothesis of research at Loma Linda University has been that TCS impairs electrical and metabolic activities of neurons and that these impairments may be linked.[2,38] Such a link is not unexpected because the central nervous system (CNS) relies almost entirely on oxidative phosphorylation of adenosine 5′-diphosphate (ADP) to provide the adenosine triphosphate (ATP) as previously mentioned[39] (**Fig. 3.7**).

One approach to understanding whether there is an oxidative metabolic consequence to TCS took advantage of the fact that reduction/oxidation (redox) shifts of the mitochondrial electron carriers (especially, the terminal carrier, cytochrome a,a_3) can be recorded in lumbosacral cord tissues noninvasively by reflection spectrophotometry (**Fig. 3.8**). In particular, gray matter occupies greater than 90% of the lumbosacral cord, and both beams of light 590 nm and 605 nm used for this technology can reach readily to the mitochondria to elicit reflection from this cytochrome.

In adapting this technology to monitor metabolic activities related to TCS, a difficulty was that the optical field to be studied was deformed by any procedure that moved or elongated the spinal cord, such as tethering or untethering procedures. To circumvent this complication, effects of spinal cord tethering in animal models and humans were evaluated by comparing redox shifts of cytochrome a,a₃ under two types of stresses: (1) transient hypoxia, which provoked transient increases in reduction of cytochrome a,a₃,[2] and (2) stimulus-induced increases in neuronal activity.[39,40]

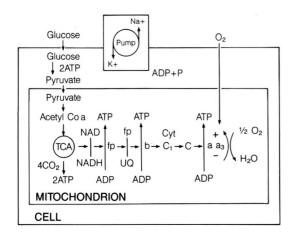

Fig. 3.7 The diagram shows high-energy production at three sites in the respiratory chain. Rapid electron transfer from nicotinamide adenine dinucleotide (NAD) to cytochrome a,a_3 facilitates adenosine diphosphate (ADP) phosphorylation to produce adenosine triphosphate (ATP) where molecular oxygen is adequately supplied. Slow ATP use is associated with a low amount of ADP, which inhibits electron transport. TCA, tricarboxylic acid cycle; UQ, ubiquinone; P, inorganic phospher; fp, flavoprotein; a,a_3, cytochrome a,a_3; b, cytochrome b.

These comparisons were made between control responses (prior to tethering) and responses during and after tethering.

In response to hypoxemia, shifts toward reduction were diminished in tethered spinal cords. These results suggested that the cytochrome existed during tethering in a more reduced state.[2] In an early study in cats, for example, weights (1 to 5 g) were applied to produce traction to the laminectomized spinal cord. Thirty seconds after the onset of traction, the animals were made hypoxemic for 2.5 minutes by increasing the fraction of $N_2O:O_2$ in the inspiratory gas mixture from 75% to 100% through a positive pressure ventilator. This was followed by inspiration of 100% O_2 for 1 minute, then by inspiration of the control (3:1) ratio of $N_2O:O_2$. Two minutes after the animal inspired the control gas mixture, the traction was released. After a 30-minute period of spinal cord relaxation, another hypoxemic insult was given to the animal, without traction.

Redox shifts of cytochrome a,a_3 in response to hypoxia varied with the degree of spinal cord traction (**Fig. 3.9**). Shifts toward reduction of this

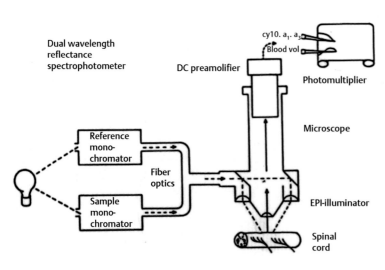

Fig. 3.8 The dual wavelength spectrophotometer utilizes two beams of light: 590 nm and 605 nm. The 605 nm light is absorbed by cytochrome a,a_3 and hemoglobin; the 590 nm light is absorbed by hemoglobin only. The amount of 590 nm and 605 nm beams absorbed by hemoglobin is exactly same; therefore 590 nm is used as a reference. The 605 nm beam is reflected from the mitochondria, the great majority of which are located in the gray matter. (From Yamada S, Zinke DE, Sanders DC. Pathophysiology of "tethered cord syndrome." J Neurosurg 1981; 54:494–503. Reprinted with permission.)

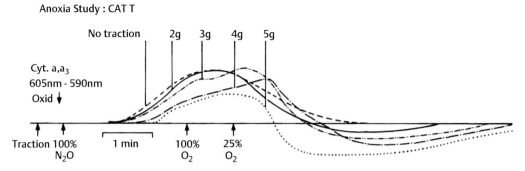

Fig. 3.9 A reduction of cytochrome a,a_3 is shown by an upward deflection in the recording. Note the differences in reduction levels depending on the traction weight. Reduction with 1 g traction is the same as control. As the weight increases, the reduction level becomes lower, indicating that cytochrome a,a_3 is basically more reduced and incapable of further reduction in response to hypoxic stress. Oxid, oxidation. (From Yamada S, Zinke DE, Sanders DC. Pathophysiology of "tethered cord syndrome." J Neurosurg 1981;54:494–503. Reprinted with permission.)

cytochrome during hypoxia under 1 g traction were not significantly different from those recorded under control conditions, but the reductive shifts were increasingly slowed and smaller as traction was increased from 2 g to 5 g.

After 1 g, 2 g, 3 g, or 4 g traction was released, reductive shifts of cytochrome a,a_3 during hypoxia were unchanged from control values. After 5 g traction was released, however, reductive shifts of this cytochrome during hypoxia remained slower and were lower in amplitude than control for more than 30 minutes. (Refer to the mechanisms of late manifestation of TCS in Chapter 15, "Tethered Cord Syndrome in Adults.") These results suggest that traction increasingly shifted the baseline redox ratio of cytochrome a,a_3 to a more reduced state.

Extrapolation of the redox activity of isolated mitochondria[41] suggests that the reduced state of mitochondria in a tethered spinal cord is due either to lack of oxygen supply or to diminished ATP use.[41] The former of these mechanisms is usually associated with diminished ATP production,[2,39,42] whereas the latter of these mechanisms would limit oxygen consumption because electron turnover within the respiratory chain is controlled by the phosphate potential (i.e., ATP/ADP + Pi).

Because evoked potential amplitudes were also diminished by spinal cord traction, these results suggest that traction-induced electrical and metabolic changes occur in the interneurons that are located in the gray matter.[2] In contrast, changes in light absorption from white matter are likely to be almost negligible. Interneurons were proved to be susceptible to anoxia and ischemia by electrophysiological[43–45] and histological studies,[46] indicating early involvement of the gray matter similar to TCS.

A link between TCS and metabolic derangements is also suggested by responses to nerve root stimulation.[37] In cats, such stimulation is normally accompanied by transient shifts toward oxidation of cytochrome a,a_3 recorded at the spinal cord segments corresponding to the stimulated nerve roots.[37] These oxidative responses to stimulation were altered when recorded during cord tethering in cats (**Fig. 3.10**). With 3 g traction, for example, the oxidative shifts in response to nerve root stimulation were decreased in amplitude by ~33%. The amplitude of these responses returned to control levels after release of the traction. With 5 g traction, however, stimulation failed to produce oxidation of cytochrome a,a_3. When the 5 g traction was released, nerve root stimulation

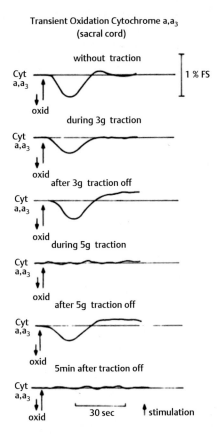

Transient Oxidation Cytochrome a,a₃
(sacral cord)

Fig. 3.10 Transient oxidation (oxid) of cytochrome a,a₃ in the S2–3 cord segments is elicited by stimulation of the corresponding nerve roots, with less amplitude during 3 g traction and no response during 5 g traction. After release of 3 g traction, transient oxidation returned to normal. After release of 5 g traction, oxidation returned but its amplitude decreased markedly within several minutes. FS, full scale.

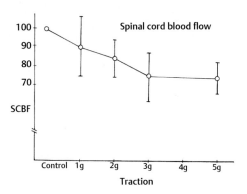

Fig. 3.11 The graph shows the blood flow of the lumbosacral cord. A linear decrease in the spinal cord blood flow (SCBF) occurred from 0 g to 3 g traction, but the blood flow with 5 g traction was the same as with 3 g traction.

then to 3 g (90%, 83%, and 75% or normal, respectively). However, blood flow was similar at 3 g and 5 g traction (**Fig. 3.11**). When the weights were released, blood flow returned to normal.

These data are compatible with the suggestion that increased reduction of cytochrome a,a₃ during mild to moderate traction is mediated, at least in part, by decreased blood flow and perhaps by a limited supply of oxygen to mitochondria. However, there was dissociation between blood flow and cytochrome a,a₃ reduction with the high-grade (5 g) traction. The cytochrome became further reduced by this traction (versus reduction at 3 g traction), whereas blood flow was similar in each condition. This suggests that an additional factor modulates metabolic changes.

In humans, Schneider et al[22] showed that blood flow was lowered during tethering but was significantly increased after untethering. Neurological improvement followed untethering. It is likely that these human cases correspond to the experimental model of low- to moderate-grade traction. The experimental results of Kang et al[47] and Turnbull et al[48] suggested a similar circulatory and neurological relationship.

Although the blood flow results suggest that tethering-induced effects may involve hypoxia, it is not yet possible to define whether hypoxia

again produced some oxidation of cytochrome a,a₃, but the amplitude of this response was markedly decreased within several minutes.

Spinal Cord Blood Flow

To provide insight into TCS and into the apparent mitochondrial dysfunction produced by cord traction, blood flow was monitored on the dorsal surface of the cat spinal cord by hydrogen clearance.[37] Blood flow decreased gradually as a traction weight was increased from 1 g to 2 g, or decreased ATP use directly underlies the apparent change in mitochondrial activity during spinal cord tethering. Either of these mechanisms could explain why cytochrome oxidase was highly reduced and why this cytochrome was limited in its capability to become further reduced in response to declines in the fraction of inspired oxygen. Additional findings that suggest a link between spinal cord tethering and impairments in oxidative metabolism include the following:

1. In cats under 3 g and 5 g traction, cytochrome a,a_3 was relatively more reduced in the S2-3 cord segments than in the L7-S1 segments, where traction produced less elongation. The reductive shifts under 3 g traction in the S2–3 segments were relatively greater than those observed during the same traction in the L7–S1 segments. These metabolic changes correlated with the percentage increases in the length of lumbosacral segments versus those in sacral segments.[7,49]

2. After release of low-grade (3 g) traction, cytochrome a,a_3 began to reoxidize, but it returned quickly to the original redox state. However, after release of 5 g traction, the cytochrome remained reduced. The residual reduction of cytochrome a,a_3 was greater in sacral than in lumbosacral segments. This correlates with findings that after release of 5 g traction, the sacral segments remained more elongated than the lumbar segments, which quickly returned to the original length.[35]

3. The redox state of cytochrome a,a_3 was not affected by traction with any weight when measured above the L6 level. Traction produced no elongation above the lowest pair of dentate ligaments (L6–7 level).[35,50]

Glucose Metabolism

The data described above support the hypothesis that the pathophysiological mechanisms of neuronal dysfunction due to traction of the spinal cord involve an impairment of oxidative metabolism. This hypothesis was supported by findings that cytochrome a,a_3 was more reduced in a tethered cord and that the cytochrome was reoxidized to levels comparable with the control condition, following untethering of the cord. These redox changes are apparently linked to cord tethering and likely indicate that mitochondrial electron transport, and therefore ADP phosphorylation, is less active in tethered spinal cords. Two mechanisms could underlie this more reduced mitochondrial state during cord tethering: (1) the oxygen supply is inadequate to maintain the cytochrome in its normal oxidized state; and (2) ATP utilization is slowed by tethering.

Insights into the mechanisms of mitochondrial changes due to tethering were also derived in animal models by monitoring glucose metabolism via autoradiography. This technique is based on the fact that radioactive two-dimensional (2-D)-deoxyglucose can be injected into the body and then be taken up by cells, including those in brain, as glucose. The difference between glucose and deoxyglucose is that the latter cannot be isomerized to fructose-6-phosphate, and its metabolism ceases at this point in the glycolytic pathway. Fortuitously, the distribution volume and the plasma concentration of deoxyglucose can be determined by quantitative autoradiography.[51] This procedure is quantitative because mathematical models allow calculation of local deoxyglucose uptake, which is related to local glucose utilization. Such procedures in the brain in vivo, for example, have confirmed the tight coupling between the functional state of a brain region, its local metabolic rate, and its blood flow.

In studies of cord tethering performed at Loma Linda University, the spinal cords of anesthetized cats were subjected to either no traction (controls) or 3 g or 5 g traction, and 2-D-deoxyglucose (12 nCi/kg) was given intravenously. After 15 minutes, the animals were sacrificed, and the descending aorta was cannulated for perfusion with a glutaraldehyde/formaldehyde mixture. After fixation, the lumbosacral segments were removed and stored at −70°C. The frozen cords were later sectioned into 10 20 μm thick sections from the L7 and S2 cord segments. Autoradiography was performed by standard techniques.[52] The films were developed and analyzed for relative glucose consumption using a densitometer (**Fig. 3.12**).

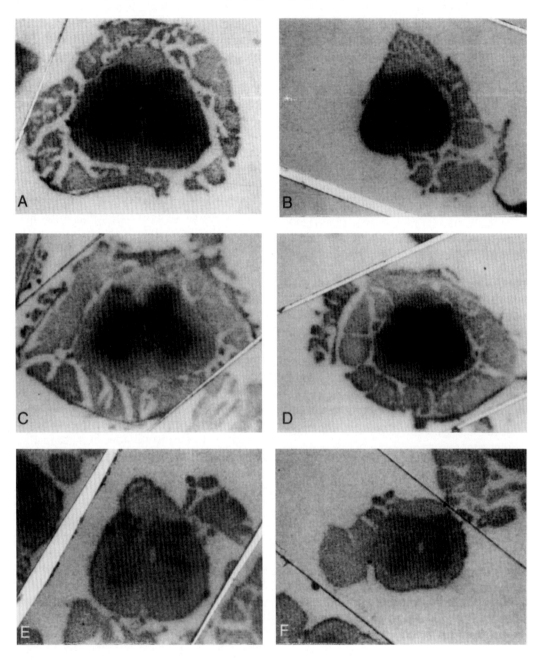

Fig. 3.12 Autoradiograms of the spinal cord without traction demonstrate normal uptake of **(A)** two-dimensional (2-D)-deoxyglucose in the L7 and **(B)** S2 cord segments, minimally decreased uptake in **(C,D)** these segments under 3 g traction, and **(E,F)** markedly decreased uptake in both segments under 5 g traction.

Compared with untethered controls, 3 g traction had only a mild effect on glucose consumption, but 5 g traction significantly decreased glucose consumption at the L7 and S2 levels.[52] These results suggest that glucose metabolism is altered in parallel to the redox alterations of cytochrome a,a_3 (see earlier discussion). The authors propose that these changes are linked to electrical suppression due to TCS. Whether the putatively linked changes in glucose consumption and electron transport are due to decreased ATP use from electrical depression or result from decreased oxygen delivery and secondarily cause electrical depression remains to be determined.

■ Is Tethering-Induced Dysfunction Reversible?

A key result from studies to determine the mechanisms of TCS dysfunction was that release of mild (2 g and 3 g) or moderate (4 g) traction was usually followed by reoxidation of cytochrome a,a_3, often to the extent that responses to transient hypoxia were not different from control responses. These studies suggest that a timely untethering procedure can promote recovery of metabolic function. This is supported by human studies on cytochrome redox activity[2] and blood flow conducted by Schneider et al.[22] The reversibility of putative metabolic dysfunction in TCS described earlier is also compatible with findings that signs and symptoms of TCS can be reversed by prompt untethering.

Despite this theoretical conclusion, neurosurgeons have encountered patients who were considered to have TCS, but neurological reversal was not complete or was delayed after what appeared to be the same procedure as performed in other TCS patients. In such a case, many other factors must be considered as to produce partially permanent neuronal damage.[53] An important goal for further research must be to understand the factors that modulate reversible or irreversible insults. A hypothesis for such research may be that sudden stretching of a tethered spinal cord with superthreshold high tension contributes to irreversible histological damage.

This hypothesis is engendered by observations that back and leg pain is accentuated by flexion and extension of the spine or by a sudden fall on the buttocks. Often motor or sensory deficit or incontinence ensues after these insults. These signs and symptoms may also be initiated or accentuated by strenuous exercises that involve repeated flexion and extension of the spine, and such signs and symptoms often become partially permanent.

The foregoing hypothesis was supported by results from studies in which cat spinal cords were placed in temporary traction with 3 g, 5 g, or 8 g weights: a histological and neurological study of experimental tethered spinal cord.[54] After this tethering, a sudden additional traction was added by dropping weights from an elevation of 1 cm. The animals were then released from traction, allowed variable times for recovery (from 24 hours to 1 week), and then sacrificed.

Additional sudden traction (with either 3 g, 5 g, or 8 g weights) to spinal cords that were already tethered produced variable results. Only the additional traction with the 5 g or greater weight resulted in observable behavioral and histological changes. In those animals, there was urinary incontinence and tail anesthesia, which continued for ~48 hours, and lymphocytic infiltration with blurring of the neuronal cell borders at 48 hours. Electron microscopic studies showed loss of cristae in mitochondria, membrane breaks, and axonal degeneration, all in gray matter. These findings clearly indicate that permanent damage to neurons can occur and that damaged cells are concentrated in the caudal spinal cord segments. However, there is a sign of regeneration mixed in the same area of degeneration. These findings may explain the weakness of distal muscles in lower limbs and the incontinence that are only partially reversible after untethering.

Chronically Tractioned Spinal Cord

The acute studies just described were conducted on cat spinal cords under isotonic traction. To relate experimental results with the signs and

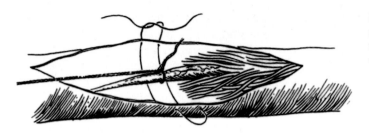

Fig. 3.13 This model of chronic tethered cord was produced by securing the ligature to the dura at the same vertebral level during traction.

symptoms of TCS and with recovery in human patients, however, studies were required in a chronic model of tethering such as that produced by isometric cord traction. This was accomplished in the following way: a 2–0 silk ligature was placed on the filum terminale, then a 4–0 silk suture to the dura was used to secure the ligature (**Fig. 3.13**) while the cord was stretched with a 3 g or 5 g weight. This isometric traction, which was equivalent to a 3 g or 5 g weight, provided constant stretching of the lumbosacrococcygeal segments. The animals were observed for 1 month, 3 months, 6 months, and 9 months under chronic traction,[20,34] and histological studies of the spinal cords were performed after the animals were sacrificed.

Such protocols showed that the hind limbs became weakened in cats that had undergone 3 g and 5 g (equivalent) traction. Weakness was more severe in the latter than in the former group. Cats with spinal cords under 3 g traction could run and jump naturally within 2 months; those animals with spinal cords under 5 g traction required from 4 to 6 months to regain the same physical ability.

In chronic studies, redox activity of cytochrome a,a_3 was sampled in the same manner as in acute studies. Increases in reductive responses to hypoxic stress in the tethered spinal cord became like control levels (i.e., their amplitudes increased) as the paralysis subsided. Restoration of the control level of redox responses of cytochrome a,a_3 to nerve root stimulation or transient hypoxia was linked to the restoration of physical activity in these animals.[20] No histological changes were produced by chronic traction, as noted in light and electron microscopy in the lumbar, sacral, and coccygeal cord.[27,34]

Incontinence was noted for several days in animals that had undergone chronic 3 g traction and for 2 to 3 weeks in animals during chronic 5 g traction. Recovery from incontinence was more rapid than from motor dysfunction. The neurological deficits (weakness, sensory changes, and a bladder dysfunction) appeared to be linked with the mitochondrial dysfunctions suggested by the acute studies, but there was no evident relationship to histologically demonstrable damage.[2,20]

The ability of cats to recover from the signs and symptoms of chronic traction, particularly incontinence, may be explained by the viscoelasticity and varying thickness of the spinal cord. As previously explained, the sacral cord segments elongated the most after initial tethering. The traction of these segments led to incontinence, weakness, and so forth. As time passed (weeks to months), however, the spinal cord compensated by allowing the elongation of more cephalic cord segments, thus relieving some tension in the sacral segments. Although the spinal cord remained stretched after a significant recovery period, the elongation was more evenly distributed, which likely permitted normal neuronal function (**Fig. 3.5**).

■ Is the Symptomatology of Tethered Cord Syndrome Reversible?

Redox Studies in Human Tethered Spinal Cord

Redox studies of cytochrome a,a_3 in patients with TCS provided data very similar to those derived from animal studies and offered new insights into TCS mechanisms and treatment.[53] Forty patients were included in these studies, ranging in age from 2 to 65 years. These patients presented with weakness or atrophy of leg muscles, sensory deficit, back or leg pain, urinary or rectal incontinence, scoliosis, leg deformity, hyporeflexia or areflexia, Babinski sign, or some combination of these signs and symptoms. Mechanical causes of tethering were a fibrous or fibroadipose filum, or a sacral lipoma attached to the conus or filum.

The sacral cord was exposed through laminectomy for untethering procedures, with the patient under anesthesia (70% N_2O and 30% O_2). Spectrophotometric studies were performed at the upper or middle sacral cord. In tests similar to those conducted in animals, the fraction of inspired oxygen gas (FiO_2) was transiently lowered from 0.3 to 0.15. After 2 minutes at 0.15, the FiO_2 was increased to 0.6 for 2 minutes, then returned to 0.3. The patients were divided into three groups depending on redox responses before and after surgery.

Type 1 Redox Changes

In this group of patients, transient hypoxemia provided mild or moderate increases in the reduction level of cytochrome a,a$_3$. After untethering, the cytochrome appeared to be shifted to a more oxidized state that became more apparent when responses to hypoxemia

were again recorded. In the latter tests, the cytochrome responded with shifts toward reduction that were larger than those recorded prior to cord untethering (what were expected in normal individuals); a similar effect of untethering occurred in cats subjected to 2 g or 3 g traction (**Fig. 3.9**). These patients had only subtle neurological signs and symptoms or musculoskeletal abnormalities before surgery, and the signs and symptoms subsided within 2 weeks to 2 months after untethering.

Type 2 Redox Changes

Other patients exhibited a moderately reduced state of cytochrome a,a$_3$ before untethering. After untethering, the cytochrome shifted to a more oxidized state in a manner consistent with that seen in cats after 4 g (moderate) traction (**Fig. 3.14**). Prior to surgery, these patients presented with definite neurological signs and symptoms or musculoskeletal abnormalities. Some of these signs and symptoms subsided within 2 months, whereas others showed delayed improvement (longer than 3 months) after untethering.

Type 3 Redox Changes

In a third group of patients, prior to untethering, the shift toward reduction during hypoxemia

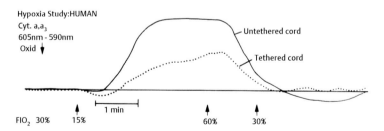

Fig. 3.14 Graph showing a reductive response to low fraction of inspired oxygen (FiO_2) (15%) in TCS patient (*dotted line*), with the reductive level equivalent to experimental tethered cord syndrome with moderate (4 g) traction, and a response to the same FiO_2 (similar to normal reductive responses) after the untethering procedure. The patient improved in motor, sensory, and bladder functions postoperatively. (From Yamada S, Zinke DE, Sanders DC. Pathophysiology of "tethered cord syndrome." J Neurosurg 1981;54:494–503. Reprinted with permission.)

was smaller than that observed in other patients. Such small responses to hypoxemia suggested that cytochrome oxidase existed in these tethered cords in a highly reduced state. After untethering in these patients, the cytochrome became only slightly more oxidized than it was prior to the untethering procedure (i.e., the response to hypoxemia was greater than prior to untethering but it was still smaller than in other patients). The authors believe that patients in group 3 are analogous to cats subjected to 5 g or greater traction. These patients showed stationary neurological signs and symptoms, with preoperative worsening that ameliorated only partially after untethering.

These data indicate that neurological deficits may parallel dysfunction of oxidative metabolism and that neurological improvement can be predicted during surgery by demonstrating improved metabolism.

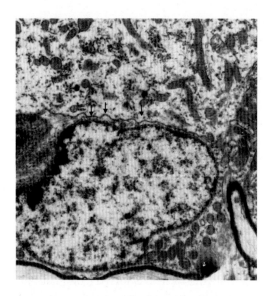

Fig. 3.15 Electron microscopy of a spinal cord that underwent fixation during 5 g traction. Wrinkling of the bilayered membrane is indicated by the *arrows*.

Histological Studies of Experimental Cord Tethering

According to the present knowledge, the CNS does not have a capacity to regenerate new cells after cell death. Therefore, studies of histopathology produced by cord tethering are important in any consideration of treatment because such injury must be considered irreversible.

Morphological changes in cat spinal neurons or glia were not evident by light microscopy after acute or chronic cord tethering. However, electron microscopic study of the spinal cord after release of 5 g traction showed wrinkling of membranes, suggesting that neuronal membranes were stretched and distorted during traction (**Fig. 3.15**)[40]

Electron microscopic (EM) studies of the spinal cord that underwent fixative infusion during traction revealed multiple membrane breaks in the dendrites and occasionally in neuronal perikarya and the glial cells.[40] Whether these membrane breaks are artifactual is not known. Sudden stiffening of these fine structures under excessive tension during arterial perfusion of fixatives (glutaraldehyde and formalin) may readily result in membrane breakage.[34] In either case of EM changes, ion channels may be altered and electrical excitability may be impaired, thereby decreasing ATP use, which in turn could decrease electron transport and glucose consumption. However, the membrane changes could also be secondary to energy failure resulting from lack of oxygen or from the direct effects of tethering on the reactions of oxidative phosphorylation. In the fetal stage where neuronal development is still immature, dyshomeostasis that resulted from these metabolic and structural changes may provoke a cascade of events, such as blocked synaptic transmission, irreversible electrical failure, lipid peroxidation, and histological change to neurons. Progressive stretching of the spinal cord parallel to vertebral growth, and repeated or sudden hard flexion and extension of the vertebral column will accentuate neuronal damage, which may lead to cell death.

■ Are Tethered Cord Syndrome Lesions Located in the Gray Matter or the White Matter?

How Is the Long Tract of the Tethered Spinal Cord Involved?

Whereas the primary lesion of TCS is located in the gray matter, in 10% of pediatric TCS patients, long tract involvement is indicated by motor dysfunction associated with hyperreflexia or Babinski sign or by sensory loss of all modalities of the distal lower limbs. To determine whether tethering effect of the long tract can cause dysfunction and histological damage, the following experiment was performed: horseradish peroxidase (HRP) was injected into the nucleus gracilis of cats, and HRP transport within axons of long tract fibers was observed 72 hours later. The numbers of HRP-labeled cells of bilateral L5, L7, and S2 sensory ganglia were unchanged by traction.[55] Therefore, these data indicate that axonal transport was unaffected by even high-grade cord traction and that acute or chronic tethering produced no histopathological changes in the long tracts.[40,55] The only possible cause of long tract damage may be a sudden traction of the spinal cord in fetal or early infant stage.

Clinical Aspects of Tethered Cord Syndrome

The foregoing experimental studies offer important insights into the mechanisms of the clinical signs and symptoms of TCS.

1. Certain clinical features of TCS indicate that the lesion is located in the gray matter: (1) motor or sensory dysfunction of the distal lower limbs; (2) extensive motor involvement in scattered or patchy distributions in lower limbs, but not following one or two myotomal or dermatomal patterns (as in patients with herniated disk); (3) sensory change only to pinprick stimuli rather than to all modalities; (4) hypoactive reflex of one or more of the lower limb tendons in greater than 95% of TCS patients; (5) mild bladder or rectal dysfunction that rapidly subsides within a few weeks; (6) extensive motor and sensory deficits that tend to occur in TCS patients with a thin elongated cord than those with a nonelongated cord.

2. Motor and sensory deficits and musculoskeletal deformities in lower limbs, and incontinence of TCS patients are reversible if untethering procedures are performed early and properly on category 1 patients (true TCS). In the category 2 patients, only if the signs and symptoms localized above the MMC neuroplaque or dorsal LMMC are relieved after surgical repair, the diagnosis would be TCS. On the other hand, neurological deficits localized at the level of anomalies is due to decompression effects or circulatory impairment.

3. White matter lesions are manifested by long tract signs: motor dysfunction associated with hyperactive deep tendon reflexes, Babinski sign, or sensory loss to all modalities (supposedly not associated with peripheral neuropathy). The Babinski signs are often seen in patients with diastematomyelia located at the L4 cord segment or above. These signs are often caused by stretching of the short cord segments between the septum (in a higher lumbar cord) and the lowest dentate ligaments or between the thoracic septum and the dentate ligament immediately above it.

4. Sudden stretch additional to chronic cord tethering may effect the axonal damage described earlier in this chapter.

5. Irreversible incontinence is the result of prolonged or repeated stretching of the conus medullaris (S2, S3, S4, and probably S5) earlier in TCS patients, progressing from the metabolic and electrophysiological derangement to the neuronal damage.

6. Signs and symptoms in cervical or thoracic TCS patients are often manifested

like the category 2. (See Chapter 10, "The Cervical Tethered Spinal Cord.")

7. The most common imaging, operative, and histological findings of "true TCS" (category 1) are an inelastic filum terminale (either with the presence or the absence of cord elongation[34] or a thick filum),[2,8,27,56] displacement of the filum posterior to the cauda equina, touching the posterior arachnoid membrane, and fibrous or fibroadipose filum.

8. The combination of an elongated (lumbosacral) cord and thickened filum is a typical form of "tethered spinal cord,"[1] but TCS patients without these features are found at a 30% rate in adults and late teenage patients[27,53] and increasingly in younger children (Knerium D and Won DJ, personal communication 2008).

9. Adult TCS patients always present with severe back and leg pain and subtle neurological signs and musculoskeletal deformities. At operation, a fibrous or fibroadipose inelastic filum is found to fasten the conus medullaris. The mechanisms underlying signs and symptoms that develop in late-teenage children and adults are described in detail in Chapter 14, "Tethered Cord Syndrome in Adults."

■ Essential Factors for Tethered Cord Syndrome

Elongated Cord and a Thick Filum

Hoffman and colleagues[1] originally described two anatomical features in patients with a tethered spinal cord: an elongated cord and a thickened terminal filum. These features are often considered to be absolute criteria in the diagnosis of this disorder. As the number of patients with a diagnosis of tethering-induced symptomatology increased, however, neurosurgeons began asking whether an elongated cord or thickened filum or both were essential. This questioning of the anatomical criteria for TCS

was brought to the forefront by the surgical experiences of Warder and Oakes,[57] who reported no cord elongation in 18% of their patients, and Yamada and colleagues,[34,40] who found that 28% of adult and late teen patients with typical signs and symptoms of TCS showed neither cord elongation nor a thickened terminal filum.[34,40] To pursue this subject, we collected relevant clinical and experimental data as follows for the development of TCS.

Diameter and Histology of the Filum

Yundt et al found that the diameter of the normal filum is 1.1 or 1.2 mm.[58] In contrast, the minimal diameter claimed for the diagnosis of tethered spinal cord varied from 1 to 2 mm.[12,59–61] This variation led us to question whether the rule of > 2 mm thick filum as a standard for the diagnosis of tethered spinal cord is absolutely necessary.[60] Selden took an intermediate position by the term "the minimally TCS" as between 1.5 mm and 2 mm.[61] It became necessary to study the viscoelasticity of the spinal cord and the filum for further analysis of the dynamic mechanisms of TCS. In addition, reports on histological studies of terminal filum removed from patients with tethered spinal cord came to our attention.[61,62] Our histological studies are described in a later section.

Embryological Origin

It was initially speculated that the elongated, thickened spinal cords in patients with TCS indicated spinal cord overgrowth, as suggested by Barry et al.[63] in patients with MMC. This theory is supported by data from the recent landmark studies conducted by Pfister et al[64] who showed stretch-induced axonal growth. This conclusion was elicited from observations of posterior ganglion cells removed from rat embryos. After continuous extreme stretching of integrated axons (by traction) for 24 hours, these axons (not the growing axons) lengthened 10-fold from baseline, and their diameters increased by 35%. Conceivably, if the newly developed caudal spinal cord and terminal filum are surrounded by mesodermal tissue and if fibrous tissue starts to grow into the terminal filum in human embryos (in the ninth week), cord tension could increase as the spine grows, and consequently the lower spinal cord and filum to grow unusually longer and thicker. In normally developing embryos, however, the coccygeal medullary vestige is isolated from the terminal filum (during the ninth to eleventh weeks), presumably preventing mesodermal tissue from growing into the filum.[34] Pfister et al[64] also found the boundary of nerve growth and disconnection. To the right of this boundary, axonal growth was accelerated as long as tension was increased, but axonal disruption occurred in the gray zone (on the left). Slightly right of the boundary, neuronal dysfunction was expected, as in tethered spinal cord. One can postulate that an elongated cord is likely to have occurred from its stretching during an embryonic period.[34] If mesodermal tissue continues to grow in the filum, the patient is likely to develop TCS.

Mechanical Dynamics of the Filum

We analyzed the dynamic features of the filum from a physiological standpoint: (1) viscoelasticity of the spinal cord and the filum, and (2) histological findings of fila terminales removed

from patients with a tethered spinal cord.[34,61,62] Our histological studies are described in the later section.

Stretch Test for Filum Viscoelasticity

Normally, natural tension exists in the thoracic cord, dentate ligaments, and dura, as reported by Tunturi[65] and Tubbs et al.[30] The vertical tension is less, however, in the lumbosacral cord and dura,[31] reflecting high viscoelasticity of the filum and lack of dentate ligaments.

In our experimental studies, the filum stretched much greater than any cord segments (**Fig. 3.3A**). When the spinal cord was directly tractioned, cord stretching became much greater. This simulated tethered spinal cord without protection of the elastic filum (**Fig. 3.3B**). In all TCS patients, stretch tests showed that the fila terminales elongated by 10% or less and returned to the original length on release of stretching (**Fig. 3.16A**, without stretch and **Fig. 3.16B**, with stretch). In contrast, the filum of each patient without TCS elongated 50% or greater, similarly to the filum of animal models. After a 1 cm segment of the filum was resected, its cephalic and caudal ends formed a 1.5 cm to 2.5 cm gap. This finding is indicative of excessive cord tension that existed before sectioning of the filum.

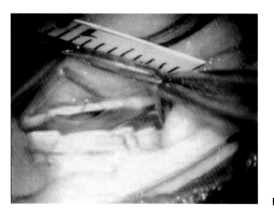

Fig. 3.16 (A) A 7 mm segment of the filum is held in place with two pairs of forceps. **(B)** The filum is pulled in opposite directions with two pairs of forceps. Only slight elongation (less than 10%) occurred concomitant with thinning of the filum.

Histological Studies of the Filum Terminale from Tethered Cord Syndrome Patients

The spinal cord consists of intermingled neurons, glial tissue and vasculature, and the surrounding pia mater tightly connected to the cord substance. Elastin in the pia, subpial tissue, and the blood vessels is probably the main source of the spinal cord elasticity. Collagen in the dentate ligaments, pia, and blood vessels resist the traction effect and prevent neuronal disruption. From our experimental traction studies on the cat spinal cord and filum, evidently the elasticity of the former is far greater than the latter.[2,35]

The specimens removed from the fila of 58 patients with TCS, with or without cord elongation and filum thickening, were studied with light microscopy. In all specimens, normal glia was replaced by fibrous tissue (**Fig. 3.17A**) or by fibroadipose tissue. Elastin staining showed only a small amount of elastin (**Fig. 3.17B**). This pathology is compatible with minimal viscoelasticity of the filum (10% elongation by stretch test) in TCS patients.

An inelastic structure continuous to the caudal spinal cord is an essential mechanical factor causing TCS. A minimal amount of elastin in the fibrosed filum provides it with some elasticity causing it to contract caudad (~10%) after a partial resection. Based on clinical and scientific evidence, we conclude that the paucity of filum viscoelasticity is the main predisposing factor for the development of TCS.

Posteriorly Displaced Filum

The spinal cords of normal individuals in supine position are located anteriorly in the thoracic spine, posteriorly in the cervical spine, and more posteriorly in the lumbar spine. Apparently the spinal cord is shifted toward the concave side of the spinal curvature. Accordingly, the subarachnoid space posterior to the spinal cord and the cauda equina is relatively narrower in the lumbosacral level than in the cervical and thoracic levels.

Normally, the posterior roots cover the entire conus and filum (**Fig. 3.2C**). Only in patients with TCS, the filum is exposed posteriomedial to the cauda equina, regardless of whether there is an elongated cord and thickened filum. Presumably, the taut inelastic filum pushed the normally relaxed posterior roots away laterally during the rapid spinal growth.[66]

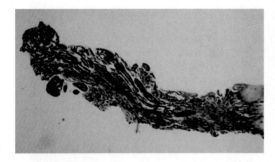

A

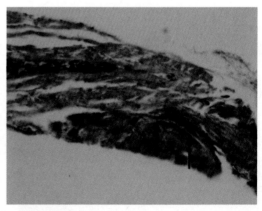

B

Fig. 3.17 (A) Photomicrograph of representative histological section of filum removed from a patient with typical tethered cord syndrome showing replacement of the entire filum with fibrous tissue. **(B)** Photograph revealing fibrotic filum with sparse, thin, and discontinuous elastin fibers (*black areas indicated by arrows*) running in between and parallel to the collagen (*pink*). Blood vessels at the left corner have abundant elastin. Malory trichrome **(A)** and elastin stain **(B)**, original magnification × 400.

The 1 mm thick filum with magnetic resonance imaging (MRI) fat signal, which is posteriorly displaced and touching the posterior arachnoid membrane, corresponds to the surgical finding (see **Figs. 15.6** and **15.7** in Chapter 15, Tethered Cord Syndrome in Adult and Teenage Patients without Neural Spinal Dysraphism).

In TCS patients, the filum is attached to the posterior arachnoid membrane, most frequently at the most lordotic spine (i.e., the L4 or L5 lamina). This shifting of the caudal spinal cord and the filum to the concave side of lumbosacral lordosis signifies their adjustment to minimize cord tension.

To visually confirm this filum displacement, intrathecal endoscopy was done before opening the dura and arachnoid widely and losing cerebrospinal fluid. This procedure was followed by tests to accurately diagnose the TCS by three steps: MRI, endoscopy, and stretch test.[34,65]

Incontinence

The lower urinary tract function is discussed eloquently in Chapters 7, 8, and 19. Readers are advised to read references in these chapters.[6,67] Recently three groups of authors discussed incontinence in patients who showed no cord elongation and filum thickening as occult TCS.[68–70] This is in contrast to the most authors that described incontinence concomitant with mild motor and sensory deficits. The reliability of MRI findings was discussed by the questionnaire.[70] It can be postulated that TCS can be manifested only by incontinence, because our experimental work has indicated that the conus medullaris is most vulnerable to traction.

These three groups of authors advocate that extensive lower urinary tract studies should be done before decision making. From our experience, however, most of the adult and late teenage patients showed negative renal and bladder tests.[70]

The frequent positive findings were the postvoid urinary residual being > 100 mL associated with decreases in residual to less than 35 mL

in all the patients with complaints of urinary incontinence.[67] After untethering surgery, more than 90% ceased to complain of incontinence within 2 days to 1 week. Yamada and Won recommended diagnostic studies including anal sphincter contraction test, which frequently shows abnormalities, coexistent with bladder dysfunction, and other studies, such as MRI, endoscopy, stretch test, and histological studies already mentioned, to enhance the diagnosis of TCS.[71]

We also suggested that additional diagnostic studies be conducted, including (1) anal sphincter diminution, (2) intra- or preoperative subarachnoid endoscopy to confirm displacement of the filum posterior to the cauda equina, (3) filum stretch test to determine the filum viscoelasticity, (4) histological studies on the resected filum, and (5) if available, in vivo reflection spectrophotometry to confirm a reduced state of cytochrome oxidase in spinal cord mitochondria. Interpolation of the data thus obtained will allow the interinstitutional studies to better interpret MRI findings.

■ Conclusion

The following correlations can be made between previous experimental results and clinical observation:

1. Cord tethering associated with stretching produces excessive tension within the spinal cord and can result in metabolic derangement, and if sudden forceful stretching occurs, there are further histological changes.
2. Impairment of oxidative metabolism is proved by the various degrees of the reduced state of cytochrome a,a_3, which indicates slow electron transport coupled with ADP phosphorylation or slow ATP use.
3. In patients with true TCS (the first category of cord tethering), wherein the caudal part of the spinal cord is anchored by inelastic filum, oxidative metabolism is impaired in the spinal cord under steady

traction, the severity of neuronal dysfunction parallels the degree of impairment in oxidative metabolism, so does the metabolic and neurological improvements deficits by surgical untethering procedures when such deficits are caused by metabolic and electrophysiological impairment.

4. A decrease in blood flow and glucose metabolic impairment is correlated with cytochrome reduction. Increases in blood flow are reported to be associated with postsurgical neurological improvement. It is likely that this human condition corresponds to the mild-to-moderate experimental cord traction.

5. Chronic cord traction may be compensated for by the plasticity of the spinal cord tissues. Spontaneous alleviation or fluctuation of a patient's symptoms may be explained by the neuronal plasticity, but these symptoms tend to recur or progress as a result of repeated cord stretching due to spine flexion and extension, as well as lateral flexion.

6. Early untethering, when minimum or mild symptoms are detected, is essential for the best treatment of TCS. This condition correlates with the experimental mild-to-moderate tethered spinal cord.

7. Irreversible neuronal damage can result from sudden stretching of the already chronically tethered cord. TCS patients who have no satisfactory surgical results may correspond to this experimental model of cord tethering. Long tract signs in human TCS may be caused by similar mechanisms.

8. Attention should be directed to category 2 or 3, if inadequate or no neurological improvement followed after the surgical procedures that appeared to be cord untethering.

In summary, the current understanding is that TCS is caused by steady excessive tension in the lumbosacral cord accentuated by repeated stretching of the spinal cord by flexion or extension movements. Histologically, demonstrable neuronal damage is associated with sudden additional violent stretching force applied to the cord, which may explain the irreversible neurological deficits in some TCS patients. Early untethering of the spinal cord is advisable in TCS patients in general.

References

1. Hoffman HJ, Hendrick EB, Humphreys RP. The tethered spinal cord: its protean manifestations, diagnosis and surgical correction. Childs Brain 1976;2: 145–155

2. Yamada S, Zinke DE, Sanders DC. Pathophysiology of "tethered cord syndrome." J Neurosurg 1981;54: 494–503

3. Al-Mefty O, Kandzari S, Fox JL. Neurogenic bladder and the tethered spinal cord syndrome. J Urol 1979;122:112–115

4. Anderson FM. Occult spinal dysraphism: a series of 73 cases. Pediatrics 1975;55:826–835

5. Bassett RC. The neurologic deficit associated with lipomas of the cauda equina. Ann Surg 1950;131: 109–116, illust

6. Blaivas JG. Urologic abnormalities in the tethered spinal cord. In: Holtzman RNN, Stein BM, eds. The Tethered Spinal Cord. New York: Thieme-Stratton; 1985:59–73

7. Churchill BM, Gilmour RF, Williot P. Urodynamics. Pediatr Clin North Am 1987;34:1133–1157

8. Fitz CR, Harwood Nash DC. The tethered conus. Am J Roentgenol Radium Ther Nucl Med 1975;125: 515–523

9. Fuchs A. Über Beziehungen der Enuresis nocturna zu Rudimentärformen der Spina Bifida Occulta (Myelodysplasie). Wien Med Wochenschr 1910;80: 1569–1573

10. Garceau GJ. The filum terminale syndrome (the cord-traction syndrome). J Bone Joint Surg Am 1953;35-A:711–716

11. Guthkelch AN, Hoffmann GT. Tethered spinal cord in association with diastematomyelia. Surg Neurol 1981;15:352–354

12. Hochhauser L, Chaung S, Harwood-Nash DS, et al. The tethered cord syndrome revisited [abstract]. AJNR Am J Neuroradiol 1986;7:543

13. Hoffman HJ, Taecholarn C, Hendrick EB, Humphreys RP. Management of lipomyelomeningoceles: experience at

the Hospital for Sick Children, Toronto. J Neurosurg 1985;62:1–8

14. Hoffmann GT, Hooks CA, Jackson IJ, Thompson IM. Urinary incontinence in myelomeningoceles due to a tethered spinal cord and its surgical treatment. Surg Gynecol Obstet 1956;103:618–624

15. James CCM, Lassman LP. Spinal dysraphism: the diagnosis and treatment of progressive lesions in spina bifida occulta. J Bone Joint Surg Br 1962;44B: 828–840

16. Jones PH, Love JG. Tight filum terminale. Arch Surg 1956;73:556–566

17. Lassman LP, James CCM. Meningocoele manqué. Childs Brain 1977;3:1–11

18. McLone DG, Naidich TP. The tethered spinal cord. In: McLaurin RL, Schut L, Venes JL, et al, eds. Pediatric Neurosurgery. 2nd ed. Philadelphia: WB Saunders; 1989:76–96

19. Naidich TP, McLone DG. Congenital pathology of the spine and spinal cord. In: Taveras JM, Ferrucci JT, eds. Radiology. Philadelphia: JB Lippincott; 1986: 1–23

20. Purtzer TJ, Yamada S, Tani S. Metabolic and histologic studies of chronic model of tethered cord. Surg Forum 1985;36:512–514

21. Rogers HM, Long DM, Chou SN, French LA. Lipomas of the spinal cord and cauda equina. J Neurosurg 1971;34:349–354

22. Schneider SJ, Rosenthal AD, Greenberg BM, Danto J. A preliminary report on the use of laser-Doppler flowmetry during tethered spinal cord release. Neurosurgery 1993;32:214–217, discussion 217–218

23. Schut L, Bruce DA, Sutton LN. The management of the child with a lipomyelomeningocele. Clin Neurosurg 1983;30:464–476

24. Scott RM. Delayed deterioration in patients with spinal tethering syndrome. In: Holtzman RNN, Stein BM, eds. The Tethered Spinal Cord. New York: Thieme-Stratton; 1985:116–120

25. Till K. Occult spinal dysraphism: the value of prophylactic surgical treatment. In: Sano K, Ishii S, Le Vay D, eds. Recent Progress in Neurological Surgery. New York: Elsevier; 1971:61–66

26. Till K. Spinal dysraphism: a study of congenital malformations of the lower back. J Bone Joint Surg Br 1969;51:415–422

27. Yamada S, Iacono R, Morgese V, et al. Tethered cord syndrome in adults. In: Menezes A, Sonntag VK, eds. Principles in Spinal Surgery. New York: McGraw-Hill; 1996:433–445

28. Yamada S, Won DJ. What is the true tethered cord syndrome? Childs Nerv Syst 2007;23:371–375

29. Yashon D, Beatty RA. Tethering of the conus medullaris within the sacrum. J Neurol Neurosurg Psychiatry 1966;29:244–250

30. Tubbs RS, Salter G, Grabb PA, Oakes WJ. The denticulate ligament: anatomy and functional significance. J Neurosurg 2001;94(2, Suppl):271–275

31. Tunturi AR. Elasticity of the spinal cord, pia, and denticulate ligament in the dog. J Neurosurg 1978;48: 975–979

32. Hawass ND, el-Badawi MG, Fatani JA, et al. Myelographic study of the spinal cord ascent during fetal development. AJNR Am J Neuroradiol 1987;8: 691–695

33. Breig A. Overstretching of and circumscribed pathological tension in the spinal cord: a basic cause of symptoms in cord disorders. J Biomech 1970;3:7–9

34. Yamada S, Won DJ, Pezeshkpour G, et al. Pathophysiology of tethered cord syndrome and similar complex disorders. Neurosurg Focus 2007;23:1–10

35. Tani S, Yamada S, Knighton RS. Extensibility of the lumbar and sacral cord. Pathophysiology of the tethered spinal cord in cats. J Neurosurg 1987;66(1): 116–123

36. Roy MW, Gilmore R, Walsh JW. Evaluation of children and young adults with tethered spinal cord syndrome: utility of spinal and scalp recorded somatosensory evoked potentials. Surg Neurol 1986;26:241–248

37. Yamada S, Knierim D, Yonekura M, Schultz R, Maeda G. Tethered cord syndrome. J Am Paraplegia Soc 1983;6:58–61

38. Yamada S, Schreider S, Ashwal S, et al. Pathophysiologic mechanisms in the tethered spinal cord syndrome. In: Holtzman RNN, Stein BM, eds. The Tethered Spinal Cord Syndrome. New York: Thieme-Stratton; 1985:29–40

39. Rosenthal M, LaManna J, Yamada S, Younts W, Somjen G. Oxidative metabolism, extracellular potassium and sustained potential shifts in cat spinal cord in situ. Brain Res 1979;162:113–127

40. Yamada S, Iacono R, Yamada BS. Pathophysiology of tethered cord syndrome. In: Yamada S, ed. Tethered Cord Syndrome. Park Ridge, IL: American Association of Neurological Surgeons; 1996:29–48

41. Chance B, Williams GR. The respiratory chain and oxidative phosphorylation. Adv Enzymol Relat Subj Biochem 1956;17:65–134

42. Jöbsis FF, Keizer JH, LaManna JC, Rosenthal M. Reflectance spectrophotometry of cytochrome aa$_3$ in vivo. J Appl Physiol 1977;43:858–872

43. Austin GM, McCouch GP. Presynaptic component of intermediary cord potential. J Neurophysiol 1955; 18:441–451

44. McCouch GP, Austin GM. Site of origin and reflex behavior of postsynaptic negative potentials recorded from the spinal cord. Yale J Biol Med 1956;28:372–379

45. Yamada S, Sanders DC, Maeda G. Oxidative metabolism during and following ischemia of cat spinal cord. Neurol Res 1981;3:1–16

46. Gelfan S, Tarlov IM. Altered neuron population in L7 segment of dogs with experimental hind-limb rigidity. Am J Physiol 1963;205:606–616

47. Kang JK, Kim MC, Kim DS, Song JU. Effects of tethering on regional spinal cord blood flow and sensory-evoked potentials in growing cats. Childs Nerv Syst 1987;3:35–39

48. Turnbull IM, Brieg A, Hassler O. Blood supply of cervical spinal cord in man: a microangiographic cadaver study. J Neurosurg 1966;24:951–965

49. Tani S, Yamada S, Fuse T, Nakamura N. Changes in lumbosacral canal length during flexion and extension: dynamic effect on the elongated spinal cord in the tethered spinal cord [in Japanese]. No To Shinkei 1991;43:1121–1125

50. Yamada S, Perot PL Jr, Ducker TB, Lockard I. Myelotomy for control of mass spasms in paraplegia. J Neurosurg 1976;45:683–691

51. Sokoloff L, Reivich M, Kennedy C, et al. The [14C]deoxyglucose method for the measurement of local cerebral glucose utilization: theory, procedure, and normal values in the conscious and anesthetized albino rat. J Neurochem 1977;28:897–916

52. Yamada S, Iacono RP, Andrade T, Mandybur G, Yamada BS. Pathophysiology of tethered cord syndrome. Neurosurg Clin N Am 1995;6:311–323

53. Yamada S, Won DJ, Yamada SM. Pathophysiology of tethered cord syndrome and clinical correlation. Neurosurg Focus 2004;16:E6

54. Yamada S, Schultz R, Mandybur G, Liwnicz BL, Adey WS. Axonal degeneration after sudden forceful traction of the spinal cord: is it the cause of permanent neurological deficit? J Neurosurg 2003;98:681

55. Fuse T, Patrickson JW, Yamada S. Axonal transport of horseradish peroxidase in the experimental tethered spinal cord. Pediatr Neurosci 1989;15:296–301

56. Pang D, Wilberger JE Jr. Tethered cord syndrome in adults. J Neurosurg 1982;57:32–47

57. Warder DE, Oakes WJ. Tethered cord syndrome and the conus in a normal position. Neurosurgery 1993;33:374–378

58. Yundt KD, Park TS, Kaufman BA. Normal diameter of filum terminale in children: in vivo measurement. Pediatr Neurosurg 1997;27:257–259

59. Pang D. Tethered cord syndrome. In: Hoffman HJ, ed. Advances in Neurosurgery. Philadelphia: Benley & Belfus; 1984:41–80

60. Greenberg MR. Handbook of Neurosurgery. New York: Thieme; 2001

61. Selden NR, Nixon RR, Skoog SR, Lashley DB. Minimal tethered cord syndrome associated with thickening of the terminal filum. J Neurosurg 2006;105 (3, Suppl):214–218

62. Selçuki M, Vatansever S, Inan S, Erdemli E, Bağdatoğlu C, Polat A. Is a filum terminale with a normal appearance really normal? Childs Nerv Syst 2003;19:3–10

63. Barry A, Patten BM, Stewart BH. Possible factors in the development of the Arnold-Chiari malformation. J Neurosurg 1957;14:285–301

64. Pfister BJ, Iwata A, Meaney DF, Smith DH. Extreme stretch growth of integrated axons. J Neurosci 2004; 24:7978–7983

65. Tunituri AR. Elasticity of the spinal cord dura in the dog. J Neurosurg 1977;47:391–396

66. Yamada S, Won DJ, Kido DK. Adult tethered cord syndrome: new classification correlated with symptomatology, imaging and pathophysiology. Neurosurg Q 2001;11:260–275

67. Yamada S, Yamada BS, Won DJ. Tethered cord syndrome. In: Corcos J, Schick E, eds. London: Informa; 2008:365–374

68. Drake JM. Occult tethered cord syndrome: not an indication for surgery. J Neurosurg 2006;104(5, Suppl): 305–308

69. Selden NR. Occult tethered cord syndrome: the case for surgery. J Neurosurg 2006;104(5, Suppl):302–304

70. Steinbok P, Garton HJ, Gupta N. Occult tethered cord syndrome: a survey of practice patterns. J Neurosurg 2006;104(5, Suppl):309–313

71. Yamada S, Won DJ. Occult tethered cord. J Neurosurg 2007;106(5, Suppl):411–413, author reply 413–414 (Letter)

4 Neurological Assessment of Tethered Spinal Cord

Sanford Schneider

A nonambulatory patient in his thirties had been a long-distance runner in college. Over a period of a dozen years he had progressively lost motor strength in his lower extremities until he became wheelchair bound. Multiple prior studies had been nondiagnostic, but on careful neurological examination, motor and sensory losses implicated the spinal cord and, subsequently, a myelogram revealed findings compatible with tethered cord syndrome (TCS). Unfortunately, surgical intervention yielded no significant improvement. TCS diagnosis had never been considered by the numerous physicians who had examined him over those many years. This scenario will, it is hoped, not repeat itself given that neurologists, internists, and urologists are now well sensitized to the existence of this disorder. Clinical awareness of TCS and its multiple clinical presentations now leads to neurological referral to "rule-out TCS." Increasingly, patients with TCS will be diagnosed prior to the onset of irreversible cord damage. However, it is important for the examining physician to be aware of the subtle historical and neurological features that warrant further diagnostic studies to establish this diagnosis.

Although widespread awareness of TCS has been a recent phenomenon, the syndrome was recognized long ago. Chute, in 1921, reported the association of urinary retention and traction on the conus medullaris.[1] In 1940, Lichtenstein utilized the all-encompassing term *spinal dysraphism* for several syndromes

associating the failure of the posterior neuropore to close, resulting in neural dysplasia both with and without mesenchymal or dermatological manifestations.[2]

Bassett in 1950 reported the association of lipomas and conus traction. He noted improvement in seven of nine patients following surgical resection of a lipomatous sac from the conus.[3] Garceau reported three teenagers with progressive paraparesis, two with scoliosis, due to a restrictive filum terminale ("cord-traction syndrome") without associated vertebral malformation.[4] Hoffman et al, several years later, described a "tethered" spinal cord after meningomyelocele repair, with significant improvement in symptoms following secondary surgical intervention.[5] Of 442 patients with spina bifida seen over a decade, six patients were diagnosed with a tight filum terminale; neurological dysfunction improved after section of the filum.[6] Anderson, in 1968, described the clinical presentation of progressive weakness and deformity of lower extremities associated with loss of bowel and bladder control in children with a tight filum terminale, either as an isolated anomaly or associated with spinal dysraphism.[7] By the 1970s, Hoffman and his associates had operated on 31 children with tethered spinal cords in a 5-year span, generally with gratifying improvement.[8] Refer to the definition of *tethered spinal cord* and *tethered cord syndrome* described in Chapter 3, Pathophysiology of Tethered Cord Syndrome.

Over the last 2 or 3 decades clinical recognition of TCS as a distinct syndrome has evolved. This diagnosis was supported by the development of imaging techniques since the mid-1970s, first initiated by computed tomography (CT), then CT myelography, to the present-day utilization of magnetic resonance imaging (MRI), which readily allows noninvasive diagnosis.[9] However, selection of patients for MRI examination must be based on careful historical and neurological features. In one series of 23 symptomatic children with refractory voiding dysfunction, 16 children (70%) had spina bifida occulta but only two children (9%) had an abnormal MRI.[10] Similar to the old axiom that an operating surgeon should occasionally remove a normal appendix when the diagnosis is suggestive, so should a certain number of spinal cord MRIs prove to be normal. However, given the expense of this technology, such imaging should be limited to those patients in whom thoughtful screening, careful history taking, and meticulous neurological examinations all suggest the possibility of TCS.

■ Patient Evaluation

History

Clinical assessment is initiated through history. The age of the patient will determine whether the pertinent history is obtained from the patient or the caregiver. A newborn presents without significant history but with clinical features: a sacral midline hair tuft ("faun's tail"), a sacral lipomatous mass, or possibly orthopedic (musculoskeletal) deformities such as shortening or atrophy of a limb or a club foot. The historical features are relatively limited and may include a poor urinary stream or urinary continuous dribbling. In the neonate the decision for further investigation is based on the clinical features, whereas historical features seldom significantly contribute to the decision-making process. The ambulatory child, however, develops a symptom complex due to the combination of upper and lower motor neuron deficits. Careful questioning will reveal whether the child has had an alteration of gait that was previously normal, impairment or awkwardness while running, and the tendency to wear out the tip or sides of generally one shoe, due to peroneus or anterior tibialis weakness. An astute parent may report that one leg seems thinner than the other (stork leg). Uncommonly, a parent may report that a child refuses to bear weight due to pain or that the child refuses to flex or rotate his or her back because of pain. Sensory loss is generally minimal in a child, so that trophic scarring is seldom noted. Rapid development of scoliosis may be the chief complaint of the adolescent child undergoing a growth spurt. Although, congenital club foot may be noted in the newborn, later development of a unilateral pes cavus or talipes may be due to TCS. The combination of scoliosis, exaggerated lumbosacral lordosis (in older children and adults), and lower extremity deformity should raise the possibility of TCS.[11] In the preteen years, the major symptoms include lower extremity weakness, gait disturbances, incontinence or reemergence of enuresis, and development of mild foot deformities. The teenager may develop a rather rapid and progressive picture of scoliosis and urinary incontinence frequently associated with gelastic leakage (often misinterpreted as due to a urinary tract infection that defies treatment with antibiotics). The urinary symptoms are frequently investigated with multiple urological studies, and even surgery to eliminate an obstruction, before a spina bifida occulta is noted on the abdominal x-ray.

Adult patients can usually be divided into two presenting groups: those with previously diagnosed and repaired spinal dysraphism and an occult group with slowly progressive and insidious symptomatology or a catastrophic acute precipitating event. This acute event may have been precipitated by the sudden stretching of the conus or lumbosacral cord (during childbirth, intercourse, vigorous sporting events, or extensive exercise) or direct trauma. Pain is the most common presenting symptom in adults, usually in the perineal-saddle region.[11,12] Lower extremity sensory loss, leg weakness, and bladder disturbances often accompany the pain.[13] Many of the patients with TCS will have a spina bifida occulta in the lumbosacral region noted on spine x-ray; however, the vast majority of patients with spina bifida occulta do not have TCS. Most patients with urinary dysfunction will have a hypotonic bladder secondary to lower motor neuron dysfunction. Although a small spastic bladder can result from cord dysfunction above the conus medullaris, spasms are often caused by bladder wall irritation in the presence of the lesion in the conus, which still preserves an adequate number of functional neurons for spinal reflex. Despite urinary dysfunction being common in this population, urinary tract infection is relatively rare in the adult but common in children.[14]

Patients with a prior history of repaired spinal dysraphism have at least a 15% chance of a TCS developing later in life.[14] Patients with prior meningomyelocele repairs should be frequently monitored for development of TCS by inquiries as to whether changes in bowel or bladder function have occurred, walking is more difficult, or new motor or sensory disturbances have developed.

Physical Examination

Careful visual examination of the lumbosacral region may reveal a hair tuft, a dermal sinus, a lipomatous mass, a midline nevus, or hypertrichosis, which may the only suggestion of embryonic failure of differentiation between the midline ectoderm and mesoderm occurring in the first trimester of pregnancy. Cutaneous manifestations occur in ~40% of patients with TCS. Orthopedic deformities, particularly if they are asymmetrical, are also common. Scoliosis, a high-riding asymmetrical hip while standing, pes cavus, and equinovarus skeletal abnormalities may be the presenting feature of TCS. A unilateral stork leg is very uncommon, but subtle asymmetries of the lower extremities are quite common. Careful measurements of the midthigh and midcalf circumferences should be made by marking the midpatella bilaterally, then measuring similar distances above and below the mark with the patient preferably standing; a 10% or 3 cm difference (be aware that the dominant limb is usually slightly greater in bulk) is suggestive of lower extremity atrophy. Differences greater than 3 cm should be considered abnormal, suggesting TCS. In the nonstanding patient, the recumbent position is satisfactory if both legs are flat and equally relaxed. If the measurements are abnormal, it is important to similarly measure the arms because a minimal hemiatrophy of cerebral origin will have asymmetrical measurements. Such subtle circumferential differences as 3 cm are virtually nondetectable by visual inspection. The technique should be routinely performed as part of the assessment of TCS, and the measurement differences should be reproducible on several repeat measurements. This simple test has proven, on many patients, to be a sensitive indicator of TCS.

With a patient of any age, the neurological examination has to be meticulously performed when there is a possibility of TCS, with modification of the exam for the infant or very young child who is nonambulatory. Observation of gait is mandatory and can be assessed watching the child at play while estimating spasticity or weakness. Generally, it is possible to cajole children as young as 3 to heel and toe walk by mimicking the examiner. Emphasis needs to be placed on the motor and sensory examination of the lower extremities. Presentations of TCS are notorious for asymmetrical motor and sensory examinations with "skip areas" of normalcy. The gastrocnemius, anterior tibialis, peroneus, quadriceps, hamstring, and hip rotators and adductor muscle groups need to be individually assessed. Sensation measured by pin and light touch, as well as posterior column function, vibration, and joint position sense are readily performed in patients above the age of 4. As noted earlier, sensation, particularly pinprick, may involve noncontiguous dermatomes, so that each dermatome needs to be examined. The anal wink must be assessed for presence and symmetry. TCS generally produces lower or upper motor neuron signs or a mixture of these signs. Accordingly, deep tendon reflexes are usually reduced or absent, particularly at the ankles, or brisk and asymmetrical. A Babinski sign may be present in one or both extremities but can be normal or silent. In patients with upper motor neuron signs, the concomitant syrinx or diastematomyelia in a higher-lumbar or thoracic level must be considered. Thus clinical suspicion depends on a combination of orthopedic deformity, sacral cutaneous manifestations, asymmetrical lower extremity atrophy, hypotonia or hypertonia, and deep tendon reflex asymmetries, all combined with a history of gait disturbance, bladder dysfunction, and a frequent description of pain in the older child or adult.

Laboratory Studies

The neurodiagnostic capability of MRI noninvasive imaging does not relieve the clinician of thoroughly evaluating the patient by history and careful neurological examination. In one study of 23 children with chronic urological dysfunction, 16 had spina bifida occulta, but MRI spine studies in all 23 patients yielded only one patient with symptomatic TCS and one patient with a syrinx.[10] Indiscriminate MRI studies as a screening tool would result in an unacceptably low yield for a relatively expensive study. Many patients with TCS will have radiological demonstration of lumbar, lumbosacral, or sacral incomplete neural arch deformities, generally at L4, L5, or S1. The older literature relates that nearly all pediatric patients with TCS will have a neural arch deformity.[15,16] Newer studies report that the syndrome can often occur in the absence of bony defects,[4,17] particularly in adults and older children.[11] The presence of an occult spina bifida is now only suggestive of TCS because 22% of the total population have an occult spina bifida and only an extremely small fraction of that population will have TCS.[15,18] As CT metrizamide myelography replaced myelography as the diagnostic tool of choice; MRI has largely supplanted CT myelog-

raphy. The normal range of the filum thickness has been established during posterior rhizotomy procedures for control of cerebral palsy–related spasms in children who showed no signs of TCS.[19] Multiple studies have confirmed the diagnostic sensitivity of MRI in children.[20] Rarely, high-resolution MRI studies may be necessary to confirm the diagnosis. In the newborn with lipoma, meningomyelocele, and spina bifida, ultrasonography by knowledgeable radiologists is a useful screening tool in determining the extent of the malformation.[21] The majority of newborns with a low-lying conus can be diagnosed by ultrasound.[22]

In the author's opinion, electromyography and nerve conduction studies are seldom of much practical clinical value in patient assessment of TCS. Often, electromyographic studies are normal, which may mislead the clinician into believing the patient is also normal. Somatosensory evoked studies of the posterior tibial nerve have frequently been useful as a screening procedure and may be a useful tool for following postoperative long-term outcome.[23]

Occasionally, urological symptoms, including incontinence, impotence, urgency, and rarely infection may be the heralding symptoms of TCS. Awareness of the typical urodynamic features of typically hypotonic and the less common hypertonic bladder due to TCS should be understood by the urological clinician.

■ Differential Diagnosis

Although, the classic presentation, as described earlier, may occur, it is the rare patient who presents with a complete constellation of historical and neurological dysfunction. Prior to MRI, the diagnosing physician had to have an extremely high probability of TCS before submitting the patient to an invasive myelogram. However, even with the ease of obtaining a spine MRI, the neurologist should be reasonably certain that TCS is a possibility.

In the infant or younger child TCS can be confused with a subtle hemiparesis due to cerebral palsy. Brain damage in the superior distribution of the anterior cerebral artery may result in weakness and spasticity primarily of the lower extremity. Eighty to 90% of children with cerebral palsy have no history of birthing difficulty, so often a difficult delivery history may not be present. However, a history of prematurity should alert the clinician to the possibility of cerebral palsy. Careful history taking may reveal that the child has had a marked hand preference early in infancy and that motor and language milestones are delayed. Examination of the child with hemiparetic cerebral palsy generally demonstrates unilateral spasticity and hyperreflexia of both the upper and the lower extremities and unilateral long tract signs such as an extensor plantar response. Spastic diplegic patients will have corticospinal tract spasticity limited to the lower extremities and Babinski sign, generally bilaterally symmetrical. In contrast, patients with TCS usually present with lower motor rather than upper motor neuron signs, and sometimes with their combination, manifested by asymmetrical dysfunction in the lower extremities.

Friedreich ataxia, particularly in the young child, can be difficult to diagnose because of the child's inability to describe a loss of posterior column function. Deep tendon reflexes can be brisk with bilateral extensor plantar responses. A positive family history of progressive weakness, ending by being wheelchair bound in middle age, aids in distinguishing between the two disorders. A DNA study for the expanded nucleotide is diagnostic. The many other forms of spinocerebellar degenerative disorders have a very slow progression, a cerebellar and peripheral neuropathy component, and a positive family history. Chronic polyneuropathy syndromes should be readily distinguished by distal weakness and absent deep tendon reflexes. The static spinomuscular atrophies, such as spinal musculature atrophy III disease, generally have marked lower extremity atrophy, fasciculations, absent deep tendon reflexes, intact bladder and sensory function, and a history of marked delay in walking. Although a family history is usually lacking due to its autosomal

recessive inheritance pattern, a DNA study can confirm the diagnosis.

Intrinsic spinal cord pathology can mimic the clinical presentation of TCS. A cord arteriovenous malformation, syrinx cavity, partial cord transection (Devic demyelination), and a cord tumor, such as an ependymoma or glioma, can present with both upper and lower motor neuron dysfunction and sensory disturbance. Tumors tend to be localized in the central part of the cord with sparing of the sacral sensation, whereas TCS tends to commonly involve the bladder function and anal sensation.

Poliomyelitis, now nearly eradicated worldwide, can mimic some features of TCS. An older patient who survived childhood polio is still rarely encountered. The virus attacks the anterior horn cells, which results in asymmetrical weakness and atrophy. A well-known syndrome of exacerbation of weakness may occur decades after the original insult. Careful assessment of the asymmetrical weakness, lack of sensory involvement, and absence of long tract signs should allow ready diagnosis. Rarely, other enteric viruses, particularly Coxsackie, may have an acute, poliolike presentation. A slowly progressive spinal bone infection such as tuberculosis (Pott disease) can present as a slowly evolving spinal cord epidural mass, which clinically would have some features that resemble TCS.

Congenital disorders, including diastematomyelia, can mimic TCS, particularly as functional tethering may occur. A fibroadipose filum terminale or lipomas extending from the caudal conus throughout the sacral canal are part of the symptom complex of TCS.[24] Sacral dysgenesis, occasionally found in children of diabetic mothers, may present with a symptom complex similar to TCS. A low-lying, imperforate anus is frequently associated with TCS.[25] Type 1 neurofibromatosis, due to an aberrant gene in chromosome 17, may develop a dumbbell schwannoma through a vertebral foramen, which can result in both upper and lower motor, as well as sensory, dysfunction. Extremely rare intraspinal anomalies may have similar clinical presentations.[17,26]

The adult patient, generally starting in late middle age and on, has a risk of progressive spinal stenosis. The symptoms and findings are similar to patients with TCS. Although back pain is a symptom common to both disorders,[11,12,27] spinal stenosis can be clinically distinguished from TCS by the later age of onset, the frequency of back pain as the presenting symptoms, the relatively rapid development of symptoms, the frequent episodes of precipitating trauma, and often a normal neurological examination.

■ Treatment

Following diagnosis with the aid of MRI, surgical intervention is necessary in the symptomatic patient. Complex studies, undertaken over many years by Yamada,[28] proved that the progressive motor and sensory dysfunction caused by stretching of the cord is not secondary to the histological changes but is due to the deterioration of mitochondrial midcord oxidation that occurs when the function of the lumbosacral spinal cord is compromised. The linear adolescent growth spurt would seem to be the time of greatest vulnerability. The tendency has been to divide patients in symptomatic and nonsymptomatic categories. The nonsymptomatic patients have little or no complaints and show no apparent neurological signs, and suspicion for potential TCS is based on evaluation of a lumbar hair tuft, a slightly asymmetrical gait, or a lipomatous mass. Previously in these stable children the tendency was to wait until the child was older, generally age 5 to 7, before surgical intervention. This was based on anesthetic risk, blood volume percentage loss, small operative field, and a feeling of increased vulnerability to surgical intervention in the infant and young child. Presently, with operating theaters designed for children, and improved monitoring and increasingly successful microscopic surgery, surgery is performed soon after diagnosis at any age.[29,30] However, significantly symptomatic patients, including newborns with spinal dysraphism or adults with acute onset need urgent untethering and should be treated as emergencies.

As the surgical risk lessens and surgical technique and knowledge expand there is little need for hesitation following diagnosis. Notwithstanding reports of series to the contrary,[31] this author seldom sees postsurgical improvement in patients with significant signs and symptoms. A lost neurological function tends to lack noticeable recovery; thus the earlier the surgical intervention, which almost always prevents further deterioration, the better the patient's prognosis.[14,32] Particularly in the adult population, or the rapidly growing teenager with accelerating progressive scoliosis, neurological loss can be noted in weeks and months, not years.

After untethering surgery, the patient needs to be periodically but indefinitely followed. The possibility of retethering or symptomatic retractive scarring is significant, particularly if the patient has undergone multiple surgeries at the same site.[14] Careful neurological examination, inquiry regarding bowel and bladder function, and periodic midthigh and calf measurements are necessary. Occasionally, if the patient becomes symptomatic, repeat MRI studies are indicated. Serial somatosensory studies of the posterior tibial nerve may be useful in early prediction of recurrence prior to the occurrence of clinical symptoms.[23]

Families with a child with spinal dysraphism will need specific genetic counseling because they have an increased risk of a second child with spina bifida. Additionally, the mother needs to be counseled in regard to potentially teratogenic drugs and the need for folic acid supplementation prior to another pregnancy. If the mother does become pregnant, she needs to be monitored in a high-risk clinic with periodic ultrasounds and α-fetoprotein monitoring.

■ Conclusion

It is gratifying that TCS is no longer looked upon as a rare entity, to be seen once or twice during medical training, then never again in many years of practice. It was seldom diagnosed a generation ago because it was seldom included in the differential diagnosis of a syndrome of progressive lower extremity weakness, gait deterioration, back pain, bowel and bladder dysfunction, and sensory loss. Recognition of the syndrome, ease of diagnosis by MRI, and knowledge of the etiology of spinal cord damage have remarkably improved the prognosis of patients with this disorder. Earlier diagnosis and skilled surgical intervention are the keys to successful management of the patient with TCS.

References

1. Chute AL. The relationship between spina bifida occulta and certain cases of retention. J Urol 1921; 5:317–324
2. Lictenstein BS. "Spinal dysraphism" spina bifida and myelodysplasia. Arch Neurol Psychiatry 1940;44: 792–809
3. Bassett RC. The neurologic deficit associated with lipomas of the cauda equina. Ann Surg 1950; 131:109–116, illust
4. Garceau GJ. The filum terminale syndrome (the cord-traction syndrome). J Bone Joint Surg Am 1953;35-A:711–716
5. Hoffmann GT, Hooks CA, Jackson IJ, Thompson IM. Urinary incontinence in myelomeningoceles due to a tethered spinal cord and its surgical treatment. Surg Gynecol Obstet 1956;103:618–624
6. Jones PH, Love JG. Tight filum terminale. Arch Surg 1956;73:556–566
7. Anderson FM. Occult spinal dysraphism: diagnosis and management. J Pediatr 1968;73:163–177
8. Hoffman HJ, Hendrick EB, Humphreys RP. The tethered spinal cord: its protean manifestations, diagnosis and surgical correction. Childs Brain 1976;2: 145–155
9. Roos RA, Vielvoye GJ, Voormolen JH, Peters AC. Magnetic resonance imaging in occult spinal dysraphism. Pediatr Radiol 1986;16:412–416
10. Pippi Salle JL, Capolicchio G, Houle AM, et al. Magnetic resonance imaging in children with voiding dysfunction: is it indicated? J Urol 1998;160(3, Pt 2):1080–1083
11. Yamada S, Won DJ, Kido DK. Adult tethered cord syndrome: new classification correlated with symptomatology, imaging and pathophysiology. Neurosurg Q 2001;11:260–275
12. Iskandar BJ, Fulmer BB, Hadley MN, Oakes WJ. Congenital tethered spinal cord syndrome in adults. J Neurosurg 1998;88:958–961
13. Pang D, Wilberger JE Jr. Tethered cord syndrome in adults. J Neurosurg 1982;57:32–47
14. Tamaki N, Shirataki K, Kojima N, Shouse Y, Matsumoto S. Tethered cord syndrome of delayed onset following repair of myelomeningocele. J Neurosurg 1988;69:393–398
15. Boone D, Parsons D, Lachmann SM, Sherwood T. Spina bifida occulta: lesion or anomaly? Clin Radiol 1985;36:159–161
16. Hendrick EB, Hoffman HJ, Humphreys RP. The tethered spinal cord. Clin Neurosurg 1983;30: 457–463
17. Ackerman LL, Menezes AH. Spinal congenital dermal sinuses: a 30-year experience. Pediatrics 2003; 112(3, Pt 1):641–647
18. Warder D. Tethered cord syndrome and occult spinal dysraphism. Neurosurg Focus 2001;10:E1
19. Yundt KD, Park TS, Kaufman BA. Normal diameter of filum terminale in children: in vivo measurement. Pediatr Neurosurg 1997;27:257–259
20. Zieger M, Dörr U, Schulz RD. Pediatric spinal sonography, II: Malformations and mass lesions. Pediatr Radiol 1988;18:105–111
21. Lam WW, Ai V, Wong V, Lui WM, Chan FL, Leong L. Ultrasound measurement of lumbosacral spine in children. Pediatr Neurol 2004;30:115–121
22. Hughes JA, De Bruyn R, Patel K, Thompson D. Evaluation of spinal ultrasound in spinal dysraphism. Clin Radiol 2003;58:227–233
23. Li V, Albright AL, Sclabassi R, Pang D. The role of somatosensory evoked potentials in the evaluation of spinal cord retethering. Pediatr Neurosurg 1996; 24:126–133
24. Rogers HM, Long DM, Chou SN, French LA. Lipomas of the spinal cord and cauda equina. J Neurosurg 1971;34:349–354
25. Golonka NR, Haga LJ, Keating RP, et al. Routine MRI evaluation of low imperforate anus reveals unexpected high incidence of tethered spinal cord. J Pediatr Surg 2002;37:966–969, discussion 966–969
26. Prahinski JR, Polly DW Jr, McHale KA, Ellenbogen RG. Occult intraspinal anomalies in congenital scoliosis. J Pediatr Orthop 2000;20:59–63
27. Yamada S, Siddiqi J, Won DJ, et al. Symptomatic protocols for adult tethered cord syndrome. Neurol Res 2004;26:741–744

28. Yamada S, Won DJ, Yamada SM. Pathophysiology of tethered cord syndrome: correlation with symptomatology. Neurosurg Focus 2004;16:E6

29. Schoenmakers MA, Gooskens RH, Gulmans VA, et al. Long-term outcome of neurosurgical untethering on neurosegmental motor and ambulation levels. Dev Med Child Neurol 2003;45:551–555

30. Koyanagi I, Iwasaki Y, Hida K, Abe H, Isu T, Akino M. Surgical treatment supposed natural history of the tethered cord with occult spinal dysraphism. Childs Nerv Syst 1997;13:268–274

31. McLone DG, La Marca F. The tethered spinal cord: diagnosis, significance, and management. Semin Pediatr Neurol 1997;4:192–208

32. Hüttmann S, Krauss J, Collmann H, Sörensen N, Roosen K. Surgical management of tethered spinal cord in adults: report of 54 cases. J Neurosurg 2001; 95(2, Suppl):173–178

5 Imaging of Tethered Spinal Cord

David B. Hinshaw Jr., J. Paul Jacobson, Jason Hwang, and Daniel K. Kido

■ History of Spinal Imaging

Visualization of the spine with x-ray imaging was first accomplished in the early 1900s, soon after the discovery of x-radiation by W. Roentgen. This technique improved rapidly and today allows visualization of bony lesions associated with dysraphism such as abnormal curvature of the spine (lordosis, kyphosis, scoliosis, or combinations thereof), widened interpedicular distance, posterior neural arch defects, hemivertebrae, and related segmentation anomalies. Ventral rounding of the vertebral bodies (associated with having myelomeningocele in children under 6 months of age)[1] and spinal canal bony spurs in patients with diastematomyelia may also be seen. The intraspinal soft tissues, however, are not well evaluated with this technique.[2]

Historically, myelography was the next development in evaluating the spine with x-rays. Various contrast agents were introduced into the subarachnoid space, changing the x-ray density of the cerebrospinal fluid (CSF) and thus outlining the neural elements. Currently, the popular intrathecal contrast agents are nonionic, have low osmolality, and have much higher safety profiles than those previously associated with myelography. With modern water-soluble intrathecal contrast agents, the conus, cord, nerve roots, and associated tumors are visualized as negative filling defects.

In the 1970s, x-ray computed tomographic (CT) scans provided improved contrast resolution of soft tissues by calculating axial images based on the various electron densities of the soft tissues, thus allowing muscle, fat, water, and blood to be distinguished from each other. For instance, intraspinal lipomas are readily distinguished from CSF on CT scans. However, because the thecal sac is surrounded by dense bone, visualization of nerve roots of the conus medullaris may be suboptimal due to Hounsfield artifact. Intrathecal contrast material is often used in combination with CT to evaluate the nerve roots, filum terminale, and conus medullaris with greater accuracy.

In the mid- and late 1980s, magnetic resonance imaging (MRI) developed to a degree that allowed visualization of the spinal anatomy without the use of x-radiation or subarachnoid injection of contrast agents. It has emerged as the most useful noninvasive modality, providing excellent detail of anatomy and characterization of soft tissue anomalies. The advantages of MRI also include its ability to obtain direct sagittal, coronal, oblique, and three-dimensional (3-D) images. MRI has become the primary imaging modality for tethered cords and has both facilitated earlier diagnosis and tailored treatment of these disorders.[3,4]

■ Techniques

Magnetic Resonance Imaging

Using MRI, radiofrequency (RF)-excited protons in the spine can be analyzed by a computer to produce images of the spinal cord and the nerve roots. With this technique, much better contrast between intrathecal soft tissues and CSF is available when compared with CT without intrathecal contrast. However, the patient must remain still for a much longer period of time than for CT while the images are being acquired.

Although the physical principles of MRI are beyond the scope of this chapter, numerous books and articles on the subject provide excellent discussions of these principles.[5–7] However, explanations of some MRI principles may be useful. Images may be weighted toward longitudinal (T1) relaxation, proton density, or transverse (T2) relaxation. In the T1-weighted images, signal from fat appears bright, CSF dark, and spinal cord, nerves, and muscle intermediate (**Fig. 5.1A**). With proton density-weighting, fat loses relative signal whereas CSF and spinal cord gain relative signal. With T2-weighting, fat loses even more relative signal, becoming dark, and CSF gains more relative signal, becoming bright; the cord (becomes hypointense) relative to CSF (**Fig. 5.1B**). Cortical bone has few mobile protons and is dark on all sequences. In older children and adults, vertebral marrow is relatively fatty and therefore brighter on T1-weighted sequences. Sagittal MRI shows the CSF and neural structures, although the conus is not always precisely identified because the nerve roots of the cauda equina tend to layer posteriorly due to gravity and may appear relatively continuous with the conus (**Fig. 5.1B**). Coronal views may provide additional information, although transverse images much more accurately identify the conus termination when correlated with sagittal views. Electrical stimulation of the conus at surgery is probably still the most definitive test of conus position when cord tethering produces an elongated conus tip.[8]

Computed Tomography

For CT of the spine, as is done for MRI, the patient is placed supine on a couch and moved into a gantry where an x-ray source and receptors rotate around the patient. The radiation passing through the patient is measured, and calculations are performed by a computer to

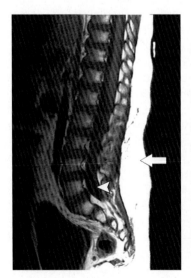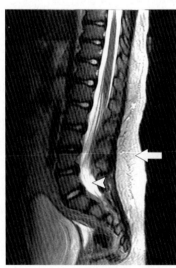

A   B

Fig. 5.1 Normal sagittal magnetic resonance images of the spine. **(A)** T1-weighted image. Cerebrospinal fluid (CSF) is low signal (*arrowhead*). Fat is high signal (*arrow*). **(B)** Turbo T2-weighted image. CSF has gained signal (*arrowhead*). Fat continues to have high signal because of averaging (*arrow*). The fat can be suppressed to appear like conventional T2-weighted images as in **Fig. 5.6B, D**.

form axial images of the soft tissues (**Fig. 5.2A**). In addition, if these scans are obtained with thin continuous slices, reconstructions can be performed in other directions (**Fig. 5.2B, C**). With the introduction of multichannel, spiral CT scanners, the patient needs to be in the scanner for only 1 to 2 minutes. During the time of the scan, the patient must not move. Following myelography, a short delay prior to CT is often indicated to allow for distribution and dilution of the intrathecal contrast material throughout the subarachnoid space.

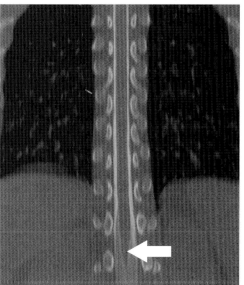

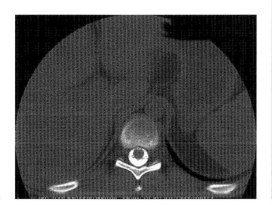

A

B

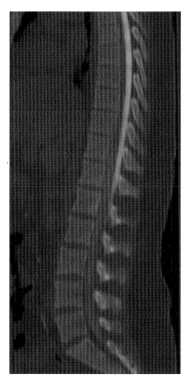

C

Fig. 5.2 Normal postmyelographic computed tomographic (CT) scan. **(A)** The axial CT scan demonstrates the conus, which is surrounded by opacified cerebrospinal fluid (CSF) and a few nerve roots. **(B)** Reconstructed coronal scan from the axial scans demonstrates the conus (*arrow*). **(C)** Reconstructed sagittal scan demonstrates the difficulty of locating the conus without additional projections.

Myelography

Myelography is an invasive radiographic spine examination technique. A spinal needle is placed into the subarachnoid space under fluoroscopic guidance. A water-soluble nonionic iodinated contrast agent is injected, then the needle is withdrawn and radiographs are obtained with the patient in appropriate positions (**Fig. 5.3**). In patients suspected of having a tethered cord, supine radiographs are often helpful because the filum tends to be stretched along the posterior aspect of the canal. Myelograms are almost always followed by CT scans (**Fig. 5.2**).

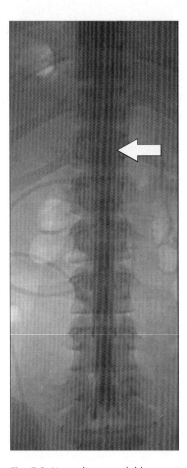

Fig. 5.3 Normal water-soluble contrast-enhanced myelogram. An anteroposterior projection taken with the patient supine shows the conus (*arrow*).

Ultrasound

A detailed discussion of the technique of ultrasound examinations is presented in Chapter 6, Ultrasound Evaluation of Tethered Cord Syndrome.

■ Anatomy and Imaging Findings

Normal Anatomy

Position of the Normal Cord

During in utero life, the bony spine grows faster than the spinal cord, thus the spinal cord effectively "ascends" in the spinal canal. The ascension occurs rapidly between 8 and 25 weeks of gestation, with the conus generally being located opposite L2 at birth.[9] It reaches the adult level at age 2 months postnatally.[10,11] There is evidence that the conus does not ascend further during childhood[12] and that the conus terminates near the L1–2 disk space in the majority of normal individuals. Conus termination may normally vary from the mid-T12 to the mid-L3 level, although 94 to 97.8% terminate above the L2–3 disk.[13,14] Thus, although some consider a conus terminus below L1–2 to be abnormal, it is probably prudent to consider a conus termination at L2–3 or above as normal at any age. A conus level terminating at or below L3–4 is abnormal (except possibly in premature infants and full-term newborns), and the significance of an L3 conus level must be determined by means other than its position.

Filum Terminale

There is some controversy as to how thick the filum may be and still be "normal." Some have said that filum thickening occurs by definition when it is wider than 2 mm,[15] whereas others claim that a filum diameter greater than 1 mm is abnormal.[16]

A fatty filum can be an incidental finding and is not considered diagnostic of tethered cord[17] because it is reportedly present in 5.8%

of the normal population on postmortem examination.[18] The fat appears as low attenuation (dark) on CT and bright (or white) on T1-weighted MRI sequences.

Vertebral Column

Occult defects in the posterior elements have been extensively studied, and the reported incidence in the general population has varied from 1.2 to 50%.[19,20] In patients with cord tethering, there is a high incidence of spina bifida occulta according to Hendrick et al,[21] who reported 100% incidence in a series of 86 patients. However, in another series, a tight filum with relief of neurological symptoms following division of the filum was found in only six of 442 cases of spina bifida occulta.[22] Therefore, even though patients with occult spinal dysraphism may have associated lesions such as congenital dermal sinus, lipomyelomeningocele, fibrous traction bands, and abnormal filum terminale,[23]

additional studies to evaluate for tethered cord are not generally recommended unless they have neurological deficits. In fact, classic neurological deficits suggestive of a tethered cord indicate the need for modern imaging examination regardless of whether spina bifida occulta is present on plain films.

Cord Tethering Associated with Spinal Bifida Occulta

Low Cord Termination

Cord tethering is often assumed when the conus is below the normal L2–3 level.[24] MRI is able to demonstrate the level of conus termination with reasonable certainty in the great majority of cases (**Fig. 5.4**). Some patients with tethered cord syndrome show a normally positioned conus that is also normally shaped at myelography, CT myelography, or MRI.[25–27] In such cases, it might be appropriate to obtain additional prone and

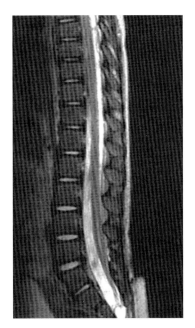
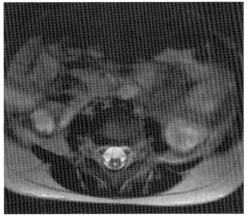

A   B

Fig. 5.4 Magnetic resonance image shows the cord terminating at the L4 level. **(A)** Sagittal T2-weighted image shows the difficulty of precisely locating the conus and evaluating the size of the filum. **(B)** Axial T2-weighted image through the tethered cord at the level of L3–4. A syrinx is located in the conus. *(Continued on page 56)*

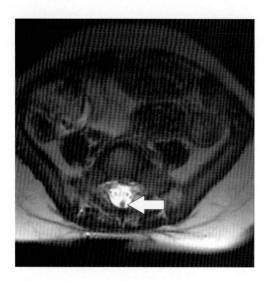

Fig. 5.4 *(Continued)* **(C)** Axial T2-weighted image through the cauda equina at the level of L5 demonstrates a posteriorly thickened filum (*arrow*).

C

supine images to determine whether the cord shows normal movement (**Fig. 5.5**). The spinal cord normally exhibits anteroposterior and craniocaudal movement when the patient has changed from the supine to the prone position, whereas the tethered spinal cord exhibits decreased or no movement.[28] Certain open MRI scanners, depending on the configuration of the magnet, allow patients to stand upright while images are taken. Images taken during flexion and extension can help determine whether there is normal craniocaudal movement.

Thick Filum

Cord tethering is usually associated with a shortened, thickened filum terminale (**Fig. 5.4C**). Fatty infiltration of the filum may be seen as a

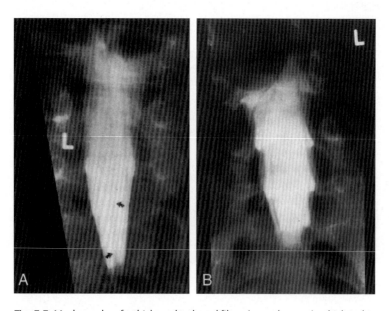

Fig. 5.5 Myelography of a thickened tethered filum (*curved arrows*), which is demonstrated **(A)** in the supine position but **(B)** not in the prone image.

We appreciate your feedback

Please mail us your completed feedback card.

Author/Book title _____

Best features _____

_____

Areas to improve _____

_____

First Name _____ Last Name _____ Title _____

Address _____

City/Postal Code/Country _____

Email _____@_____ Phone _____

Profession/Specialty _____

I am a: ☐ Faculty Member ☐ and I would recommend this book   ☐ Physician

☐ Student, Year of Graduation _____ _____   ☐ Other _____

Thieme does not sell or rent customer contact details.

We appreciate your feedback

Please mail us your completed feedback card.

Author/Book title _____

Best features _____

_____

Areas to improve _____

_____

First Name _____ Last Name _____ Title _____

Address _____

City/State/ZIP _____

Email _____@_____ Phone _____

Profession/Specialty _____

I am a: ☐ Faculty Member ☐ and I would recommend this book   ☐ Physician

☐ Student, Program (MD, DDS, DPT, other) _____   ☐ Other _____

Thieme does not sell or rent customer contact details.

Please affix
sufficient
postage

Dear Customer,

We welcome and encourage your feedback. Please share your thoughts by sending us this postcard or submitting your comments online at **www.thieme.com/feedback**. As a "thank you," we will enter your name into a raffle for a chance to win a Thieme gift certificate. Raffle drawings will be held four times a year.

We look forward to hearing from you.

Sincerely,

Thieme Publishers

Thieme Publishers
ATTN: Marketing Department
P.O. Box 30 11 20
70451 Stuttgart

GERMANY

NO POSTAGE
NECESSARY
IF MAILED
IN THE
UNITED STATES

BUSINESS REPLY MAIL

FIRST-CLASS MAIL   PERMIT NO. 7654   NEW YORK, NY

POSTAGE WILL BE PAID BY ADDRESSEE

Attn: Marketing Department
Thieme Publishers
333 Seventh Avenue
New York, NY 10017-2214

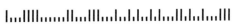

clue to cord tethering (**Fig. 5.6A, B**). This finding is present in 29% of patients with a thickened filum.[15] The thickened, shortened filum seeks the shortest distance between the tethering site and the lowest pair of dentate ligaments and may tent the dura posteriorly, resulting in a triangular shape of the thecal sac. This posterior placement of the filum often with the conus is

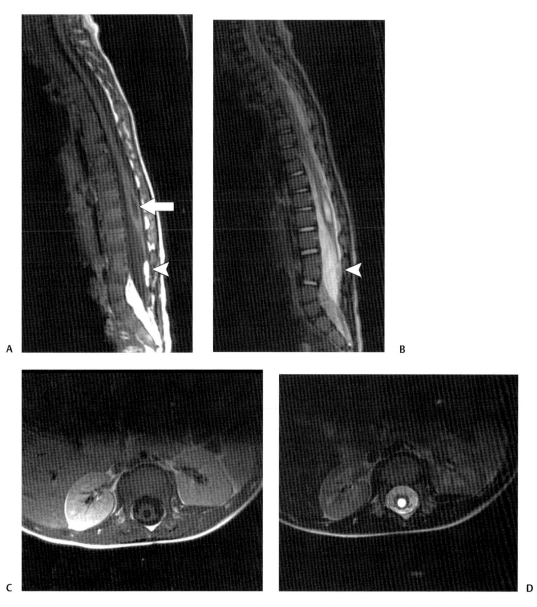

Fig. 5.6 Magnetic resonance images showing low cord termination associated with a syrinx, fatty filum, and bony anomalies. (**A**) Sagittal T1-weighted image demonstrates a syrinx (*arrow*) and fatty filum (*arrowhead*). There is also fusion of T10–11, and L4–5, and S1–2 vertebral bodies. (**B**) Sagittal turbo T2-weighted image with fat saturation shows increased signal in the syrinx. The fat saturation decreases fat signal in the subcutaneous soft tissues as well as in the fatty filum (*arrowhead*). (**C**) Axial T1-weighted image through the midportion of the syrinx. (**D**) Axial T2-weighted, fat-saturated image through the midportion of the syrinx.

well seen on MRI.[29] The thick filum appears as a small round filling defect extending through multiple sections. The thick filum has higher signal than CSF on relatively T1- or proton density-weighted MRI scans. Lesions frequently associated with tethered cord are distal cord syrinx (**Fig. 5.6A–D**) and the caudal regression syndrome. An associated dermoid or lipoma can also be seen and, rarely, even a sacral teratoma.

Dermal Sinus Tracts

Dermal sinus tracts may be visualized on MRI as a subcutaneous line of decreased signal (relative to fat) on T1-weighted images (**Fig. 5.7**) and may be associated with sacral and intraspinal lipomas. Careful attention to the contrast and brightness settings may be necessary to see these tracts because they may not be visible on routine MRI scans due to the intense signal of the sacral fat or the lipoma that they may traverse.

Diastematomyelia

The word *diastematomyelia* is derived from the Greek terms *cleft* and *marrow* (in this case,

marrow refers to the spinal cord). This term is applied when there is a congenital sagittal splitting of the spinal cord. The clefting produces symmetric or asymmetric hemicords, each with one dorsal horn and one ventral horn, which give rise to the ipsilateral dorsal and ventral nerve roots. There may be a single arachnoid and dura with a fibrous septum or bone spur (**Fig. 5.8A, B**). The variety that is most significant surgically has a septum that intervenes between the two hemicords, which are covered by a double arachnoid and dura (**Fig. 5.9**). The septum may be bony, cartilaginous, or fibrous. The cord is united above the septum and usually reunites below the septum. This configuration tethers the cord and may result in traction; which in turn may interfere with the vascular supply to the cord.[30] Associated lesions that may be seen on plain films or 3-D reconstructed CT scans include spina bifida, hemivertebrae, butterfly vertebrae, block vertebra, hypoplastic vertebra, bony spurs, and narrow intervertebral disk spaces (**Fig. 5.10A, B**). Rarely, there is an associated hemimyelocele or lipomyelomeningocele. These two lesions are discussed in more detail elsewhere in this chapter.

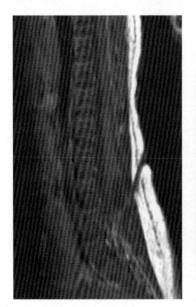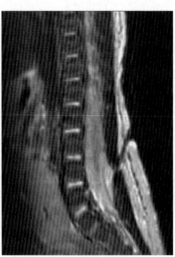

A   B

Fig. 5.7 Dermal sinus tract. **(A)** Sagittal T1- and **(B)** T2-weighted images demonstrate an oblique tract from the skin to the dorsal thecal sac, which is slightly tented.

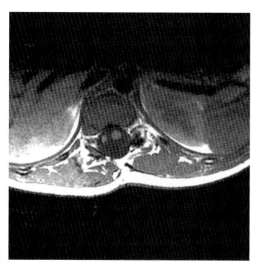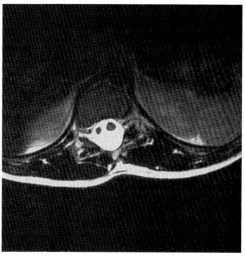

A B

Fig. 5.8 Diastematomyelia. **(A)** Axial T1- and **(B)** T2-weighted images demonstrate asymmetric hemicords with a single arachnoid and dura. Note partial lack of posterior vertebral structures.

The term *diplomyelia* is used when there is complete duplication of the spinal cord, with each having a central canal, two dorsal and two ventral horns, and four segmental nerve roots at each level.[15]

Lipomas

Lipomas that are not associated with myelodysplasia account for 1% of intraspinal tumors and

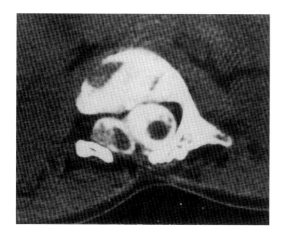

Fig. 5.9 Postmyelography computed tomography demonstrates fibrous separation between duplicated thecal sacs in a patient with diastematomyelia.

are not included in the present discussion. Lipomas associated with myelodysplasia are typically composed of fatty elements and fibrous tissue. Naidich et al[31] describe lipomas in myelodysplasia as being intimately associated with the dorsal aspect of the tethered cord, which retains the shape of the embryonal neural placode. There is a partial dorsal myeloschisis of the placode, with dorsal and ventral nerve roots originating in nearly the same coronal plane. The nerve roots extend anteriorly and typically do not become involved in the lipoma. The lipoma extends to the cord through a dehiscence in the dura, which is reflected onto the edges of the placode just lateral to the dorsal nerve root origins. Therefore, the lipoma is usually totally extradural. Lipomas may extend upward along the dorsal myeloschisis or may enter the central spinal canal and form an isolated "intradural" lipoma at a higher level (**Fig. 5.11**). Lipoma size varies considerably; lipomas may be quite small (**Fig. 5.11**), or they may be very large, causing expansion of the spinal canal.

Dermoids

Skin and skin appendages may become entrapped in the spinal canal during embryonic

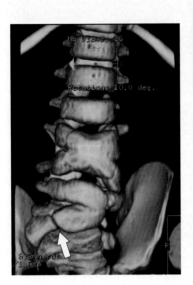
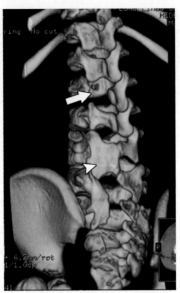

A

B

Fig. 5.10 Three-dimensional computed tomographic (3-D CT) reconstruction of the vertebral column of the patient imaged in **Fig. 5.7**. **(A)** Anteroposterior view shows fusion of the L4–5 and S1–2 vertebral bodies. Note a cleft in the right side of the S2 vertebral body. **(B)** Oblique posterior view shows absence of the right side of the L2 lamina (*arrow*). In addition, the right side of the L5 lamina has been incorporated into the adjacent L4 lamina (*arrowhead*). The right sacral laminae are absent.

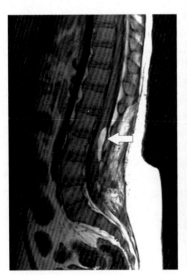
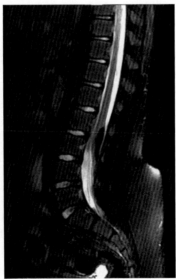

A

B

Fig. 5.11 Lipoma of the conus (*arrow*) appears **(A)** bright on the T1-weighted image, but **(B)** dark on the turbo T2-weighted image due to fat suppression added to this sequence.

development or following surgery, resulting in epidermoids or dermoid inclusion cysts. The difference between the two is based on the histological finding of skin appendages seen with dermoids. The appearance of these lesions is quite varied, but they may have a simple cystic appearance. A dermal sinus tract is generally associated with these lesions.

Cord Tethering with Spina Bifida Cystica

Spina bifida cystica includes entities such as myeloceles, meningoceles, meningomyeloceles, lipomyelomeningoceles, and hemimyeloceles.

Myeloceles

Myeloceles are herniations of the spinal cord through a defect in the bony spinal canal. They are a form of spina bifida that has a primary deficiency of skin in the midline, a placode of exposed neural tissue that is flush with the dorsal surface of the body, and a midline cleft with widely everted dorsal halves of the cord. The midline cleft is continuous with the central spinal canal located superiorly.[15] The dorsal exposed neural tissue composes what normally would be the central portion of the spinal cord, and the ventral neural tissue would normally form the periphery of the spinal cord. The dorsal surface is continuous with the skin of the back and thus forms a tethering of the cord. This lesion is usually repaired before imaging studies are done.

Meningoceles and Meningomyeloceles

Meningoceles are herniations of meninges through a defect in the bony spinal canal and by definition contain no neural tissue. They may be located in the sacral, lumbar, thoracic, or cervical region and may project anteriorly, posteriorly, or laterally.

Meningomyeloceles are herniations of meninges and spinal cord through a defect in the bony spinal canal. The lesion is similar to

the myelocele except that the placode is elevated from the dorsal surface of the body, with an underlying expansion of the subarachnoid space. There is fusiform widening of the interpedicular distances spanning several vertebral bodies and outward rotation of the axes of the pedicles and laminae toward the coronal plane. In severe defects, the laminae may become so rotated that the laminar surface, which normally faces posteriorly, is directed anteriorly. These bony changes can be seen on plain films. Kyphoscoliosis is present 30 to 35% of the time due to severe segmentation anomalies and 65% of the time due to neuromuscular imbalance. The muscles that would normally lie posteriorly and oppose the psoas muscles may lie anterior to the spinal canal and contribute to the kyphosis.[32] In a study of 194 patients with repaired myelomeningoceles, Nelson et al[33] reported that 98% were attached to the surgical closure, and inclusion dermoids were present in 16% of cases surgically treated for the release of a tethered neural placode. An example of a repaired myelomeningocele is seen in **Fig. 5.12**.

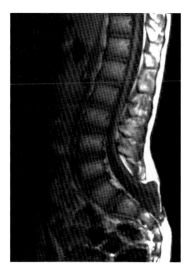

Fig. 5.12 Sagittal T1-weighted magnetic resonance imaging of a repaired myelomeningocele. Note the tethered cord and lack of subcutaneous fat.

Lipomyelomeningocele

In lipomyelomeningoceles, there is posterior herniation of meningocele, spinal cord, and lipoma into the subcutaneous tissues. According to Naidich and associates,[31] as the lipomyelomeningocele herniates through the canal, its superior aspect is notched by a fibrovascular band. This band is continuous with the periosteum, joins the laminae of the most cephalic vertebra with widely bifid laminae, and appears to tether the neural tissue and meningocele because they relax after surgical transection of the band. If the spinal canal reforms inferiorly, there is a similar fibrovascular band that kinks the inferior aspect of the meningocele (**Fig. 5.13**).

Other Cord Tethering Lesions Associated with Spina Bifida Cystica

A hemimyelocele occurs when there is a diastematomyelia with one of the hemicords being "normal" and the other hemicord involved in a meningomyelocele. In patients with myelomeningocele, 8% will have this type of configuration, and both hemicords may be affected at very different levels. Other rare lesions include double discontinuous lipomyelomeningoceles[34] (two separate lipomyelomeningoceles at different levels, without diastematomyelia) and the so-called lipomeningomyelocystocele[35] (lipomyelomeningocele with a separate associated cyst that is continuous with the central spinal canal).

Complex Malformation Associations

There are reports in the literature of complex malformations associated with tethered cord. Tank and Lindenauer[36] reported that meningoceles are seen in 40% of patients with cloacal exstrophy. Howell et al[37] did a retrospective review of 15 patients with cloacal exstrophy and

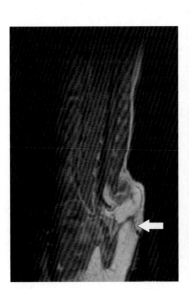
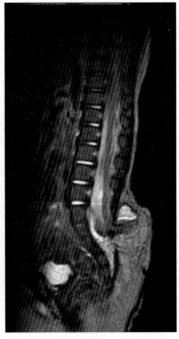

A   **B**

Fig. 5.13 Lipomyelomeningocele. **(A)** High signal fat extending through a defect in the spine. The cord is tethered. Note the fibrous band associated with the inferior portion of the lipoma (*arrow*). **(B)** The corresponding T2-weighted image shows the fat to have decreased in signal. There is also a small fluid collection superior to the subcutaneous fat posterior to the caudal spinous processes.

found seven with associated myelomeningoceles. Karrer and colleagues[38] reported 14 patients with cloacal exstrophy, or high or low imperforate anus, all of whom had a tethered cord. One example of the anomalies associated with tethered cord is the spectrum of the VATER sequence: vertebral anomalies, anal atresia, tracheoesophageal fistula, renal anomalies, and radial dysplasia. Other abnormalities sometimes associated with tethered cord include arachnoid cysts and hydronephrosis.

■ Use of Imaging Modalities

In patients with meningomyelocele or myelocele, no routine radiological evaluation is required unless the patient has postoperative deterioration of neurological deficits or there are initially marked asymmetric neurological deficits.[15] In these instances, MRI should be helpful in evaluating for retethering of the spinal cord, associated syringomyelia or hydromyelia, or in evaluating complex underlying congenital pathology such as a hemimyelocele, lipomyelomeningocele, or diastematomyelia. When there are indications to study patients for myelodysplasia, the options

include ultrasonography (see Chapter 6, Ultrasonographic Evaluation of Tethered Cord Syndrome), CT with intrathecal contrast, and MRI. The advantages of CT include rapid scan time, direct visualization of bony and calcified structures, and better definition of nerve roots. The advantages of postmyelographic CT include its ease in assessing anatomy in multiple planes, its noninvasive nature, and the fact that no ionizing radiation is used. The disadvantages of MRI have included difficulty evaluating patients with severe scoliosis or those who have difficulty holding still (given that acquiring data with MRI generally requires longer scan times than with CT).

However, the availability of 3-D techniques and rapid gradient echo sequences is obviating some of these previous potential disadvantages. MRI is considered preferable to CT for viewing congenital spine malformations[39,40] and is currently considered the tool of choice for detailed anatomical evaluation of patients with spinal dysraphism.[40-44] However, once detailed anatomical imaging has been obtained, serial ultrasound is the preferred method of following neonates and very young children to determine the best time for surgical intervention (see Chapter 6).

References

1. Kramer PP, Scheers IM. Round anterior margin of lumbar vertebral bodies in children with a meningomyelocele. Pediatr Radiol 1987;17:263
2. Naidich TP, Doundoulakis SH, Poznanski AK. Intraspinal masses: efficacy of plain spine radiography. Pediatr Neurosci 1985-1986-1986;12:10–17
3. Chopra S, Gulati MS, Paul SB, Hatimota P, Jain R, Sawhney S. MR spectrum in spinal dysraphism. Eur Radiol 2001;11:497–505
4. Selçuki M, Coşkun K. Management of tight filum terminale syndrome with special emphasis on normal level conus medullaris (NLCM). Surg Neurol 1998; 50:318–322, discussion 322
5. Haacke EM, Braun RW, Thompson MR, Ventakesan R. Magnetic Resonance Imaging: Physical Principles and Sequence Design. New York: Wiley-Liss; 1999
6. Zimmerman RA, Gibby WA, Cormody RF. Neuroimaging: Clinical and Physical Principles. New York: Springer-Verlag; 2000

7. Atlas SW. Magnetic Resonance Imaging of the Brain and Spine. 3rd ed. Philadelphia: Lippincott Williams & Wilkins; 2002
8. Pang D, Wilberger JE Jr. Tethered cord syndrome in adults. J Neurosurg 1982;57:32–47
9. Kaufman BA. Neural tube defects. Pediatr Clin North Am 2004;51:389–419
10. Barson AJ. The vertebral level of termination of the spinal cord during normal and abnormal development. J Anat 1970;106(Pt 3):489–497
11. Hawass ND, el-Badawi MG, Fatani JA, et al. Myelographic study of the spinal cord ascent during fetal development. AJNR Am J Neuroradiol 1987;8: 691–695
12. Wilson DA, Prince JR. John Caffey award. MR imaging determination of the location of the normal conus medullaris throughout childhood. AJR Am J Roentgenol 1989;152:1029–1032

13. James CCM, Lassman LP. Spinal Dysraphism: Spina Bifida Occulta. New York: Appleton-Century-Crofts; 1972

14. Reimann AF, Anson BJ. Vertebral level of termination of the spinal cord with report of a case of sacral cord. Anat Rec 1944;88:127–138

15. Naidich TP, McLone DG. Congenital pathology of the spine and spinal cord. In: Taveras JM., ed. Radiology. Philadelphia: JB Lippincott; 1986:1–23

16. Hochhauser L, Chuang S, Harwood-Nash DD, et al. The tethered cord syndrome revisited [abstract]. AJNR Am J Neuroradiol 1986;7:543

17. McLendon RE, Oakes WJ, Heinz ER, Yeates AE, Burger PC. Adipose tissue in the filum terminale: a computed tomographic finding that may indicate tethering of the spinal cord. Neurosurgery 1988;22:873–876

18. Emery JL, Lendon RG. Lipomas of the cauda equina and other fatty tumours related to neurospinal dysraphism. Dev Med Child Neurol Suppl 1969;20:62–70

19. Fidas A, MacDonald HL, Elton RA, Wild SR, Chisholm GD, Scott R. Prevalence and patterns of spina bifida occulta in 2707 normal adults. Clin Radiol 1987;38: 537–542

20. Boone D, Parsons D, Lachmann SM, Sherwood T. Spina bifida occulta: lesion or anomaly? Clin Radiol 1985;36:159–161

21. Hendrick EB, Hoffman HJ, Humphreys RP. The tethered spinal cord. Clin Neurosurg 1983;30:457–463

22. Jones PH, Love JG. Tight filum terminale. AMA Arch Surg 1956;73:556–566

23. Anderson FM. Occult spinal dysraphism: a series of 73 cases. Pediatrics 1975;55:826–835

24. Page LK. Occult spinal dysraphism and related disorders. In: Wilkins RH RS, ed. Neurosurgery. New York: McGraw-Hill; 1985:2053–2058

25. Khoury AE, Hendrick EB, McLorie GA, Kulkarni A, Churchill BM. Occult spinal dysraphism: clinical and urodynamic outcome after division of the filum terminale. J Urol 1990;144(2, Pt 2):426–428, discussion 428–429, 443–444

26. Tortori-Donati P, Rossi A, Cama A. Spinal dysraphism: a review of neuroradiological features with embryological correlations and proposal for a new classification. Neuroradiology 2000;42:471–491

27. Tubbs RS, Oakes WJ. Can the conus medullaris in normal position be tethered? Neurol Res 2004;26: 727–731

28. Witkamp TD, Vandertop WP, Beek FJ, Notermans NC, Gooskens RH, van Waes PF. Medullary cone movement in subjects with a normal spinal cord and in patients with a tethered spinal cord. Radiology 2001; 220:208–212

29. Yamada S, Won DJ, Kido DK. Adult tethered cord syndrome: new classification correlated with symptomatology, imaging pathophysiology. Neurosurg Q 2001;11:260–275

30. Guthkelch AN. Diastematomyelia with median septum. Brain 1974;97:729–742

31. Naidich TP, McLone DG, Mutluer S. A new understanding of dorsal dysraphism with lipoma (lipomyeloschisis): radiologic evaluation and surgical correction. AJR Am J Roentgenol 1983;140:1065–1078

32. Piggott H. The natural history of scoliosis in myelodysplasia. J Bone Joint Surg Br 1980;62-B:54–58

33. Nelson MD Jr, Bracchi M, Naidich TP, McLone DG. The natural history of repaired myelomeningocele. Radiographics 1988;8:695–706

34. Gorey MT, Naidich TP, McLone DG. Double discontinuous lipomyelomeningocele: CT findings. J Comput Assist Tomogr 1985;9:584–591

35. Vade A, Kennard D. Lipomeningomyelocystocele. AJNR Am J Neuroradiol 1987;8:375–377

36. Tank ES, Lindenauer SM. Principles of management of exstrophy of the cloaca. Am J Surg 1970;119: 95–98

37. Howell C, Caldamone A, Snyder H, Ziegler M, Duckett J. Optimal management of cloacal exstrophy. J Pediatr Surg 1983;18:365–369

38. Karrer FM, Flannery AM, Nelson MD Jr, McLone DG, Raffensperger JG. Anorectal malformations: evaluation of associated spinal dysraphic syndromes. J Pediatr Surg 1988;23(1, Pt 2):45–48

39. Osborn RE, Byrd SE, Radkowski MA, et al. MRI preferable to CT to view spine malformations. Radiol Today 1989; 6.

40. Roos RA, Vielvoye GJ, Voormolen JH, Peters AC. Magnetic resonance imaging in occult spinal dysraphism. Pediatr Radiol 1986;16:412–416

41. Davis PC, Hoffman JC Jr, Ball TI, et al. Spinal abnormalities in pediatric patients: MR imaging findings compared with clinical, myelographic, and surgical findings. Radiology 1988;166:679–685

42. Jaspan T, Worthington BS, Holland IM. A comparative study of magnetic resonance imaging and computed tomography-assisted myelography in spinal dysraphism. Br J Radiol 1988;61:445–453

43. Wippold FJ, Citrin C, Barkovich AJ, Sherman JS. Evaluation of MR in spinal dysraphism with lipoma: comparison with metrizamide computed tomography. Pediatr Radiol 1987;17:184–188

44. Zimmerman RA, Bilaniuk LT. Applications of magnetic resonance imaging in diseases of the pediatric central nervous system. Magn Reson Imaging 1986; 4:11–24

6 Ultrasonographic Evaluation of Tethered Cord Syndrome

Marvin D. Nelson Jr.

Real-time ultrasonography is an imaging tool that is useful for evaluating neonates with suspected congenital spinal cord malformations and patients with repaired lipomyelomeningocele or myelomeningocele at risk for spinal cord tethering. Ultrasonography provides inexpensive high-resolution images, usually without sedation.

■ How Ultrasonography Works

The ultrasonic image is produced by transmitting a high-frequency sound beam into the tissue of interest, then "listening" for the reflections (echoes) produced at the interfaces of tissues of different densities. The echoes are usually depicted as shades of white on a black background. A large difference in density between the two tissues produces a stronger returning echo and a brighter area on the image. Interfaces with bone or air reflect 99% of the sound beam, causing a very bright echo at the interface, with no through transmission distal to that point. By using multiple sound sources fired in sequence, a computer can time the echoes and separate them in a rapid series of images, similar to a motion picture, producing a "real-time" image depicting the movement of structures within the field of view of the transducer.

■ Imaging the Spinal Canal and Contents

At birth, the posterior vertebral arch has yet to ossify in the midline, allowing a sonographic "window" to image the spinal canal and contents in great detail. However, within 8 weeks, the posterior arch is no longer sonolucent. Thereafter, attempts to image the spinal cord are limited to angling the ultrasound beam between spinous processes.

Patients with spina bifida have permanent "windows" due to their posterior vertebral arch defects. This allows ultrasonic imaging at the involved levels at any age.

■ Technique

The patient is examined prone with the head in a neutral position. Using a 3, 5, or 7 mHz linear array transducer, both longitudinal and transverse static images are made of the spine from the foramen magnum to the coccyx. The spinal cord is then observed for evidence of normal pulsatile movement at all levels and documented by saving the cine clip.

■ Findings

Ultrasonographic Findings for Normal Anatomy[1–3]

Within the spinal canal, the dura (thecal sac) appears as a thin echogenic line around the spinal cord (**Figs. 6.1, 6.2**). The cerebrospinal fluid (CSF) produces no echoes (anechoic) and appears black on the images. The spinal cord has well-defined echogenic margins because

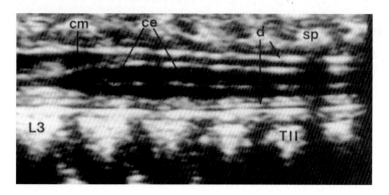

Fig. 6.1 Midline longitudinal sonogram of the distal spinal cord in a normal 1-week-old girl. Not the hypoechoic spinal cord parenchyma. The skips in the central echo (ce) are from shadowing of the overlying spinous processes (sp). d, dura; cm, conus medullaris. (From Nelson MD Jr, Sedler JA, Gilles FH. Spinal cord central echo complex: histoanatomic correlation. Radiology 1989; 170:479–481. Reprinted with permission.)

the sound beam is partially reflected off the surface of the cord (**Figs. 6.1, 6.2A**). The spinal cord parenchyma appears hypoechoic (few echoes, relatively black on the images), with no differentiation between gray and white matter. The central end of the anterior median fissure produces an echo interface that appears as a short linear or oval white dot near the center of the cord[2] (**Figs. 6.1, 6.2B**). The central canal does not produce a separate echo unless it is enlarged, as in hydromyelia.

In a few neonates, the central canal enlarges in the lumbar enlargement as a normal variant, the so-called ventriculus terminalis.[4] Nerve roots, dentate ligaments, and arachnoid septations can be defined around the spinal cord (**Fig. 6.2**). The individual layers of skin, subcutaneous fat, fascia, and paraspinal muscles are well defined and separated by continuous echogenic lines at each interface (**Fig. 6.2C**).

Most importantly, the exact position of the conus medullaris can be determined relative to the vertebral bodies.[5,6] At birth (term gestation) the conus is normally located above the lower border of L3. A spinal cord below the lower border of L3 is considered abnormal.

The filum terminale can be seen from its origin at the tapered end of the conus and followed as it courses between the nerve roots of the cauda equina to where it pierces the distal tapered end of the thecal sac at S2 (**Fig. 6.2E**). The extradural filum is not identifiable within the sacral canal as it courses to insert into the periosteum of the coccyx. The filum should not be larger than 3 mm in diameter.

Ultrasonographic Findings for Normal Physiological Motion of the Spinal Cord

The spinal cord is suspended within the thecal sac by 21 pairs of triangular fibrous bands called dentate ligaments.[7] These ligaments are continuous with the pia mater along the lateral surface of the spinal cord between the dorsal and central nerve roots. The ligaments narrow to a point and laterally insert into the dura at regular intervals. The dentate ligaments limit craniocaudal movement of the spinal cord without restricting anteroposterior (AP) movement.[7]

In real-time scanning mode, the spinal cord is seen to be centered slightly below the midpoint of the spinal canal. From this baseline, the cord intermittently deflects 2 to 3 mm in the AP direction and returns to the baseline position. In the prone position, these "pulses" of the spinal cord match the arterial pulse of the radial artery at the wrist. The movement of the spinal cord is secondary to the vascular pulsations from the radicular arteries and pulsations of the brain.[8,9]

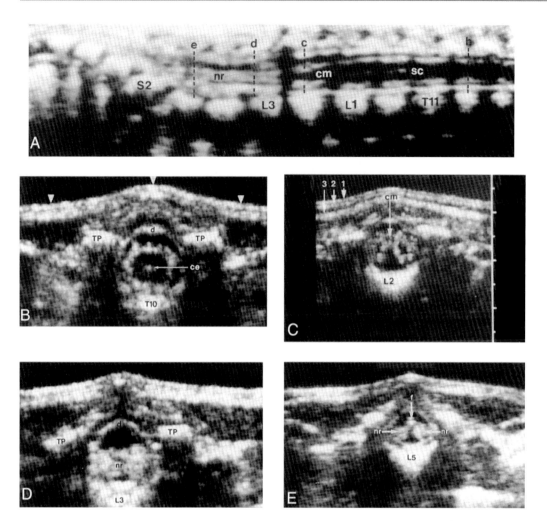

Fig. 6.2 Ultrasound study in a normal 3-day-old boy. **(A)** Midline longitudinal sonogram shows the location of the transverse images in **(B–E)**. cm, conus medullaris; sc, spinal cord; nr, nerve roots of the cauda equina. **(B)** Transverse sonogram at the T10 level. Note hypoechoic cord parenchyma and central echo (ce), and the echogenic "halo" around the cord produced by the nerve roots, blood vessels, and arachnoid septations. d, dura; TP, transverse process of the T10 vertebral arch. *Arrowheads* mark the skin surface. **(C)** Transverse sonogram at the L2 level. Note the tapered conus medullaris (cm) and "X" pattern of the surrounding nerve roots. 1, skin surface; 2, interface of skin with subcutaneous fat; 3, lumbodorsal fascia. **(D)** Transverse sonogram at the L3 level. nr, bundles of nerve roots of the cauda equina; d, dorsal aspect of the dural sac; TP, transverse process of L3. **(E)** Transverse sonogram at L5. The filum (f) is seen between the two lateral nerve root bundles (nr) of the cauda equina.

Normal respiration will change the baseline position of the cord because the thecal sac varies in size with the amount of blood in the surrounding epidural venous plexus. The venous flow is directly related to the changing intrathoracic pressure with respiration. Similarly, a Valsalva maneuver will deflect the spinal cord by the same mechanism.[10]

Postural changes of the patient also influence the baseline position of the spinal cord. Maximally flexing the neck causes the cervical and upper thoracic spinal cord to move anteriorly.

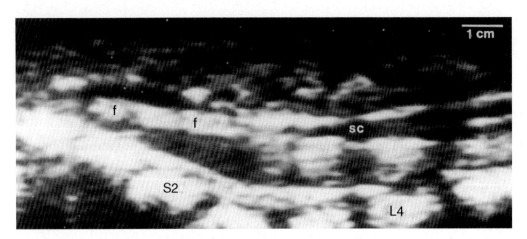

Fig. 6.3 Short, thickened filum terminale. Midline longitudinal sonogram of the distal vertebral column in a 1-month-old girl with a recently repaired imperforate anus. The spinal cord (sc) extends to the level of the L5 vertebral body. A short, thick filum terminale (f) is well visualized and measures 5 mm in diameter. The thecal sac is elongated, extending to S4. At surgery, a 5 to 6 mm fatty filum was sectioned at S2.

In the sitting position, maximally flexing the patient at the hips causes the thoracic cord to move anteriorly. The amount of spinal cord displacement varies with each individual and is probably related to the degree of curvature of each spine. Of interest, in normal controls, maximal flexion may cause the thoracic spinal cord to move anteriorly against the posterior vertebral body and cease normal pulsations.

Ultrasonographic Findings for Cutaneous Manifestations of Spinal Cord Malformation

Spinal ultrasonography is the best imaging method for evaluating neonates with hairy patches, hemangiomas, skin-covered masses, and dimples. In addition, any infant born with an imperforate anus, vertebral anomalies, or cloacal exstrophy should be examined due to the high incidence of associated spinal cord malformations.[11–16]

Figures 6.3, 6.4, 6.5, 6.6 are examples of neonates evaluated with spinal ultrasonography. As illustrated, the level of the conus medullaris and the diameter of the filum terminale are easily determined (**Fig. 6.3**).

Skin-covered masses are quickly assessed as to whether the spinal canal and contents are involved. The extent of fat, within both the spinal canal and the overlying soft tissues, is well defined in cases of lipomyelomeningocele (**Fig. 6.4**). Myelocystoceles are identified by the terminal dilatation of the central canal of the low-lying spinal cord (**Fig. 6.5**).

Dermal sinuses appear as hypoechoic tracts crossing the normally continuous planes of the dorsal soft tissues. These tracts may be followed to the dura (**Fig. 6.6**). Sinus tracts penetrating the dura cannot be separated from nerve roots; however, dermoids within the spinal canal are seen as echogenic masses.

The hemicords of diastematomyelia and the presence or absence of separate dural tubes are easily determined.

Ultrasonic study of repaired lipomyelomeningocele/myelomeningocele patients is useful to determine whether the neural placode has become attached/scarred into the closure (**Fig. 6.7**). Inclusion dermoids may be identified as homogeneously echoic masses.

One of the most difficult problems in following these patients is the determination of

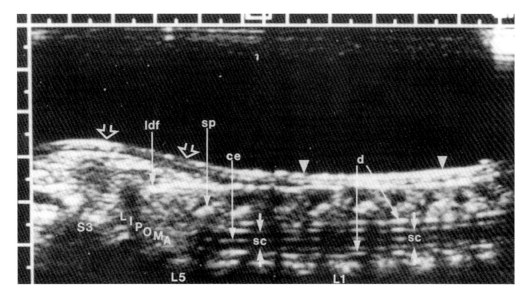

Fig. 6.4 Lipomyelomeningocele. Midline longitudinal sonogram of the distal spine in a 6-week-old girl with a large skin-covered mass above a distorted gluteal cleft. A gel pad was used to offset the transducer, allowing visualization of the skin surface (*arrowheads*). *Open arrowheads* indicate the area of the mass. The spinal cord (sc; *short arrows* mark the anterior and posterior margins of the cord) is at the L5 vertebral body level where it opens to cup the lipoma. D, dura; ce, central echo; sp, last intact spinous process; ldf, lumbodorsal fascia. Note the lipoma extending from the subcutaneous fat through a rent in the lumbodorsal fascia and dura to fill the distal spinal canal.

whether a patient's clinical deterioration is due to a tethered spinal cord.

Nelson and colleagues followed 27 myelomeningocele patients with serial ultrasonic studies from the time of repair and found that the neural placode attached dorsally at the closure in all 27[11] (**Fig. 6.7**). Nelson et al randomly studied 235 myelomeningocele patients at the time of routine renal ultrasonography and found the neural placode to be fixed into the closure in 231.[11] Therefore, because the majority of these patients have spinal cords/neural placodes fixed into the closure, the diagnosis of an attached "tethered" spinal cord, as made on both computed tomography and magnetic resonance imaging (MRI), is of questionable use in determining which patients are clinically tethered and need to be released. Real-time ultrasonic imaging for the presence or absence of normal cord pulsations provides additional physiological information that may help in the difficult decision of whether and/or when to operate on these patients.

Ultrasonographic Findings for Abnormal Spinal Cord Motion

Two factors must be present for the spinal cord to "pulse": the cord must be free to move within the dural sac and the CSF flow around the cord must be unobstructed. For instance, if there is an intra- or extramedullary mass filling the spinal canal, there will be no pulsations distal to the mass. Similarly, in hydromyelia, there will be no pulsations when the cord is expanded to fill the spinal canal. Ventriculoperitoneal shunt failure does not cause the cord to stop pulsing. If the spinal cord lies against the side of the spinal canal, as around a curve of scoliosis, the pulsations will be absent in the area of contact yet may be present proximal or distal to that area.

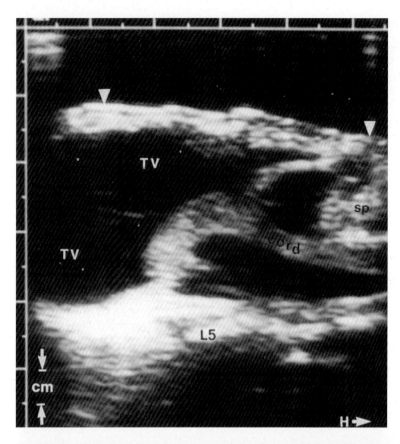

Fig. 6.5 Myelocystocele. Midline longitudinal sonogram of the distal spine in a 1-week-old boy with exstrophy of the bladder and a skin-covered mass in the lumbosacral area. In this case, the spinal cord (cord) splays open to form a large fluid-filled cavity, which is the dilated terminal ventricle (TV) of the central canal. Sp, last intact spinous process; H, head. *Arrowheads* mark the skin surface.

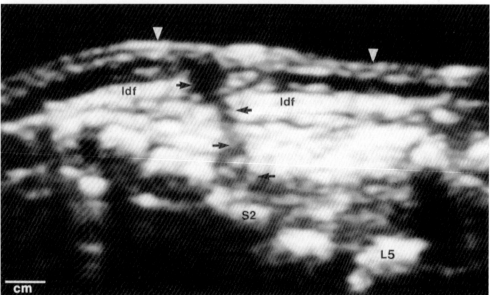

Fig. 6.6 Dermal sinus. Midline longitudinal sonogram in a 1-month-old girl with a sacral dimple. The hypoechoic dermal sinus tract (*black arrows*) interrupts the normal plane of the lumbodorsal fascia (ldf) as it passes to the tip of the thecal sac at S2. *Arrowheads* mark the skin surface.

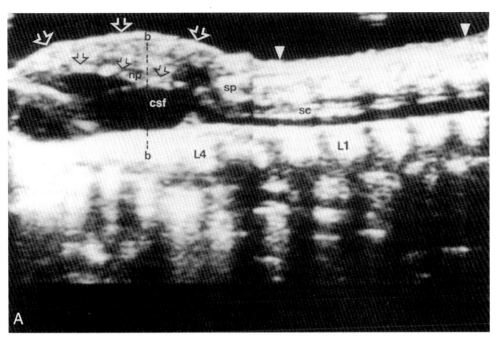

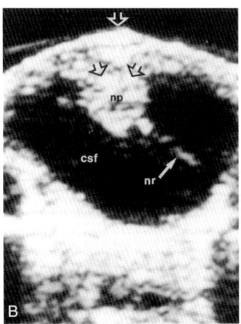

Fig. 6.7 Ultrasound study in a 1-month-old boy with a lumbosacral myelomeningocele repaired 2 days after birth **(A)** Midline longitudinal sonogram of the distal spine. **(B)** Transverse sonogram at level marked b . . . b on longitudinal sonogram in **(A)**. The spinal cord (sc) loops around the last intact spinous process (sp), where the neural placode (np) attaches into the surgical closure (*open black arrowheads*). csf, cerebrospinal fluid; nr, nerve root. *Open white arrowhead* marks the surgical scar on the skin surface.

As previously mentioned, following the initial repair of a lipomyelomeningocele or a myelomeningocele, the neural placode usually becomes fixed in the closure scar. Likewise, congenital cord malformations also fix the spinal cord by lipoma, short filum, dermal sinus, or an intracanalicular septum (as in diastematomyelia). At birth, the spinal cord in these patients is not under tension and pulses normally. However, as the patient ages, the growth of the spinal cord may lag behind that of the vertebral column, causing increasing tension and subsequent stretching and damage to the distal spinal cord. As the tension on the spinal cord increases, the pulsations dampen and finally cease. The cord pulsations usually disappear before the patient becomes clinically symptomatic, suggesting that this change from a pulsing to a nonpulsing cord may be the ideal time to release the distal attachment. This hypothesis is currently under evaluation, and preliminary results seem to validate the premise with the following qualifications:

- The significant event is the change in cord pulsations, which stresses the necessity of serial examinations. The spinal sonogram is most easily accomplished when the patient has routine renal sonography, usually every 6 months. If the cord is not pulsing when first examined, serial ultrasounds are of limited use, and MRI of the spine becomes the imaging method of choice.

- The pulseless cord must be validated as caused by increased tension on the cord. Correlation with the clinical examination and other imaging studies should sort out the question of false-positive cases due to scoliosis, severe hydromyelia, and CSF obstruction at or below the foramen magnum.

In practice, thoracic cord pulsations are useful for following lumbar and lumbosacral lipomyelomeningocele/myelomeningocele patients from the initial repair until 4 or 5 years of age. After the patient reaches 5 years of age, it becomes increasingly difficult to image the thoracic spinal cord to adequately evaluate pulsations.

In conclusion, spinal ultrasonography is a useful tool in the evaluation of the newborn with cutaneous signs of a congenital tethered spinal cord malformation, and as an aid in the evaluation of the repaired lipomyelomeningocele/myelomeningocele patient with symptoms of spinal cord tethering.

References

1. Clemente CD, ed. Gray's Anatomy of the Human Body. 30th ed. Philadelphia: Lea and Febiger; 1985:709
2. Nelson MD Jr, Sedler JA, Gilles FH. Spinal cord central echo complex: histoanatomic correlation. Radiology 1989;170:479–481
3. Gusnard DA, Naidich TP, Yousefzadeh DK, Haughton VM. Ultrasonic anatomy of the normal neonatal and infant spine: correlation with cryomicrotome sections and CT. Neuroradiology 1986;28:493–511
4. Kriss VM, Kriss TC, Coleman RC. Sonographic appearance of the ventriculus terminalis cyst in the neonatal spinal cord. J Ultrasound Med 2000;19: 207–209
5. Wilson DA, Prince JR. John Caffey award. MR imaging determination of the location of the normal conus medullaris throughout childhood. AJR Am J Roentgenol 1989;152:1029–1032
6. DiPietro MA. The conus medullaris: normal US findings throughout childhood. Radiology 1993;188: 149–153
7. Stoltmann HF, Blackwood W. An anatomical study of the role of the dentate ligaments in the cervical spinal canal. J Neurosurg 1966;24:43–46
8. Matsuzaki H, Wakabayashi K, Ishihara K, Ishikawa H, Kawabata H, Onomura T. The origin and significance of spinal cord pulsation. Spinal Cord 1996;34: 422–426
9. Bering EA Jr. Circulation of the cerebrospinal fluid: demonstration of the choroid plexuses as the generator of the force for flow of fluid and ventricular enlargement. J Neurosurg 1962;19:405–413
10. Epstein BS. The effect of increased intraspinal pressure on the movement of iodized oil within the spinal canal. AJR Am J Roentgenol 1944;52:196–199
11. Nelson MD Jr, Bracchi M, Naidich TP, McLone DG. The natural history of repaired myelomeningocele. Radiographics 1988;8:695–706
12. Karrer FM, Flannery AM, Nelson MD Jr, McLone DG, Raffensperger JG. Anorectal malformations: evaluation of associated spinal dysraphic syndromes. J Pediatr Surg 1988;23(1, Pt 2):45–48

13. Naidich TP, Fernbach SK, McLone DG, Shkolnik A. John Caffey award. Sonography of the caudal spine and back: congenital anomalies in children. AJR Am J Roentgenol 1984;142:1229–1242

14. Nelson MD Jr, Segall HD, Gwinn JL. Sonography in newborns with cutaneous manifestations of spinal abnormalities. Am Fam Physician 1989;40:198–203

15. Gerscovich EO, Maslen L, Cronan MS, et al. Spinal sonography and magnetic resonance imaging in patients with repaired myelomeningocele: comparison of modalities. J Ultrasound Med 1999;18:655–664

16. Schumacher RS, Kroll B, Schwarz M, Ermert JA. M-mode sonography of the caudal spinal cord in patients with meningomyelocele: work in progress. Radiology 1992;184:263–265

7 Urological Aspect of Tethered Cord Syndrome I: Lower Urinary Tract Dysfunction in Tethered Cord Syndrome

H. Roger Hadley, Herbert C. Ruckle, Brian S. Yamada, and Gideon D. Richards

Bladder dysfunction occurs in ~40% of patients affected by tethered cord syndrome. It is the exclusive complaint in 4%.[1] The most common urological symptom is incontinence; in some patients, it may be the earliest sign of the syndrome. Management of patients with voiding dysfunction secondary to tethered cord syndrome requires a basic understanding of bladder physiology and voiding mechanisms. This chapter provides an understanding of these principles.

■ Principles of Normal Bladder Function

Bladder function has a twofold purpose: to store urine and to empty when socially acceptable. Despite the apparent simplicity of these two functions, storage and emptying of the bladder requires a complex interplay between the central nervous system, peripheral nervous system, urethra, and bladder.

Normally, the bladder is a highly compliant structure accommodating continuous production of urine from the kidneys while maintaining low intravesical pressure. This low pressure protects the kidneys and ureters from hydronephrosis, urine reflux, and damage from transmitted pressure, and it permits urine storage without high urethral sphincter resistance. Continence of urine is dependent upon a competent urethral mechanism that can both maintain passive continence at rest and can almost instantaneously increase tone in response to the increases of intravesical pressure that occur throughout daily life. The process of bladder emptying is not a simple neuromuscular reflex; it requires a sophisticated coordination of urethral sphincter relaxation and bladder contraction. This process begins on command and continues to completion automatically, without further conscious neural input unless these pathways are voluntarily interrupted.

The lower urinary tract receives efferent impulses from both the autonomic and somatic nervous systems via several pathways (**Fig. 7.1**). Sympathetic fibers exit the thoracolumbar spinal cord and descend via the superior hypogastric plexus and then bifurcate into the bilateral hypogastric nerves. The parasympathetic fibers emanate from the sacral spinal cord and become the pelvic nerves, which join the hypogastric nerves and form the pelvic plexus (inferior hypogastric plexus). Nerve fibers within this plexus reach their targets within the bladder and urethra, ensuring both sympathetic and parasympathetic innervation. The somatic efferent nerves, in contrast, travel through the corticospinal tracts to synapse on lower motor neurons in the pudendal nuclei of the sacral spinal cord. Motor impulses travel from these nuclei to their destination in the urethral sphincter muscle via the pudendal nerve.

The pelvic, hypogastric, and pudendal nerves all route afferent impulses from the urethra and bladder to the central nervous system (**Fig. 7.2**). Upon entering the spinal cord, some

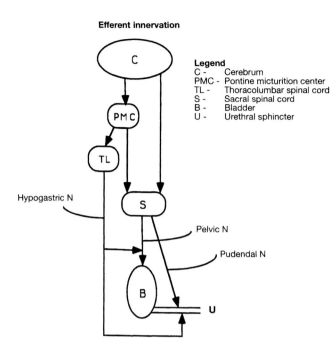

Fig. 7.1 This diagram depicts efferent pathways from the cerebrum, pontine micturition center, and spinal cord centers to the detrusor and urethral sphincter mechanism.

nerve impulses travel along fibers destined for segmental reflex arcs with spinal nuclei, whereas others synapse upon nerves ascending within the spinal cord to convey the information to the supraspinal and conscious levels.[2-5]

The concept of micturition reflex, in which coordinated detrusor muscle contraction and urethral sphincter relaxation are triggered by bladder distension, was introduced in 1900.[6] Since that time, many models of reflex pathways have been proposed. The majority of the experimental evidence supports a supraspinal organization of the micturition reflex.[7-9] The supraspinal region that serves to organize this reflex is the pontine mesencephalic micturition center (PMC).[2,3,10] Conscious neurological control

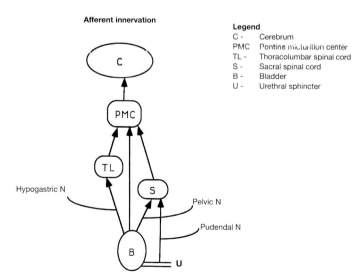

Fig. 7.2 This diagram depicts afferent pathways from the bladder and urethra to the spinal cord, pontine micturition center, and cerebrum.

of the detrusor and urinary sphincters is provided by discrete cortical regions and is mediated via the PMC and directly through corticospinal pathways to motor nuclei in the sacral spinal cord. Neural connections of these pathways with pathways involving the midbrain, cerebellum, and other centers have been identified, but their functional significance is not yet clear.[10,11]

Current understanding divides the micturition cycle into two functional phases: the phase of bladder storage and the phase of micturition. The viscoelastic properties of the bladder wall afford high compliance during filling and storage, thus allowing low-pressure filling without neural input.[12] After reaching a threshold volume, afferent impulses travel through the pelvic nerves up the spinal cord to the PCM and higher centers. This orchestrates the sympathetic efferent discharge from the hypogastric nerves to activate α-adrenergic receptors contracting the smooth muscle of the urethral sphincter and to inhibit parasympathetic perivesical ganglia via β receptors, thereby decreasing bladder tone and contractility. This sympathetic activity is coupled with cortical inhibition of the PMC and stimulation of the striated sphincter via the pudendal nerve. Together these actions are responsible for the appropriately contracted, continent urethral sphincter muscle and detrusor muscle quiescence that characterize the storage phase of bladder function.[4,5,10,13,14]

The micturition phase of bladder function is triggered in normal urinary systems by the progressive distension of the bladder and increasing afferent activity through the hypogastric nerves and pelvic nerves that occur as the bladder fills. The impulses reach the PMC and cortical centers, which produces a conscious sensation of a full bladder and the need to void. The PMC coordinates the transition into the voiding phase. Decreased activity in the pudendal nerve results in a relaxation of the urethral sphincter muscle. Efferent sympathetic discharge also decreases, thereby relieving the inhibition on the parasympathetic ganglia and allowing the smooth muscle of the bladder neck to relax. An increase in sacral parasympathetic outflow causes a coordinated contraction of the detrusor, and voiding ensues. Voluntary interruption of voiding can occur when somatic efferent impulse from frontal cortex contracts the voluntary sphincter, which increases bladder outlet resistance, and the detrusor muscle contraction reflexively abates.[4,5,8,10,14]

■ Patient Evaluation for Neurogenic Bladder Dysfunction

Like most aspects of medicine, a careful history and physical exam are essential to diagnose and treat a neurogenic bladder. It is vital to investigate other potential neurological symptoms. The patient's urinary symptoms must be placed within the framework of both the bladder's micturition and storage functions. Furthermore, it is important to elicit from the patient a clear picture of the patient's normal diurnal and nocturnal voiding patterns and habits. One must ask specifically about symptoms of nocturia, urgency, frequency, hesitancy, straining, sensation of fullness, sensation of complete emptying, dysuria, ability to interrupt or inhibit micturition, urinary incontinence, bowel habits, ability to achieve erection and ejaculation, paralysis, weakness, numbness, paresthesias, or seizures. The patient's past medical history should be probed for any spinal, pelvic, or neurological problems, trauma, or surgery. The possibility of the patient's use of medications that affect the autonomic pathways that mitigate bladder function (α agonists and antagonists, anticholinergics, β blockers, opioids, caffeine, and other methylxanthines) should be explored.

The physical exam should include a thorough evaluation of neurological and urological systems. The anal wink and the bulbocavernosus reflex are particularly useful because they correspond to the S2–4 levels where the somatic and parasympathetic efferent and afferent pathways intersect with the spinal cord.[13,15–17]

Urodynamic Testing

Urodynamic testing has emerged as the quintessential evaluation to explicitly identify, document, and quantify the effects of neurological dysfunction on the urinary system. Urodynamic parameter improvement has become a quantifiable outcome that is used to gauge the effectiveness of treatment for tethered cord syndrome. The evaluation consists of some combination of cystometry, uroflometry, and electromyelography performed during the phases of filling and micturition, with the goal of reproducing and evaluating a patient's typical voiding cycle.

Cystometry

Cystometry is the measure of pressure changes in the bladder throughout the voiding cycle. A pressure transducer is placed transurethrally into the bladder to measure intravesical pressure (pves). Both the tone of the detrusor muscle and intraabdominal pressure combine to produce the measured pves. To determine the actual pressure of the detrusor another pressure transducer is introduced to measure abdominal pressure (pabd). This transducer is typically placed in the rectum. A subtraction of the abdominal pressure from the intravesicular pressure results in the pressure contribution of the detrusor (pdet) (i.e., pves − pabd = pdet). The relationship of pdet and the patient's sensation of bladder filling with bladder volumes (**Fig. 7.3**) during the filling cystometrogram and voiding allows the measurement of bladder compliance, bladder contractility, and maximum cystometric capacity. The patient's subjective report of the first sensation of filling, first desire to void, and strong desire to void during bladder filling are used to evaluate the patient's sensation and characterize it as normal, reduced, increased, or absent. The compliance of the bladder is a quantification of the viscoelastic properties of the bladder wall. Compliance is equal to the change in volume divided by the change in pressure during filling and is expressed in mL/cm H_2O. The normal bladder has a high compliance during passive filling and the pressure volume curve of the cystometrogram (CMG) is relatively flat until the cystometric capacity is approached. A bladder with decreased compliance (**Fig. 7.4**) will exhibit a filling CMG with a steady rise in the pressure–volume curve. Contractility refers to the ability of the detrusor to increase the pdet during detrusor contraction. Involuntary detrusor contractions can be demonstrated on the CMG (**Fig. 7.5**), and this is referred to as detrusor overactivity (formerly detrusor instability).

Stable detrusor

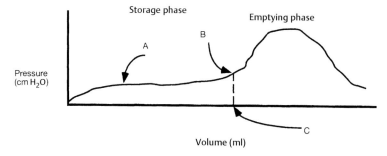

Fig. 7.3 Normal cystometrogram depicting the relationship between detrusor muscle pressure and intravesical volume during the storage and emptying phases of voiding. A, first sensation of filling; B, sensation of maximum fullness; C, bladder capacity.

Detrusor instability (Tonic)

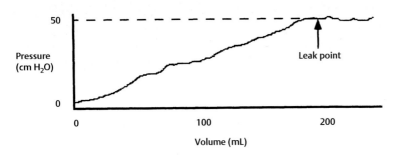

Fig. 7.4 Tonic detrusor instability describes a poorly compliant bladder with steeply rising filling pressures at low bladder volumes. The leak point pressure is important in evaluating the risk of upper tract deterioration.

If detrusor overactivity is present and can be attributed to a neurological cause, the term *neurologic detrusor* overactivity is used (formerly *hyperreflexia*). If the detrusor does not contract during the CMG it is referred to as an acontractile bladder, and if it can be attributed to a neurologic cause, the term *bladder areflexia* applies (**Table 7.1**).

Uroflowmetry

Uroflowmetry measures the volume of urine expelled per unit of time, typically mL/s. The urine flow is determined by a combination of the effects of detrusor pressure and urethral resistance during micturition. Maximum and average flow rates can be determined. The voiding pattern can be displayed graphically, which allows its characteristics to be evaluated (e.g., interrupted flow versus continuous flow). Flow can be reduced by poor detrusor tone or bladder outlet obstruction as in the case of detrusor-sphincter dyssynergia (DSD) (**Fig. 7.6**).

Electromyography

The external urethral sphincter is composed of skeletal muscle. Electromyography (EMG) employs a needle electrode to measure the

Detrusor instability (Phasic)

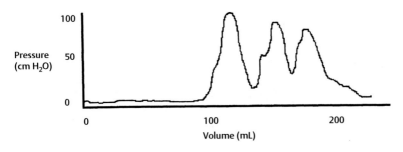

Fig. 7.5 Phasic detrusor instability describes an overactive detrusor muscle with spontaneous or provoked involuntary detrusor muscle contractions.

Table 7.1   Terminology

- *Acontractile detrusor*: Detrusor that cannot be demonstrated to contract during urodynamic evaluation
- *Areflexia*: A contractile detrusor due to an abnormality of neural control
- *Detrusor-sphincter dyssynergia (DSD)*: Involuntary contraction of the external urinary sphincter muscle during an involuntary detrusor contraction
- *Bladder compliance*: The relationship between change in bladder volume and change in bladder pressure
- *Postvoid residual*: The volume of urine that remains in the bladder immediately after voiding
- *Maximum cystometric capacity*: The volume at which the patient feels he or she may no longer delay micturition and has a strong desire to void
- *Urgency*: A sudden compelling desire to void, which is difficult to defer
- *Overactive bladder*: Urgency with or without urge incontinence often with frequency and nocturia
- *Detrusor overactivity*: Involuntary detrusor contractions during the filling phase of urodynamics, which may be either provoked or spontaneous
- *Neurogenic detrusor overactivity*: Detrusor overactivity due to a neurological cause (formerly detrusor hyperreflexia)
- *Clean intermittent catheterization (CIC)*: Aspirating or draining the urinary bladder with a catheter and subsequently removing the device. All performed with clean (not sterile) technique

Source: [8,43–45]

bioelectrical activity of urethral skeletal muscle. Quiescent at rest, as more muscle cells are recruited into contraction, the EMG tracing demonstrates increasing electrical activity. In normal micturition, the external sphincter relaxes, and the activity on the EMG drops immediately before detrusor contraction begins and tone returns after the completion of voiding.

DSD describes the situation where the coordination of these events is lost and an involuntary external sphincter contraction persists during detrusor contraction, resulting in decreased flow, obstruction, and, often, increased intravesical pressure and kidney damage. DSD is a common finding in patients with neurological causes of bladder dysfunction.

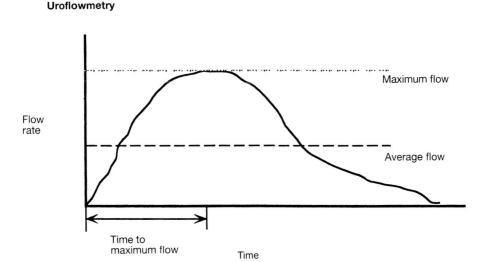

Uroflowmetry

Fig. 7.6 Normal uroflow pattern mimics a bell-shaped curve, with maximum flow rates of 20 to 25 and 25 to 30 mL/s for men and women, respectively, given a minimum voided urine volume of 150 mL.

■ Neurogenic Bladder Dysfunction in Tethered Cord Syndrome

Normal Voiding Cycle

During a normal urodynamic voiding cycle the bladder is filled slowly with water. During the filling phase the pdet remains low (below 10 cm H$_2$O), and there are no involuntary detrusor contractions. This low pressure is mediated by both the viscoelastic properties of the bladder wall and the increasing sympathetic outflow from the PMC in response to increasing afferent inflow from bladder distension. Somatic sacral output increases and the EMG activity increases throughout filling as more skeletal sphincter motor units are recruited. The patient reports subjective sensations of bladder fullness, and after the strong desire to void is reached, the maximum cystometric capacity is noted and the patient is permitted to void. The EMG activity drops as the external sphincter relaxes and the detrusor contracts, producing a curve on the pdet recording. Uroflometry records the flow rate and characteristics. When the bladder is empty, the pdet returns to baseline and EMG activity resumes (**Fig. 7.7**).

Multichannel urodynamic study

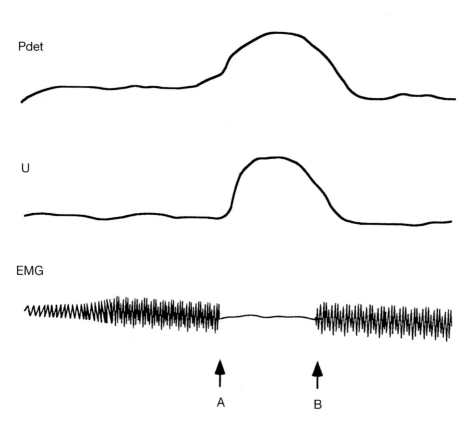

Fig. 7.7 This schematic represents a normal multichannel urodynamic tracing. Simultaneous recording of the urodynamic modalities during the cycle allows the examiner to observe the characteristics of each parameter and evaluate the relationship between them. Pdet, detrusor muscle pressure; U, overflow; EMG, pelvic floor electromyelogram; A, command to void; B, command to stop.

Pathophysiology of Incontinence in Tethered Cord Syndrome

Studies of experimental models of spinal cord traction and reports of human tethered cord syndrome (TCS) indicate that the conus medullaris is highly susceptible to traction.[18–20] Accordingly, alterations in the control of bladder function often occur early in TCS and often precede the loss of motor or sensory function of the lower limbs. The principle neurological lesion in TCS is located in the spinal cord gray matter[18] and not the long tracts of the cord.[21] Because of this, it is likely that the loss of spinal synaptic reflexes, which depend on transmission from pelvic and pudendal afferent neurons to the efferent neurons located in the intermediolateral cell column and in the anterior horn, is responsible for the loss of the normal micturition reflex in TCS. The parasympathetic motor outflow is affected. The sympathetic reflex arcs, passing higher in the cord passing through the T10–L2 levels, are not involved in the TCS lesion. Patients with TCS and abnormal urodynamic findings will typically have either areflexia or neurogenic detrusor overactivity with or without DSD.[22,23]

Urine leakage is experienced in those with areflexic bladders, most often as a result of overflow incontinence. The normally or near normally compliant bladder fills to its capacity where the compliance of the bladder wall falls sharply. Upon further filling, the pressure exceeds the urethral sphincter's capacity and urine leaks. More commonly the urethral sphincter has some degree of incompetence, and urine leaks at much lower bladder pressures. Those with decreased compliance, however, produce a persistently elevated intravesical pressure, placing the upper urinary tracts at risk for hydronephrosis and kidney damage. McGuire and Denil found that 80% of myelodysplastic children with intravesical filling pressures of 40 cm H_2O or above developed significant upper urinary tract dilation.[24]

Those with neurogenic detrusor overactivity can experience symptoms of urgency and urge incontinence. The bladder has an exaggerated response to filling and contracts involuntarily, which is responsible for these symptoms.

Reports of Bladder Dysfunction in Tethered Cord Syndrome

Hellstrom et al and Kondo et al reviewed separate case series of 18 and 15 patients with tethered cord syndrome and urological complaints, respectively. Their combined rate of areflexia was found to be 55%, neurogenic detrusor overactivity to be 18%, mixed lesions (i.e., decreased compliance with involuntary contractions) to be 12%, urgency with decreased cystometric capacity in 6%, and normal studies in 6%.[25,26]

A later report of 24 TCS patients that had urodynamic studies found a 71% areflexia rate and a 29% neurogenic detrusor overactivity rate.[27]

Giddens et al reported a series of 21 adults with tethered spinal cords; 13 primary and eight secondary to previous spinal procedures.[28] Urgency was the most common symptom (62%), and urge incontinence (50%) the second most common. Of the 21 patients only two had demonstrated areflexia before intervention.

A series of 20 patients that underwent untethering for category 2 (see Chapter 1, Introduction to Tethered Cord Syndrome) tethered cord syndrome was reviewed by Abrahamsson et al. Seven had postoperative improvement to a milder level of dysfunction after the procedure. There was one patient where the level of function deteriorated after the procedure. The investigators also reported that six patients had a documented worsening degree of urodynamic findings, 10 had no change, and four patients had improvement in these findings in the preoperative period. All six patients that were found to have clinical deterioration prior to untethering and nine out of 10 that had stable findings before surgery had urodynamic improvement following surgical intervention.[29]

Fone et al[30] reviewed the records of 39 patients with TCS and found a marked difference in outcomes between patients undergoing detethering for primary tethered cord and those undergoing the procedure for secondary causes. Eleven patients had primary tethered cord, and 28 were secondary to previous spinal surgery. Of the 11 with primary tethered cord, seven were found to have neurogenic detrusor overactivity, three had normal studies on preop urodynamics, and one was not evaluated with a preoperative urodynamic study (UDS). Improvement or resolution of the overactive detrusor was noted in five. Two had areflexia postoperatively, two voided normally postoperatively, four used clean intermittent catheterization (CIC), and five were too young for toilet training and remained in diapers. One had improved postoperative bladder compliance, and one had worsened postoperative bladder compliance.

Of the 28 patients with secondary tethered cord, all had voiding dysfunction and all had UDS abnormalities. Seventeen had decreased compliance, 15 had neurogenic detrusor overactivity, and 12 had areflexia. After a detethering procedure, 15 had decreased compliance, 13 had neurogenic detrusor overactivity, and eight had areflexia. Of all the patients, nine had no change in UDS findings postoperatively, six had worsened neurogenic overactive bladder, and four had resolution of preoperative neurogenic overactive bladder. Postoperative compliance was worse in five and improved in three of the patients. Two patients are able to void, three have vesicostomies, 17 were successfully using CIC at the conclusion of the study, and five have had surgical reconstructions.

Though the data from the Fone et all series suggest a better outcome with primary tethering of the cords, the aforementioned Giddens et al series[28] also reported urodynamic outcomes after untethering the spinal cord in these two classes of patients. Of the 13 patients with primary tethered cord, nine had neurogenic overactive detrusor, two had a normal UDS, and one demonstrated areflexia. One had improved postoperative urodynamics (no longer with neurogenic detrusor overactivity), eight had no change, and the rest were unable to be evaluated. Among the eight patients with secondary tethered cord, four had findings of DSD, four had neurogenic detrusor overactivity, and one

had areflexia on the preoperative UDS. There was reported urodynamic improvement in three and no change in three postoperatively. Three had findings of areflexia, postoperatively (one unchanged from preop). Four had findings of neurogenic detrusor overactivity postoperatively (two of these where not evaluated preoperatively with UDS), and one had persistent DSD. The data from this series suggest that tethering secondary to a previous surgical treatment of a spinal cord malformation may be associated with a better outcome.

Yamada et al[31] reported a series of 50 adult and late-teenage patients with TCS who underwent untethering. Of these, 36 (72%) complained of urinary incontinence. Urge or stress incontinence was reported in 28 of these, and of these 11 had a postvoid residual (PVR) > 35 mL and in 17 PVR was > 80 mL. All regained continence and had a PVR ≤ 10 mL after surgical intervention. The remaining eight incontinent patients in this series had overflow incontinence with a PVR > 45 mL. Six of them regained continence and had their PVR decrease to < 35 mL, and the remaining two required CIC after surgery. The 14 patients who did not experience incontinence had little or no PVR both pre- and postoperatively. All 50 had decreased anal sphincter tone on exam, which was improved after the surgery.

The medical records of 17 children undergoing a detethering procedure with both preoperative and postoperative urodynamics were reviewed by Hsieh et al.[32] Ten were found to have abnormal preoperative urodynamic studies, and of these, two had urological symptoms. Also of those 10, five showed improvement in or normal postop urodynamics. The preoperative urodynamic abnormalities included open bladder neck, low bladder capacity, high bladder capacity, VUR, high PVR, retention of urine, poor bladder compliance, high pressure voiding DSD, and uninhibited bladder contractions. Furthermore, there were seven with demonstrated preoperative VUR. Three patients had complete VUR resolution, one had persistent grade 3 reflux, and another had persistent grade 1 in a ureteral stump (after nephroureterectomy for a contralateral nonfunctional kidney with duplicated collecting system and history of febrile urinary tract infections). One patient had a worse grade of reflux after the procedure, and another developed postoperative contralateral reflux. The seven with normal urodynamics had normal UDS postoperatively with the exception of one where the urodynamics improved by the time of repeat examination 6 months later.

A score that quantified and assigned relative weight for four separate urodynamic findings was proposed by Meyrat et al to help identify and evaluate children with tethered cord reproducibly in the pre- and postoperative periods. The score combines the following parameters into a single number: percent of normal bladder volume, compliance, detrusor activity, and vesicosphincter synergy assessments.[33] In 15 children with TCS the mean score was 8.9, and in a control group of children (under urodynamic evaluation for anorectal malformations or enuresis) the mean score was 3.5.

Taskinen et al evaluated 30 children with a history of anorectal malformation repair and fecal or urinary incontinence with urodynamics and magnetic resonance imaging (MRI).[34] Of these children, 13 were found to have TCS by MRI and 12 had normal spinal MRI (the remaining five had other spinal abnormalities). Forty-six percent of the children with tethered cord and 46% of children with a normal MRI had normal UDS, 31% of the children with tethered cord and 31% of the children with normal MRI had overactive detrusor, and 15% of patients with tethered cord and 15% of children with normal MRI exhibited DSD. The result failed to demonstrate an association between anorectal malformation and type of spinal anomaly and also failed to suggest that spinal cord anomalies are responsible for abnormal UDS findings in patients with anorectal malformations.

Among the 17 children reported by Hsieh et al, three had anorectal malformations. One had normal UDS before and after untethering, one had abnormal UDS that normalized after untethering, and one had abnormal UDS that persisted after untethering.

Recently, three groups of authors[35-37] have discussed incontinence in patients with radiologically occult TCS. These patients lack evidence of filum thickening and cord elongation. When the reliability of MRI findings was discussed by a questionnaire, all polled neurosurgeons agreed the presence of elongated cord, thick filum, and fat signal in the filum would all warrant surgical intervention in incontinent patients with motor and sensory dysfunction. However, without such MRI signs, the neurosurgeons' opinions were divided. Extensive lower urinary tract evaluation should be undertaken prior to offering a surgical intervention in this population.[38]

Management of Neurogenic Bladder Dysfunction in Tethered Cord Syndrome

It is clear from the review of the case series presented that the treatment of TCS requires intervention beyond detethering of the cord in a significant number of cases. Complete resolution of urodynamic abnormalities is uncommon, but the abnormalities can be improved or changed to more manageable ones. As discussed earlier in the chapter, the three most common UDS abnormalities among patients with tethered cord syndrome are areflexic bladder, neurogenic overactive detrusor, and DSD. It is often helpful to view these each in terms of the two functional roles of the bladder—storage and emptying. For those with failure to empty (i.e., areflexia), a CIC routine is most effective. Often patients attempt to augment emptying with abdominal straining and a Crede maneuver (manual suprapubic compression). This technique should be avoided because it will rarely empty the bladder and generates high intravesical pressures, which may ultimately be detrimental to renal function.[39] In those unable to perform self-catheterization, an indwelling catheter, urinary diversion, or a catheterizable stoma that is anatomically more accessible to the patient is a potential option. There is a theoretical benefit to the use of cholinergic agonists to augment the contractility of the bladder; this has not, however, been found to be supported by experimental evidence.

When the bladder is poorly compliant the intravesical pressure and risk of damage to the upper urinary tracts is higher. To prevent this outcome strategies aimed at increasing bladder compliance or sphincter resistance are employed. There has been some success in addressing this situation with α-adrenergic antagonism to enhance bladder compliance and decrease outlet resistance, simultaneously.[40,41] Improved compliance has also been described following mechanical urethral dilation.[42] If these measures with or without intermittent catheterization fail to adequately control intravesicular pressure, then a sphincterotomy may rarely be required to allow lower-pressure urine leakage and protect the upper tracts. Protection of the upper tracts may also be achieved with bladder augmentation or urinary diversion to increase the compliance or capacity of the reservoir.

Storage failure due to neurogenic detrusor overactivity can be addressed with a variety of pharmacological agents directed at decreasing detrusor muscle contractility, but anticholinergic and antispasmodic agents are the most commonly used.

■ Conclusion

TCS can occur at any age but commonly occurs during periods of rapid growth, spinal cord stretching due to postural changes, and weight gain. The syndrome often complicates known cases of spinal dysraphism, but it may also be the first sign of radiologically occult disease. As a lower motor neuron lesion of the conus medullaris, voiding dysfunction is a common complaint. Unexplained incontinence or other alterations in an otherwise stable neurological state should raise concerns and prompt a full neurourological evaluation. Although techniques do exist to manage voiding dysfunction, prompt detection of cord tethering and surgical correction in the earlier state of TCS may benefit large numbers of patients.

References

1. French BN. Midline fusion defects of formation. In: Youmans JR, ed. Neurological Surgery. Philadelphia: WB Saunders; 1990:1182–1185
2. Blaivas JG. The neurophysiology of micturition: a clinical study of 550 patients. J Urol 1982;127: 958–963
3. De Groat WC. Nervous control of the urinary bladder of the cat. Brain Res 1975;87:201–211
4. Elbadawi A. Neuromuscular mechanisms of micturition. In: Yalla SV, McGuire EJ, Elbadawi A, eds. Neurology and Urodynamics. New York: Macmillan; 1988:1–28
5. Wein AJ, Raezer DM. Physiology of micturition. In: Krane RJ, Siroky MB, eds. Clinical Neurology. Boston: Little, Brown; 1979:11–29
6. Guyon JF. Role de nerf erecteur sacredans la micturition normal. CR Soc Biol 1900;52:712
7. Denny-Brown D, Robertson EG. On the physiology of micturition. Brain 1933;56:149–190
8. Yoshimura N, Chancellor MB. Physiology and pharmacology of the bladder and urethra. In: Wein AJ, Kavoussi LR, Novick AC, Peters CA, eds. Campbell-Walsh Urology. Philadelphia: WB Saunders; 2007:1937–1966
9. McLellam FC. The Neurogenic Bladder. Springfield, IL: Charles C Thomas; 1939:56–57,116–117
10. Bradley WE, Timm GW, Scott FB. Innervation of the detrusor muscle and urethra. Urol Clin North Am 1974;1:3–27
11. Ruch TC. The urinary bladder: physiology and biophysics. In: Ruch TC, Patton HD, eds. Circulation, Respiration, and Fluid Balance. Philadelphia: WB Saunders; 1974:525–546
12. Klevmark B. Motility of the urinary bladder in cats during filling at physiological rates, II: Effects of extrinsic bladder denervation on intramural tension and on intravesical pressure patterns. Acta Physiol Scand 1977;101:176–184
13. Elbadawi A. Neuromorphologic basis of vesicourethral function: histochemistry, ultrastructure and function of intrinsic nerves of the bladder and urethra. Neurourol Urodyn 1982;1:3–50
14. Satchell P, Vaughan C. Efferent pelvic nerve activity, ganglionic filtering, and the feline bladder. Am J Physiol 1989;256(6, Pt 2):R1269–R1273
15. Bors E, Comarr AE. Neurological Urology: Physiology of Micturition. Neurological Disorders and Sequella. Baltimore: University Park Press; 1971

16. Diokno AC. Neurologic examination. In: Yalla SV, McGuire EJ, Elbadawi A, eds. Neurology and Urodynamics. New York: Macmillan; 1988:150–154

17. Sax DS. The history and examination in neurology. In: Krane RJ, Siroky MB, eds. Clinical Neurology. Boston: Little, Brown; 1979:63–67

18. Yamada S, Zinke DE, Sanders D. Pathophysiology of "tethered cord syndrome." J Neurosurg 1981;54: 494–503

19. Tani S, Yamada S, Knighton RS. Extensibility of the lumbar and sacral cord: pathophysiology of the tethered spinal cord in cats. J Neurosurg 1987;66: 116–123

20. Tubbs RS, Oakes WJ. Can the conus medullaris in normal position be tethered? Neurol Res 2004;26: 727–731

21. Fuse T, Patrickson JW, Yamada S. Axonal transport of horseradish peroxidase in the experimental tethered spinal cord. Pediatr Neurosci 1989;15:296–301

22. Blaivas JG. Urological abnormalities in the tethered spinal cord. In: Holtzman RN, Stien BM, eds. The Tethered Spinal Cord. New York: Thieme-Stratton; 1985:41–46

23. Kuru M. Nervous control of micturition. Physiol Rev 1965;45:425–494

24. McGuire EJ, Denil J. Adult Myelodysplasia. American Urological Association Update Series. American Urological Association; 1991:10

25. Hellstrom WJ, Edwards MS, Kogan BA. Urological aspects of the tethered cord syndrome. J Urol 1986;135:317–320

26. Kondo A, Kato K, Kanai S, Sakakibara T. Bladder dysfunction secondary to tethered cord syndrome in adults: is it curable? J Urol 1986;135:313–316

27. Flanigan RC, Russell DP, Walsh JW. Urologic aspects of tethered cord. Urology 1989;33:80–82

28. Giddens JL, Radomski SB, Hirshberg ED, Hassouna M, Fehlings M. Urodynamic findings in adults with the tethered cord syndrome. J Urol 1999;161:1249–1254

29. Abrahamsson K, Olsson I, Sillén U. Urodynamic findings in children with myelomeningocele after untethering of the spinal cord. J Urol 2007;177:331–334, discussion 334

30. Fone PD, Vapnek JM, Litwiller SE, et al. Urodynamic findings in the tethered spinal cord syndrome: does surgical release improve bladder function? J Urol 1997;157:604–609

31. Yamada S, Won DJ, Yamada BS, Colohan AR, Siddiqi J. Post-void urinary residual for evaluation of TCS. Poster presented at the Annual Meeting of the American Association of Neurological Surgeons; April 26–31, 2008; Chicago, IL

32. Hsieh MH, Perry V, Gupta N, Pearson C, Nguyen HT. The effects of detethering on the urodynamics profile in children with a tethered cord. J Neurosurg 2006;105(5, Suppl):391–395

33. Meyrat BJ, Tercier S, Lutz N, Rilliet B, Forcada-Guex M, Vernet O. Introduction of a urodynamic score to detect pre- and postoperative neurological deficits in children with a primary tethered cord. Childs Nerv Syst 2003;19:716–721

34. Taskinen S, Valanne L, Rintala R. Effect of spinal cord abnormalities on the function of the lower urinary tract in patients with anorectal abnormalities. J Urol 2002;168:1147–1149

35. Drake JM. Occult tethered cord syndrome: not an indication for surgery. J Neurosurg 2006; 104(5, Suppl):305–308

36. Selden NR. Occult tethered cord syndrome: the case for surgery. J Neurosurg 2006; 104(5, Suppl): 302–304

37. Steinbok P, Garton HJ, Gupta N. Occulta tethered cord syndrome: a survey of practice patterns. J Neurosurg 2006;104(5 Suppl Pediatrics):309–313

38. Yamada S, Won DJ. Neurosurgical forum. Letters to the editor. Occult tethered cord syndrome. J Neurosurg 2007;160:411–414

39. Barbalias GA, Klauber GT, Blaivas JG. Critical evaluation of the Crede maneuver: a urodynamic study of 207 patients. J Urol 1983;130:720–723

40. Norlén L, Sundin T. Influence of the adrenergic nervous system on the lower urinary tract and its clinical implications. Int Rehabil Med 1982;4:37–43

41. Andersson KE, Ek A, Hedlund H, Mattiasson A. Effects of prazosin on isolated human urethra and in patients with lower motor neurons lesions. Invest Urol 1981;19:39–42

42. Bloom DA, Knechtel JM, McGuire EJ. Urethral dilation improves bladder compliance in children with myelomeningocele and high leak point pressures. J Urol 1990;144(2, Pt 2):430–433, discussion 443–444

43. Abrams P, Cardozo L, Fall M, et al; Standardisation Subcommittee of the International Continence Society. The standardisation of terminology of lower urinary tract function: report from the Standardisation Subcommittee of the International Continence Society. Neurourol Urodyn 2002;21:167–178

44. Wein AJ. Pathophysiology and classification of voiding dysfunction. In: Wein AJ, Kavoussi LR, Novick AC, Peters CA, eds. Campbell-Walsh Urology. Philadelphia: WB Saunders; 2007:1978–1985

45. Peterson AC, Webster GD. Urodynamic and videourodynamic evaluation of voiding dysfunction. In: Wein AJ, Kavoussi LR, Novick AC, Peters CA, eds. Campbell-Walsh Urology. Philadelphia: WB Saunders; 2007:1986–2005

8 Urological Aspect of Tethered Cord Syndrome II: Clinical Experience in Urological Involvement with Tethered Cord Syndrome

Antoine E. Khoury

With the acceptance of tethered cord syndrome (TCS) as a true and important medical problem a multidisciplinary approach has allowed us to gain a better understanding of its pathophysiology and the complex ramifications of this anomaly on other organs and systems. Along with other manifestations such as lower extremity sensory and motor disturbances, the lower urinary tract (LUT) shares the potentially affected nervous system pathways and is commonly involved. The abnormal interplay between bladder and urethra, along with abnormalities in urine storage and elimination, leads to changes that may have significant effects in patients' quality of life and that could also lead to irreversible kidney damage. The impact on the urinary tract ranges widely depending on the timing of the diagnosis, the severity of the process, and the other associated neurological problems besides the tethered cord.

The common physical feature among these patients is the abnormal anchoring of the spinal cord at its end by an inelastic structure.[1] As shown in experimental models, the lumbosacral cord is markedly susceptible to hypoxic stress generated by constant or intermittent traction between the attachments of the lowest pair of dentate ligaments and caudal fixation.[2,3] These metabolic and electrophysiological changes are at least in part due to stretch-mediated distortion of vascular structures, with progressive impairment of oxidative metabolism,[2] and are prevented or improved by surgical release of the cord, which halts the noxious injury and possibly facilitates neuronal reparative mechanisms. The nerve cells located in the gray matter of the tethered spinal cord have a higher metabolic demand than surrounding axons.[3] This and the fact that the conus medullaris is most vulnerable to traction because of its vicinity to the caudal fixation point *may explain the sometimes early and isolated appearance of bladder dysfunction as the initial manifestation of a tethered spinal cord.* It also raises the possibility that a minimal degree of traction applied to the cord can result in the aforementioned impaired oxidative metabolism and electrophysiological changes without actual displacement of the cord caudally. The progressive deterioration of symptoms and signs in patients presenting with primary incontinence or the appearance of secondary incontinence may presumably be the result of repeated and/or longstanding metabolic insults. These include further intermittent cord stretching by flexion-extension of the spine, relative systemic hypoxia during strenuous exercises, local hypoxia secondary to venous congestion caused by Valsalva maneuver or abdominal straining, or during periods of growth spurts, which may aggravate the traction on the cord because of disproportionate elongation of the vertebral column.

■ Clinical Presentation of Urological Dysfunction Secondary to Tethered Cord Syndrome

TCS presents to the urologist as (1) patients with a history of open spinal dysraphism, (2) patients with urinary tract dysfunction as part of a constellation of other neurological or orthopedic abnormalities, (3) children with isolated refractory LUT symptoms, (4) asymptomatic children with lumbosacral cutaneous abnormalities, or (5) patients with other abnormalities associated with an increased risk of TCS. Even though there may be some overlap, following are highlights of the clinical characteristics of these groups:

1. *Children with myelomeningocele/open spinal dysraphism* Patients with spina bifida aperta usually present with obvious neuromuscular and/or urological dysfunction and are diagnosed prenatally or the defect is evident soon after birth. For the most part, these patients are evaluated following repair of the myelomeningocele and prior to discharge from the hospital. These children are followed closely to promptly detect any changes in their urological status, especially during growth spurts possibly due to tethering of the cord, and to treat the commonly associated neurogenic bladder dysfunction.[4] The encountered neurological defects are sometimes complex, resulting not only from stretch injury but also related to other noxious events such as compression and neuronal maldevelopment or agenesis.
2. *Children with abnormal neurological exam or orthopedic problems* This group includes patients with occult lesions, such as lumbosacral lipoma, lipomeningomyelocele, or a fibro-adipose tight filum terminale, who commonly present initially with musculoskeletal and neurological manifestations, and the urological involvement is either secondary or is discovered following investigation. Patients who present with neurosurgical or orthopedic complaints and are subsequently found to have a tethered cord are usually referred for urological assessment to uncover any subtle involvement of the bladder that has not yet given rise to clinical symptomatology, and to obtain baseline studies before intervention. These patients can present at any age but are more commonly seen in late childhood or adolescence.
3. *Children with refractory or difficult to treat dysfunctional bladder or bowel function* Occasionally, TCS is found to be the underlying etiology for patients who present solely with urological dysfunction. It is this group of patients that may escape diagnosis for the longest period of time because the underlying neurological etiology is discovered only after thorough evaluation and empirical treatment for other more common conditions that might be responsible for the incontinence. Their urinary symptoms are frequently blamed on behavioral and/or developmental factors. The diagnosis becomes a difficult one, especially when one considers that a very large group of patients present to the urologist with similar complaints but have no neurological lesion, currently referred to as dysfunctional bladder or dysfunctional elimination disorder.[5,6] Maintaining a high index of suspicion allows the clinician to select patients that need further evaluation. Based on our previously reported experience,[7] this subgroup can be defined based on the following criteria:

   1. No other cause for the urinary incontinence could be detected.
   2. Patients exhibit either prolonged or secondary diurnal or nocturnal incontinence.
   3. The incontinence is refractory to all conventional conservative measures of management, including anticholinergic medications and behavioral modifications.

4. The incontinence becomes progressively worse despite aggressive conservative therapy, especially in relation to growth spurts.

5. Patients commonly have associated fecal incontinence.

4. *Asymptomatic child with lumbosacral cutaneous abnormalities* The common ectodermal origin of the intertegumentary and nervous systems helps explain the association between malformations of the spinal cord and midline cutaneous lesions. Affected children either present for evaluation of a possible neurological defect after an abnormality is found during a thorough physical exam, or the lesion is detected during evaluation triggered by LUT symptoms. In contrast to spina bifida aperta where dorsal herniation of the spinal contents is usually obvious, the findings in spina bifida occulta can be very subtle, ranging from small back masses to dimples or pits, dermal sinuses, hair tufts, dyschromic lesions, polypoid lesions (i.e., skin tags), soft tissue masses (i.e., lipomas), and/or hemangiomas.[8] The early diagnosis of a sacral cutaneous abnormality may not only help diagnose occult dysraphism, but may also lead to early correction potentially preventing recurrent or difficult to treat meningitis due to the abnormal communication between the spinal canal and the skin surface. Due to the relatively high prevalence (up to 3%) of *simple* isolated sacral dimples (defined as < 5 mm in diameter, located in the midline, < 25 mm from the anus or within the natal cleft) in "normal" infants, some have called into question the need for further evaluation in patients with negative prenatal studies and no associated anomalies.[9]

5. *Children with conditions associated with increased incidence of spinal cord abnormalities* Some congenital abnormalities present with a relatively high incidence of associated anomalies involving the spinal cord and genitourinary tract. For example, neurovesical dysfunction should be suspected in children with anorectal malformations (ARMs), including boys with rectourethral fistulae and patients with cloacal anomalies and the VATER association (vertebral anomalies, anal atresia, tracheoesophageal fistula, renal anomalies, and radial dysplasia).[10] The prevalence of spinal cord tethering has been detected in children with different degrees of ARM severity and even in patients without sacral anomalies,[11] suggesting that early investigation may be desirable to achieve prompt recognition and appropriate management. This gains even further importance for patients who undergo surgical correction for ARM because this carries an inherent risk of iatrogenic nerve injury.

■ Patient Evaluation

History and Physical Exam

The clinical findings and symptomatology that patients present with is secondary to the stretch-induced functional disorder in the *lumbosacral* cord. Therefore, the examination should be directed toward motor and sensory deficits in the lower limbs, urinary or fecal elimination problems, and musculoskeletal deformities.[12] Some of these symptoms may be difficult or even impossible to evaluate because urinary and fecal incontinence is part of normal development up to a certain age. Urinary dribbling or incontinence, sensation of incomplete emptying, urinary frequency, recurrent urinary tract infections, difficulty initiating or sustaining the urinary stream, fecal incontinence, constipation, unexplained lower extremity pain or pain that is triggered/aggravated by flexion-extension of the spine or prolonged sitting, and propensity to stumble or fall should all be investigated. Intractable or severe constipation must not be overlooked because it has been determined that up to 9% of these patients may have spinal cord abnormalities, most commonly TCS.[13]

From a urological perspective, it is important to develop a high index of suspicion in patients presenting with secondary incontinence (i.e., incontinence that presents in a child previously toilet trained for > 6 months) and refractory primary incontinence. The early diagnosis and detection of an underlying tethered cord as the responsible etiological factor for incontinence could potentially result in complete reversal of the bladder dysfunction, especially when corrected promptly. When a neurogenic cause for the incontinence is suspected, a careful physical evaluation should be performed. The lumbosacral area should be examined for deformities and for any of the stigmata of spina bifida occulta that are associated with a tethered spinal cord. The lower extremities should also be evaluated for discrepancy in size, presence of muscle wasting, foot deformities, or foot drop. Some findings on physical exam, such as lower-extremity hyperreflexia or spasticity,[3] should raise the possibility of associated higher cord lesions (i.e., syringomyelia, tumors, multiple sclerosis). As part of the initial evaluation a urinalysis and urine culture are obtained to rule out any other underlying abnormalities, such as a urinary tract infection, that may be responsible for the patient's symptoms.

Lumbosacral X-ray and Voiding Cystourethrogram

Patients suspected of having an underlying neurogenic cause for their urinary incontinence are usually screened with a lumbosacral spine x-ray. It has been suggested that a carefully evaluated plain x-ray of the lumbosacral spine may help detect patients with complicated enuresis who deserve a more extensive evaluation.[14] This test may also help establish the possibility of neurogenic bowel by disclosing a significant amount of fecal material in the colon.

Radiological evaluation of the LUT is typically obtained by voiding cystourethrography. Even though invasive, a great deal of information may be gained from this relatively inexpensive study. A voiding cystourethrogram (VCUG) is ordered to study the posterior urethra in males (for evidence of posterior urethral valves or stricture), the bladder neck (for elevation and hypertrophy), the presence of vesicoureteral reflux (VUR), the thickness of the bladder wall, the presence of trabeculation or diverticulae, and changes in the shape of the bladder, such as elongation as seen classically in the "Christmas tree" form that signifies a neurogenic bladder (**Fig. 8.1**).

Ultrasonography

Under the age of 3 months, ultrasonography of the spinal canal is the screening investigation of choice for the evaluation of infants suspected of having TCS. Abnormal findings include a low or blunt conus medullaris, a thickened or fatty filum terminale, fixed dorsal position of the cord in the thecal sac, and lack of pulsatile movement of the cord.[9] As the child's spine undergoes normal skeletal maturation ultrasonography quickly looses its usefulness for this purpose.[15] If ultrasonographic examination is abnormal or technically inadequate, magnetic resonance imaging (MRI) is indicated as an accurate secondary examination to clearly define the malformation.

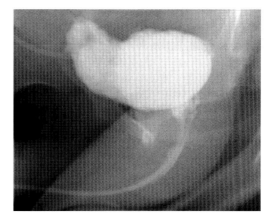

Fig. 8.1 Voiding cystourethrogram (VCUG) on a patient with neurogenic dysfunction. Note abnormal bladder contour and shape.

Abdominopelvic ultrasonography allows for effective and noninvasive evaluation of the urinary tract and permits estimation of postvoid residual (PVR) urine in the bladder. Helpful information such as kidney size and presence of hydronephrosis can be obtained without the need for sedation or ionizing radiation.

Magnetic Resonance Imaging

The diagnosis of TCS is primarily based on neurological and musculoskeletal signs and symptoms. Imaging features are in general obtained to *support* rather than make the diagnosis.[3] MRI has revolutionized the noninvasive evaluation of spinal cord lesions. The major obstacle to obtaining an MRI in children is the need for sedation or general anesthesia. Patients with tethered cord have displacement of the conus and elongation of the cord, with a sometimes thickened or fatty density in the filum. Proper imaging not only helps establish the diagnosis but also allows for identification of associated anomalies before and after treatment (such as scar formation, tumors, syrinx, or bony abnormalities within the spinal canal).

Role of Urodynamics in Evaluating Lower Urinary Tract Function

Urodynamic testing allows for a *functional* evaluation of the LUT. A full urodynamic evaluation is obtained in those patients with a known tethered cord who are referred for urological assessment or in an incontinent patient when an underlying neurological etiology is suspected. To understand and apply the results of this test, a comprehensive understanding of the LUT physiology is required.

The LUT is composed of the bladder (including the ureterovesical junction area), the urethra, and the pelvic floor/urinary sphincter mechanism. The detrusor muscle is responsible for storage and voiding, whereas the urethra is responsible for control and conveyance of urine for elimination. The normal bladder should allow for low-pressure storage of urine delivered

from the kidneys via the ureters. Normal innervation of the LUT allows for this phenomenon to occur. The efferent pathways consist of parasympathetic fibers from the sacral spinal cord (S2, S3, and S4), sympathetic fibers from the thoracolumbar cord (mainly T12, L1, and L2), and somatic efferents, including the pudendal nerve, which innervates the striated sphincter muscle. Together they promote detrusor muscle contraction or relaxation with coordinated sphincter activity, a process that involves different neurotransmitters, including acetylcholine, norepinephrine, and nitric oxide. The afferent sensory nerves from the bladder transmit information via the lumbosacral spinal cord through axons in the pelvic, hypogastric, and pudendal nerves. Their proper function senses bladder fullness, responds to changes in bladder wall stretch, and triggers nociception to overdistention. The fiber types involved (A and C fibers) have recently sparked interest in new concepts for managing neurogenic states, yet to be described here.

The complex innervation of the bladder and urethral control mechanism aims at achieving low-pressure storage and periodic voluntary complete expulsion of urine. As proposed by Wein,[16] this can be better understood by dividing the LUT function into two phases: filling/storage and emptying/voiding. Normal function occurs by accommodating increasing volumes of urine at low pressures, with appropriate sensation, in the absence of involuntary contractions, and with a closed bladder outlet (i.e., the bladder should be *compliant, capacious,* and *stable*). Storage pressures higher than the net glomerular filtration pressures are associated with a detrimental effect on renal function, deterioration of upper tract morphology, interference with ureteral transport of urine to the bladder, and VUR. Bladder emptying, on the other hand, must involve a coordinated contraction of the detrusor muscle that is of adequate magnitude and duration to effectively empty the bladder, with an appropriate decrease in resistance at the bladder outlet level without distal functional or anatomical obstruction. The urethral control mechanism should be coordinated with the detrusor muscle.

Normally, sphincteric relaxation slightly precedes detrusor muscle contraction, which in turn causes continued sphincteric relaxation. This is termed by some as the detrusor-sphincter reflex and is sacral cord mediated.

The urodynamic evaluation of the LUT consists of three basic studies: (1) urinary flow rate and estimation of PVR urine; (2) cystometrography; and (3) outlet resistance and coordination.[17] In conjunction, this functional assessment aims at evaluating urine storage (by addressing the "3 Cs": capacity, compliance, and contractility), voiding function, and bladder outlet activity. In selected cases the addition of fluoroscopic real-time imaging along with the use of hydrosoluble contrast media allows for evaluation of anatomical features of the LUT and may aid in better understanding of the functions of the LUT, specifically the interaction between the bladder and its outlet.

Evaluation of Voiding Function

Urinary Flow Rate and Estimation of Postvoid Residual Urine

A urinary flow rate (or *uroflow*) is the initial phase of urodynamic testing. It consists of a voiding study that plots the volume of urine expelled from the urethra per unit time and is expressed in milliliters per second.[17] The main parameters evaluated are the maximum flow rate (Qmax), the voided volume, the flow time, and the shape of the curve or flow pattern. Peak flow rates are graphically displayed against the voided volume and then plotted on a nomogram, allowing for estimation of normal values based on the patient's age and sex. The PVR urine volume can then be measured by bladder ultrasonography or catheterization.

The Qmax should be attained in the first one third of the voided volume, and the uroflow curve should be uninterrupted, "bell-shaped," leading to complete bladder emptying (see **Fig. 8.2**). *A normal uroflow curve with an adequate voided volume and with minimal or no PVR urine indicates that the bladder capacity is satisfactory and that the coordination between the detrusor muscle and the urethral control mechanism is likely normal.* It also excludes any significant functional or mechanical outflow obstruction. Intermittent, fractionated, or "staccato" flow patterns, prolonged "plateau" curves, and persistently elevated PVR volumes (i.e., > 10% of the estimated bladder capacity), should be considered abnormal in most clinical settings.[17]

Evaluation of Storage Function

Cystometrogram

The cystometrogram constitutes the measurement of intravesical pressure during bladder filling, allowing for study of the relationship between pressure and volume during the storage and emptying phases. The bladder capacity, contractility, compliance, and sensation are recorded or calculated. The medium is infused through a urethral or suprapubic triple lumen catheter, which allows simultaneous filling and

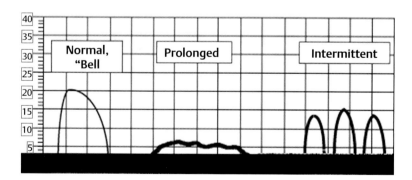

Fig. 8.2 Urinary flow rate curve patterns.

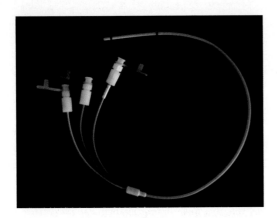

Fig. 8.3 Picture of cystometrogram catheter with channels for measurement of intravesical pressure during bladder filling, allowing for study of the relationship between pressure and volume during the storage and emptying.

pressure recording through separate channels as shown in **Fig. 8.3**. The bladder is filled at a rate equal to the square root of the expected bladder capacity for age using the formula (age in years + 2) × 30 = capacity in mL). While filling the bladder real-time measurement of the intravesical pressure (pves) is monitored. The total pressure inside the bladder (pves) represents the sum of the pressure generated by the detrusor muscle (pdet) and external events such as abdominal straining (pabd). A transducer is placed in the rectum (or infrequently in the vagina) to measure the intraabdominal pressures. The net pressure generated

by the bladder wall (detrusor muscle) (pdet) is then automatically calculated by subtracting the intraabdominal pressure (pabd) from the measured intravesical pressure (pves), as shown in the formula:

$$pdet = pves - pabd.$$

A normal cystometrogram is a flat curve throughout filling as a result of the highly compliant nature (i.e., accepts additional volume without a significant increase in intravesical pressure) of a normal detrusor muscle (see **Fig. 8.4**). Numerically, this compliance is measured by dividing the volume change (ΔV) by the change in pdet (Δpdet) during bladder filling ($\Delta V/\Delta$pdet). Abnormally low compliance is observed in patients with a hypertrophied detrusor muscle, or when the normally more elastic type I collagen is replaced by the stiffer type III collagen in the connective tissue between the detrusor bundles, or as a result of detrusor spasticity secondary to the neurogenic dysfunction of the bladder.

In a neurologically intact child detrusor muscle contractions can usually be suppressed during filling even with provocation (previously defined as a "stable" bladder). Close to bladder capacity the sensation of bladder fullness occurs, and this may lead to a detrusor contraction. Abnormalities detected on urodynamics include detrusor overactivity (DOA), either spontaneous or provoked, characterized by phasic involuntary elevations in pdet during bladder filling (also referred to as an "unstable"

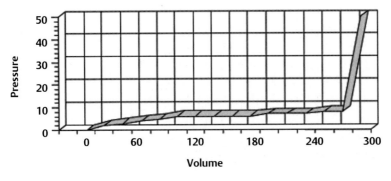

Fig. 8.4 Normal cystometrogram. Note pressure elevation at the end of the tracing caused by volitional voiding.

bladder). Gradual (nonphasic) increases in pdet with no subsequent decrease are better described as abnormal compliance rather than overactive bladder activity. During the voiding phase the bladder may not demonstrate an effective detrusor contraction. In this regard, detrusor underactivity is defined as a contraction that is insufficient in magnitude and/or duration leading to incomplete or inefficient bladder emptying. The term *detrusor hyperreflexia* (better referred to as neurogenic DOA[18]) is reserved to describe overactivity arising from a neurological disorder. Likewise, *detrusor areflexia* is reserved for acontractility arising from abnormalities of the nervous system.

Evaluation of Bladder Outlet Function

The urethral occlusion mechanism is composed of a striated muscle component, a smooth muscle component, and the elastic properties of the periurethral connective tissues. Measurement of the pelvic floor musculature and sphincter mechanism activity is achieved by simultaneous electromyography through patch or needle electrodes during bladder filling and voiding. The normal sphincter complex response is to increase the occlusive pressure in reaction to both bladder filling (with a gradual increase in activity noted, a phenomenon know as recruitment) and increases in intraabdominal pressure such as with coughing or straining (the "guarding" reflex). Under normal conditions reflex relaxation of the urethral control mechanism occurs only in response to detrusor muscle activity, preceding the effective bladder contraction and lasting for the duration of the voiding phase (i.e., electrical silence of the pelvic floor is observed). A discoordinated sphincter contraction during micturition leads to a functional obstructive state. This may be encountered in neuropathic states, termed detrusor-sphincter dyssynergia (DSD), or more commonly in neurologically normal children, a phenomenon that is described as dysfunctional voiding.

When the occlusion mechanism fails during storage the patient clinically presents with urinary incontinence. Although this is certainly a social inconvenience and mostly impinges on the child's quality of life, the incompetent urinary sphincter may be acting as a safety "pop-off valve" (i.e., when the pressures within the bladder raise above certain levels, urine leaks per urethra and the pdet decreases transiently). Urodynamically this is measured by determining the lowest pressure in the bladder, at any given volume during filling, at which urine leaks per urethra (defined as the leak point pressure). In patients with a neuropathic bladder, safe leak point pressures should be well bellow 40 cm H_2O.[19] Above this value there is interference with the normal ureterovesical junction mechanism, pressure is transmitted to the upper tracts, and kidney damage may occur.

Urethral Pressure Profile

The urethral pressure profile (UPP) is a graphic recording of the intraluminal pressure along the length of the urethra with the bladder at rest (static UPP) or during a period of intermittent stress (stress UPP). A mechanical arm pulls the urodynamic catheter at a rate of 1 mm/s while saline is infused through. The pressure required to displace the urethral wall is recorded and plotted. It assesses the continence length and the maximum urethral closing pressure. The clinical value of the UPP is limited because it only records the intraurethral pressure at rest, and this may not correlate with the events that take place during bladder filling/storage or during voiding. Furthermore, not uncommonly its measurement triggers a strong reflex contraction of the pelvic floor muscles. Despite these limitations, it may be useful in specific circumstances such as patients with suspected sphincter incompetence in the presence of electromyographically normal pelvic floor activity and in evaluating the success of medical and surgical therapy of sphincteric incontinence.

■ Management Principles

All together, the goals of treatment include the following:

1. Preservation of the upper urinary tracts and kidney function
2. Achievement of low pressure bladder storage and coordinated emptying with improvement of urinary incontinence and lower urinary tract symptoms. The mechanism behind urinary incontinence is better understood by visualizing this problem utilizing Wein's practical classification (see **Fig. 8.5**).
3. Complete and regular bladder emptying, preventing recurrent urinary tract infections
4. Early detection of neurological dysfunction to achieve reversal of the neurological deficits or prevent further deterioration

Treatment is tailored to correct the urinary storage or emptying problem; individualized therapeutic strategies are therefore essential. An outline of the most useful therapeutic modalities follows (see **Fig. 8.6**), with a concise discussion of some of the more frequently used therapies. Neurosurgical intervention remains the only means of addressing the etiology of TCS. Urological interventions, with the aforementioned aims, are valuable throughout the spectrum of severity of TCS and apply to patients awaiting definitive neurosurgical procedures, patients who have failed surgery, or patients with residual or progressive deficits despite tethered cord correction.

One of the key objectives of therapy is the protection of the upper tracts against damage by high intravesical pressures and infection. *This must never be compromised to achieve urinary continence.* A relatively simple and clear understanding of the mechanisms of incontinence and the principles of management can be achieved by viewing the cause of bladder dysfunction and urinary incontinence as due to (1) failure to store urine due to causes in the bladder, the urethra, or both; or (2) failure to empty the bladder due to causes in the bladder, the urethra, or both. Some patients do not have a distinct storage or emptying failure but rather have a combination deficit, which must be recognized to properly manage their condition. It is also important to note that failure in either category is usually relative and not absolute.

Based on this, the deficit in bladder function can be treated or circumvented using a variety of nonsurgical and surgical modalities. The choice of treatment options depends on the severity of the dysfunction, the relative risk of renal injury, and the patient's satisfaction with his or her quality of life.

Independent of the form of treatment elected, one key intervention that has brought a significant improvement in the management of patients with ineffective bladder emptying or and overtly active dyssynergic sphincter is based on the concept of clean intermittent

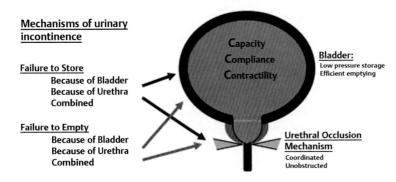

Fig. 8.5 Wein's functional classification.

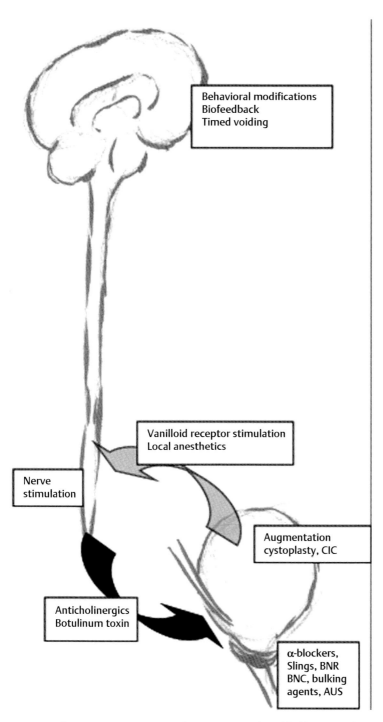

Fig. 8.6 Schematic representation of most commonly used interventions for patients with neurogenic bladder dysfunction. BNR, bladder neck reconstruction; BNC, bladder neck closure; AUS, artificial urinary sphincter; CIC, clean intermittent catheterization.

catheterization (CIC). This simple yet effective means to assist with bladder empting revolutionized the management of patients with neuropathic dysfunction after it was introduced and popularized by Lapides in the 1970s.[20] Either through the use of medications or by surgical intervention, the detrusor muscle can be rendered inefficient, albeit more compliant and capacious. It is through CIC that these patients can easily and safely manage their LUT with significant improvement in their quality of life.

Pharmacological Therapy

Interventions Aimed at Improving Bladder Storage Function

Several reviews have been published evaluating the effects of the different pharmaceutical agents available.[21] Currently, the most commonly used pharmacotherapy is to some degree restricted to anticholinergic agents, having widespread clinical use and a long track record for a favorable safety profile. As previously mentioned, acetylcholine plays a major role as one of the key neurotransmitters involved in stimulation of the detrusor muscle for contraction. In patients with neurogenic DOA, anticholinergic agents acting on the postganglionic parasympathetic cholinergic receptors reduce the amplitude of the detrusor muscle contractions, increase the volume to the first contraction, increase the functional bladder capacity, decrease urgency in patients with sensate tracts, and possibly improve bladder compliance. Oxybutynin chloride remains one of the most commonly used oral anticholinergic agents worldwide, although the market has recently expanded to include others such as tolterodine (Detrol, Pfizer, Inc., New York, NY) and the upcoming M3 muscarinic selective receptor antagonists (solifenacin and darifenacin).[21,22] In addition to having similar anticholinergic activity, one advantage oxybutynin has is its strong smooth muscle relaxant properties associated with local anesthetic activity[23]. Unfortunately, these agents are not without side effects, which occasionally limit their clinical usefulness in individual patients. The most common of these include mouth dryness, blurry vision, constipation, heat intolerance, and flushing. With the recent introduction of long-acting/prolonged-release oxybutynin and tolterodine tablets (Ditropan XL [Ortho-McNeil, Raritan, NJ] and Detrol LA [Pfizer, Inc., New York, NY]), as well as oxybutynin transdermal delivery patches (Oxytrol, Watson Urology, Morristown, NJ), the incidence of these side effects is reportedly lower as a result of the slower release of active metabolites into the bloodstream. Each agent may vary slightly in the degree and incidence of adverse effects, and individual patients may be able to tolerate or become tolerant to one drug preferentially over the others. This is achieved in most settings by a trial-and-error process.

In recent years, new innovative treatment strategies have been developed exploiting the intravesical approach to medication delivery.[24] By acting on the afferent arc of the bladder or by direct activity on the detrusor muscle, this allows for a more direct modulation of the neurogenic overactive bladder with absent or low systemic absorption. Besides anticholinergics, two other important groups of drugs can be delivered this way. The first group, composed of vanilloid receptor agonists, directly activates nociceptive type C fibers and interrupts pathological reflex activity by desensitization. Clinical trials support improvements in cystometric bladder capacity with a decrease in detrusor pressure and DOA by means of the administration of capsaicin[25] or the more potent, less painful, and perhaps superior agent, resiniferatoxin.[26] The second group consists of botulinum neurotoxins. After injection into the bladder wall, botulinum-A toxin or Botox (Allergan, Inc., Irvine, CA), the most potent known natural toxin, binds the presynaptic nerve endings of cholinergic neurons, disrupts the protein mechanism crucial for synaptic vesical fusion, and effectively inhibits neuronal acetylcholine release leading to temporary chemodenervation. Even though there are limited data available, this intervention seems to be relatively safe, with a favorable short-term symptomatic and urodynamic response.[27] The duration of this response appears to be between 4 and 14 months (average 9 months), with subsequent need for reinjection. Unclear to this date is the likelihood and rate at which tolerance is developed in patients subjected to multiple injections.

Interventions Aimed at Improving Bladder Outlet and Voiding Function

Another drug class that has found its way into the treatment of neurogenic conditions is the α-blockers. Initially limited by their side effect profile, selective (i.e., doxazosin) and superselective (tamsulosin) α-blockers have been slowly introduced into the pediatric clinical practice, with promising results in selected children particularly affected by functional bladder outlet obstruction.[28]

Surgical Interventions

It should be reemphasized, however, that once the diagnosis is made progressive signs and symptoms should lead in most situations to quick definitive surgical correction of the tethered cord, especially for patients with incontinence, because the condition may quickly become irreversible.[12] The prognosis might not always be straightforward because surgical untethering may not lead to improvement (and may even progress to deterioration) either because of an inaccurate preoperative diagnosis, late intervention after severe redox changes or significant histological damage has already occurred, or surgical damage to and/or entrapment of healthy adjacent nervous structures within scar tissue. With improvements in microsurgery and intraoperative monitoring by means of somatosensory evoked potentials, continuous electromyography, and maybe even intraoperative urodynamics,[29] this latter problem should be reduced to a minimum.

Keeping in mind that long-term or randomized trials are lacking, division of the filum terminale leads to varying degrees of improvement in daytime incontinence, nocturnal enuresis, stool incontinence, detrusor hyperreflexia, bladder compliance, VUR, and back or leg pain after short- and intermediate-range follow-up.

From a urological perspective, the management of patients with neuropathic bladder disorders must be based on a thorough evaluation to identify the resultant effects of the neurological lesion on the whole urinary tract. Armed with information about the status of the upper tracts, the bladder storage characteristics, the effectiveness of the urethral control mechanism, and the degree of coordination between the detrusor muscle and the urethral sphincter, the urologist can design a therapeutic plan to correct or improve bladder function.

Depending on the severity of the defect in detrusor storage ability, patients at low risk may respond to simple pharmacological manipulation to improve bladder capacity and compliance, sometimes assisted with frequent timed voiding or with the aid of CIC to achieve complete bladder emptying. On the other hand, the high-risk group generally requires more aggressive and sometimes more invasive intervention to attain low-pressure storage, protection of the upper tracts, and complete bladder emptying. A risk stratification scheme is suggested in **Table 8.1**.

In most cases, urinary diversion with the aid of an external collection appliance is no longer an option in the management of children with a neurogenic bladder. Also, the destruction of the urethral control mechanism to cause incontinence and low-pressure voiding (i.e., sphincterotomy or placement of urethral stents such as the UroLume, American Medical Systems, Inc., Minnetonka, MN) is not required because CIC will accomplish low-pressure emptying in the absence of complete voiding. The direct and indirect stimulation of the sacral nerve roots and peripheral nerves by external or implantable stimulation devices (e.g., InterStim, Medtronic, Inc., Minneapolis, MN) is not widely used and is still considered by many to be an experimental procedure in patients with neurogenic dysfunction secondary to TCS. Dorsal rhizotomies and other nerve destruction procedures are also rarely, if ever, employed in these children.

Table 8.1 Risk of Hydronephrosis and Renal Injury

Parameter	Low Risk	Intermediate	High Risk
Leak point pressure	< 40 cm H_2O	> 40 cm H_2O	> 40 cm H_2O
Intravesical pressure at capacity	< 40 cm H_2O	> 40 cm H_2O	> 40 cm H_2O
Maximum urethral closing pressure on urethral pressure profile	< 40 cm H_2O	40–70 cm H_2O	> 70 cm H_2O
Bladder capacity under 35 cm H_2O pressure	> mean standardized for age	< mean standardized for age	< mean standardized for age
Detrusor-sphincter dyssynergia	Absent	Present	Present
Vesicoureteric reflux	Absent	Grades 1–2*	Grades 3–5*
Thickened, trabeculated bladder wall	Absent	Present	Present
Hydronephrosis	Absent	Moderate	Severe

*International system of radiographic grading of vesicoureteric reflux.

Interventions Aimed at Improving Bladder Storage Function

Surgical augmentation of the bladder is the best described and most successful surgical procedure devised to achieve a low pressure high compliance urine reservoir. The bowel segment to be used for the augmentation is isolated and then opened along its antimesenteric border to disrupt the circular muscle fibers and abolish peristalsis (principle known as detubularization). A long sagittal incision is subsequently made in the bladder, extending from the bladder neck anteriorly to the trigone posteriorly ("clamshell" opening), permitting for a wide anastomosis between the bowel segment and the bladder, and guarding against stenosis at the suture line with consequent diverticulum formation. The choice of bowel segment to be used is less important than the fashion by which it will be applied. Two points to remember are (1) the loss of an excessive amount of terminal ileum may be associated with disruption of the enterohepatic circulation of bile salts and may result in diarrhea, which can be difficult to manage in patients who also have a neurogenic bowel, and (2) in patients with borderline renal function the absorptive capacity of the bowel segment used for augmentation taxes the patient's residual functional kidney mass by reabsorption of acids and metabolites from the urine, and this may accelerate the onset of end-stage renal failure and the need for dialysis or transplantation. In selected circumstances these patients are offered augmentation with a portion of the stomach instead of or in addition to small bowel. The obvious advantage is the excretion of acid by the stomach segment into the urine, with a resultant reduction in acid load and an actual decrease in the oral bicarbonate supplementation required. Unfortunately, this is a technically more demanding intervention and is associated with its own set of complications, such as the hematuria dysuria syndrome, which can be seen in up to 35% of patients.[30]

The majority of patients require CIC following augmentation cystoplasty to completely empty the bladder. To avoid potential postoperative difficulties with bladder emptying, all candidates for bladder augmentation must be sufficiently facile with CIC before being considered for surgery. Those who have difficulty with this procedure because of urethral stricture, false lumens, or severe pain with catheterization can be provided with a continent catheterizable stoma on the abdominal wall. These channels are created by connecting the appendix or a reconfigured segment of bowel to the bladder in a nonrefluxing fashion, using the Mitrofanoff[31] or the Monti[32] principles, respectively. The low intravesical pressures achieved following augmentation cystoplasty render more than 85% of the patients continent, even if urethral occlusion pressures are marginal preoperatively.

Interventions Aimed at Improving Bladder Outlet and Voiding Function

In some cases the sphincter mechanism is so inefficient that no matter how low the intravesical pressures are the child will have varying degrees of incontinence, usually worsened by sudden increases in pressure such as during transferring in and out of a wheelchair. In such patients, augmentation cystoplasty has been safely combined with procedures to increase urethral resistance. These include minimally invasive injection of bulking agents [Macroplastique (Uroplasty, Inc., Minnetonka, MN), collagen, or Deflux (Q-Med Scandinavia, Inc., Princeton, NJ)], urethral suspension procedures, bladder neck/proximal urethra sling placement, bladder neck reconstruction, insertion of an artificial urinary sphincter, and, generally as a last resort, bladder neck closure. The decision to proceed with these interventions in the setting of bladder augmentation should not be taken lightly. The price of continence in these children may be a high one because absence of a pop-off valve to avoid overdistention may lead to rupture of the augmented bladder with subsequent peritonitis, sepsis, and even death.

without LUT symptoms[35]) may escape the need for urodynamic evaluation, it is a reasonable clinical rule to always err on the side of obtaining this study.

Unfortunately, postoperative neurological recovery is neither fast nor predictable, and several months may pass before any improvement is noted. With the always present possibility of retethering and the sometimes long-lasting persistence of neurological deficits, these patients require lifelong urologic monitoring. As patients mature certain aspects of the neurourological history and exam may gain importance, such as erectile function in males[36] and genital sensation. Infants and young children being an obvious exception, patients are typically able to describe even subtle changes in symptoms, sometimes to the point that they may seem trivial to the clinician. Reevaluation should be initiated soon thereafter because early detection may lead to intervention and prevent further neurological deterioration. As we continue to learn about the natural history of this disorder, the benefit of repetitive surgical untethering in the long-term outcome of patients with otherwise progressive symptoms will be better defined.[37]

■ Follow-up Evaluation

The effects of the neurological lesion may vary with time and growth; therefore, patients must be followed closely on a long-term basis to recognize any changes in bladder behavior that may require corresponding adjustments in management. Each institution has adopted different protocols for evaluation after diagnosis and treatment. In general, it is desirable to obtain a full urological assessment (including urodynamics) before surgical intervention. These "baseline" studies are very helpful because they can uncover abnormalities that precede clinical manifestations and serve as a comparison test that can be contrasted with studies obtained thereafter.[33,34] Even though it has been suggested that certain patients (such as those with isolated orthopedic problems

■ Conclusion

The implication of spinal cord pathology as the underlying etiology for urinary incontinence is usually made by exclusion. A more sensitive and specific modality for the diagnosis of early tethering of the cord is desirable because a timely diagnosis appears to be critical to prevent further deterioration and to improve existing deficits. Such a test is currently lacking. Because the presence of a low-lying conus on imaging studies may represent a relatively late finding in the disease process,[3] the need for better diagnostic *functional* tools becomes apparent.

Clearly, one of the current challenges for the urologist is to devise diagnostic algorithms and screening techniques that would allow us to diagnose patients at an earlier stage while avoiding unnecessary tests in children without TCS.

Even though imperfect, the currently applied urological interventions do allow for successful treatment of most patients with neurogenic bladder dysfunction—renal failure is preventable in all but the rare patient born with severe kidney damage, urinary continence is readily achievable, and urinary tract infections and sepsis are easily treated under most circumstances.

References

1. Yamada S, Won DJ, Siddiqi J, Yamada SM. Tethered cord syndrome: overview of diagnosis and treatment. Neurol Res 2004;26:719–721
2. Yamada S, Zinke DE, Sanders D. Pathophysiology of "tethered cord syndrome." J Neurosurg 1981;54: 494–503
3. Yamada S, Knerium DS, Mandybur GM, Schultz RL, Yamada BS. Pathophysiology of tethered cord syndrome and other complex factors. Neurol Res 2004;26:722–726
4. Phuong LK, Schoeberl KA, Raffel C. Natural history of tethered cord in patients with meningomyelocele. Neurosurgery 2002;50:989–993, discussion 993–995
5. Farhat W, Bägli DJ, Capolicchio G, et al. The dysfunctional voiding scoring system: quantitative standardization of dysfunctional voiding symptoms in children. J Urol 2000;164(3, Pt 2):1011–1015
6. Koff SA, Wagner TT, Jayanthi VR. The relationship among dysfunctional elimination syndromes, primary vesicoureteral reflux and urinary tract infections in children. J Urol 1998;160(3, Pt 2):1019–1022
7. Khoury AE, Hendrick EB, McLorie GA, Kulkarni A, Churchill BM. Occult spinal dysraphism: clinical and urodynamic outcome after division of the filum terminale. J Urol 1990;144(2, Pt 2):426–428, discussion 428–429, 443–444
8. Soonawala N, Overweg-Plandsoen WC, Brouwer OF. Early clinical signs and symptoms in occult spinal dysraphism: a retrospective case study of 47 patients. Clin Neurol Neurosurg 1999;101:11–14
9. Robinson AJ, Russell S, Rimmer S. The value of ultrasonic examination of the lumbar spine in infants with specific reference to cutaneous markers of occult spinal dysraphism. Clin Radiol 2005;60: 72–77
10. Uehling DT, Gilbert E, Chesney R. Urologic implications of the VATER association. J Urol 1983;129:352–354
11. Mosiello G, Capitanucci ML, Gatti C, et al. How to investigate neurovesical dysfunction in children with anorectal malformations. J Urol 2003;170(4, Pt 2): 1610–1613
12. Yamada S, Won DJ, Siddiqi J, Yamada SM. Tethered cord syndrome: overview of diagnosis and treatment. Neurol Res 2004;26:719–721
13. Rosen R, Buonomo C, Andrade R, Nurko S. Incidence of spinal cord lesions in patients with intractable constipation. J Pediatr 2004;145:409–411
14. Pippi Salle JL, Capolicchio G, Houle AM, et al. Magnetic resonance imaging in children with voiding dysfunction: is it indicated? J Urol 1998;160(3, Pt 2): 1080–1083
15. Korsvik HE, Keller MS. Sonography of occult dysraphism in neonates and infants with MR imaging correlation. Radiographics 1992;12:297–306, discussion 307–308
16. Wein AJ. Pathophysiology and categorization of voiding dysfunction. In: Walsh PC, Retik AB, Vaugham ED, and Wein AJ, eds. Campbell's Urology. 8th ed. Philadelphia: WB Saunders; 2002: 887–899
17. Nørgaard JP, van Gool JD, Hjälmås K, Djurhuus JC, Hellström AL; International Children's Continence Society. Standardization and definitions in lower urinary tract dysfunction in children. Br J Urol 1998; 81(Suppl 3):1–16
18. Abrams P, Cardozo L, Fall M, et al; Standardisation Sub-Committee of the International Continence Society. The standardisation of terminology in lower urinary tract function: report from the standardisation sub-committee of the International Continence Society. Urology 2003;61:37–49
19. McGuire EJ, Woodside JR, Borden TA, Weiss RM. Prognostic value of urodynamic testing in myelodysplastic patients. J Urol 1981;126:205–209
20. Lapides J, Diokno AC, Silber SJ, Lowe BS. Clean, intermittent self-catheterization in the treatment of urinary tract disease. J Urol 1972;107:458–461
21. Chapple CR, Yamanishi T, Chess-Williams R. Muscarinic receptor subtypes and management of the overactive bladder. Urology 2002;60(5, Suppl 1) 82–88, discussion 88–89
22. Hashim H, Abrams P. Drug treatment of overactive bladder: efficacy, cost and quality-of-life considerations. Drugs 2004;64:1643–1656
23. DeWachter S, Wyndaele J. Intravesical Oxybutynin: A local anesthetic effect on bladder C afferents. J Urol 2003;169:1892–1895

24. Reitz A, Schurch B. Intravesical therapy options for neurogenic detrusor overactivity. Spinal Cord 2004; 42:267–272

25. de Sèze M, Wiart L, Ferrière J, de Sèze MP, Joseph P, Barat M. Intravesical instillation of capsaicin in urology: a review of the literature. Eur Urol 1999;36: 267–277

26. Giannantoni A, Di Stasi SM, Stephen RL, et al. Intravesical capsaicin versus resiniferatoxin in patients with detrusor hyperreflexia: a prospective randomized study. J Urol 2002;167:1710–1714

27. Riccabona M, Koen M, Schindler M, et al. Botulinum-A toxin injection into the detrusor: a safe alternative in the treatment of children with myelomeningocele with detrusor hyperreflexia. J Urol 2004;171(2, Pt 1): 845–848, discussion 848

28. Austin PF, Homsy YL, Masel JL, Cain MP, Casale AJ, Rink RC. Alpha-adrenergic blockade in children with neuropathic and nonneuropathic voiding dysfunction. J Urol 1999;162(3, Pt 2):1064–1067

29. Schaan M, Boszczyk B, Jaksche H, Kramer G, Günther M, Stöhrer M. Intraoperative urodynamics in spinal cord surgery: a study of feasibility. Eur Spine J 2004;13:39–43

30. Mitchell ME. Bladder augmentation in children: where have we been and where are we going? BJU Int 2003;92(Suppl 1):29–34

31. Mitrofanoff P. Trans-appendicular continent cystostomy in the management of the neurogenic bladder [in French]. Chir Pediatr 1980;21:297–305

32. Monti PR, Lara RC, Dutra MA, de Carvalho JR. New techniques for construction of efferent conduits based on the Mitrofanoff principle. Urology 1997;49: 112–115

33. Vernet O, Farmer JP, Houle AM, Montes JL. Impact of urodynamic studies on the surgical management of spinal cord tethering. J Neurosurg 1996;85: 555–559

34. Meyrat BJ, Tercier S, Lutz N, Rilliet B, Forcada-Guex M, Vernet O. Introduction of a urodynamic score to detect pre- and postoperative neurological deficits in children with a primary tethered cord. Childs Nerv Syst 2003;19:716–721

35. Nogueira M, Greenfield SP, Wan J, Santana A, Li V. Tethered cord in children: a clinical classification with urodynamic correlation. J Urol 2004;172(4, Pt 2): 1677–1680, discussion 1680

36. Boemers TM, van Gool JD, de Jong TP. Tethered spinal cord: the effect of neurosurgery on the lower urinary tract and male sexual function. Br J Urol 1995;76: 747–751

37. van der Meulen WD, Hoving EW, Staal-Schreinemacher A, Begeer JH. Analysis of different treatment modalities of tethered cord syndrome. Childs Nerv Syst 2002; 18:513–517

9 The Cervical Tethered Spinal Cord

Kenji Muro, Arthur J. DiPatri Jr., and David G. McLone

Tethered cord syndrome (TCS) is a well-established and recognized disease entity whose protean manifestations were first described by Hoffman, Hendrick, and Humphreys in 1976.[1] That study cohort included cases of caudal TCS caused by a thickened filum terminale with or without associated lipomas. Since this initial report, other investigators have recognized similar clinical scenarios originating from pathological entities in the cervical spinal cord. A spectrum of underlying etiologies has been described in the literature but only case reports and case series exist at present. In addition to the clinical and radiographic features that cervical TCS shares with the more common caudal TCS, other characteristics also deserve mention. The definition, historical perspective, and pathophysiology of TCS as a whole are discussed in greater detail in other chapters within this text.

The hallmarks of TCS are a progressive and often subtle deterioration in motor, sensory, bowel, and bladder function. Evidence of both upper- and lower-extremity involvement may be present with cervical tethering, but the sequence of involvement is unpredictable. Pain along the spinal axis and radicular pain are common presenting complaints,[1-3] whereas bladder and bowel involvement are the most variable. Even though cervical TCS is a less common clinical entity than caudal TCS, prompt recognition and appropriate management of cervical TCS is warranted to avoid potentially irreversible morbidity. This chapter highlights features unique to TCS of the cervical region, with comparison to the more common caudal TCS, where appropriate.

■ Etiology and Embryology

In our own experience and through a review of the published literature, tethering of the cervical spinal cord occurs much less frequently than at the more caudal levels. Many of the well-described lesions responsible for caudal TCS such as intradural lipomyelomeningocele, fibrous adhesions, split cord malformation, dermal sinus tract, and adhesive arachnoiditis after myelomeningocele repair also apply to the cervical region. One of the more common causes of caudal TCS, the tight filum terminale, for obvious reasons is not relevant to the cervical region; however, we believe like others that the pathophysiology by which the filum terminale effects the onset of caudal TCS also applies to lesions of the cervical spine.[4] In addition to the pathological entities already listed, other etiologies such as postsurgery spinal arachnoiditis and adhesions that occur following intramedullary spinal cord tumor surgery or after penetrating or nonpenetrating spinal cord injury are being increasingly recognized as a cause for delayed neurological deterioration among these select cohorts. Although cervical spine TCS does seem to be a distinct entity, it shares with caudal TCS the most salient feature, that is, clinical improvement following surgical untethering.[3,5-19]

In general there are two broad two categories of lesions that may lead to the development of TCS—congenital and acquired. The cutaneous stigmata associated with congenital lesions are often noted at birth and typically the symptoms associated with TCS manifest early in life, depending on the degree of traction[20] on the spinal cord. The acquired forms occur more frequently in adults. After the initial insult the time that it takes for symptoms attributable to TCS to develop may vary considerably, with reported cases occurring up to 37 years[3] after injury.

Congenital Lesions

Almost all of the lesions responsible for tethering of the cervical spinal cord in young patients are congenital. Most occur as a result of defective neurulation. The embryogenesis of these lesions dictates that the epicenter of the tethering structure generally occurs at the dorsal raphe of the spinal cord, and this is an important consideration for preoperative planning and for intraoperative intervention. The defect in primary neurulation that leads to the formation of the cervical myelomeningocele has been well described. This example of disordered embryogenesis ultimately leaves the spinal cord in the form of the neural plate of the embryo. The split cord malformation also originates from defective neurulation, but as detailed by Pang[22] in his unified theory, its genesis is from the persistence of an "accessory" or "anomalous" neurenteric canal.[21] Usually, the neurenteric canal is a developmentally transient communication between the endoderm and ectoderm layers of the embryo. Failure of the accessory neurenteric canal to involute leaves a structure that transfixes the developing neural tube. The resulting fibrous band or bony spur divides and ultimately tethers the spinal cord.[22]

Both the lipomyelomeningocele and dermal sinus are defects that occur later in neurulation, at the time when the neural tube undergoes disjunction from the superficial ectoderm. Premature disjunction prior to closure of the neural tube allows mesenchymal cells access to the central portions of the neural tube. Lying in apposition to these mesenchymal cells, the luminal surface of the neural tube induces the mesenchyme to form adipose and connective tissues resulting in a lipoma. In contrast, it is incomplete disjunction, resulting in a persistent connection between the neural and superficial ectoderm, that forms a dermal sinus. Other forms of spinal dysraphism reported to cause cervical TCS include the cervical myelocystocele[18] and meningoceles.[7,8,12] In general cervical meningoceles are not directly responsible for causing the symptoms of a TCS, but rather their presence may indicate the existence of an associated intraspinal lesion such as a lipomyelomeningocele or a split cord malformation,[8,12] which may not necessarily be found at the level of the meningocele.

Acquired Lesions

Among the acquired forms of TCS, the posttraumatic TCS is the most frequently encountered clinicallly and in the literature. A prerequisite for the occurrence of an acquired TCS is some form of intradural pathology. Intradural spinal tumor resections, spinal cord injuries, and previously operated degenerative spine conditions[14] are some of the more common examples. Radiographically, the posttraumatic spinal cord manifests diverse morphological patterns of myelomalacia, namely, progressive posttraumatic myelomalacic myelopathy (PPMM) and progressive posttraumatic cystic myelopathy (PPCM).[3,12,16,17,23] These two entities are considered by some to be a continuum of the same posttraumatic pathophysiology,[24] and risk factors that may increase a patients' likelihood of developing symptomatic tethering are not clearly defined. It has been hypothesized that in addition to the primary injury to the spinal cord and intradural contents, posttraumatic arachnoiditis and scarring, which are felt to be responsible for the eventual tethering, are promoted by the locally hemorrhagic environment, the chronic recumbent position of many trauma patients, changes in the local cerebrospinal fluid (CSF) dynamics, and chronic ischemia.[3]

There has not been a correlation between the level of cervical spinal tethering and the time to symptom onset. Furthermore, to explain the variable time period between the initial injury and the onset of TCS, it is likely that the degree of tethering and tension among these patients differs, which results in the variable time to presentation, a theory that Pang and Wilberger proposed in their study of adult patients with caudal TCS.[25]

■ Clinical Presentation

The presence of cutaneous stigmata suggestive of an underlying dysraphic lesion is present in almost all congenital lesions. As is frequently the case with the more caudal forms of TCS, it is not uncommon for these structural abnormalities that occur with the congenital etiologies of tethered cervical cord to be noted at birth but ignored until the onset of symptoms later in life. Dermal pits, hemangiomas, meningoceles, lipomas, and a short neck are markers of underlying pathology. Those cases of TCS that are due to spinal injury or are related to prior surgery become apparent after the history and physical exam is obtained.

Regardless of the etiology, the development of symptoms may involve all or relatively few of the neurological modalities traversing the tethered segment. In a caudal tethered cord, onset and worsening of symptoms appear to correlate with periods of rapid growth when it is theorized that increased traction is applied to the spinal cord.[1] Among adult patients, the signs and symptoms of caudal TCS may be aggravated by prolonged sitting or forward bending. No such description exists in cervical TCS except in the posttraumatic literature, where Lee at al[17] describe their patients' symptoms as "positional" but do not elaborate further. The signs and symptoms of the caudal TCS may also develop acutely after trauma as was noted in 61% of patients in one series.[25] In cervical TCS the association with trauma preceding the onset of symptomatic TCS has only been described in one case report of a 34-year-old adult with a split cord malformation of the cervical spine.[6] Unlike adults, who are able to specify and indicate symptoms, a cautionary note must be voiced in the young infant whose lack of achieving motor and/or sphincter milestones may be perceived as individual variance.

Individuals often give a long history of clumsiness, abnormal gait, and patchy numbness in all four extremities, although initially the symptoms may be limited to only the lower extremities. Bladder and bowel involvement or spinal axis pain is frequently the reason these patients finally seek medical care. Unlike caudal TCS, patients with cervical TCS may also present with involvement of other neurological signs or symptoms, including autonomic dysreflexia, hyperhydrosis, respiratory insufficiency, or even Horner syndrome.[3,17]

Neurological examination of the patient often reveals, in addition to the cutaneous manifestation, atrophy of the upper extremity musculature,[15] especially the intrinsic muscles of the hands. Complaints may involve all four limbs, with quadriparesis being a common finding, An asymmetrical motor exam or possibly a hemiparesis may occur. Sensory symptoms may vary from a patchy or asymmetrical sensory loss to a well-defined cervical sensory level. Deep tendon reflexes may range from hypoactive to brisk, and pathological reflexes are not uncommon. A neurogenic bladder can occur as the sole manifesting complaint.

■ Diagnostic Studies

Magnetic resonance imaging (MRI) has become the first-line modality for screening purposes when concern exists for a tethered spinal cord. Conventional roentgenograms and computed tomographic (CT) scans are indicated for the analysis of the patient's bony anatomy and may show anomalies such as spina bifida, fused laminae, the bony spur of a split cord malformation, or the segmentation abnormalities of Klippel-Feil syndrome. In most cases, MRI is sufficient to determine the cause and extent of the tethering lesion, and the decision to operate and the design of the procedure can often be made utilizing this study alone. Water-soluble contrast-enhanced CT myelography may be helpful in situations where the MRI is equivocal, and postmyelography tomographic images can sometimes demonstrate the tethering bands and clefts in the spinal cord.[20,23,25] This is especially useful in the situation of prior spinal instrument implantation, which may make MRI difficult to interpret.

Several studies have addressed the co-occurrence of cervical meningoceles with an intraspinal tethering lesion. In five patients with cervicothoracic meningocele, Chaseling et al found "deep extension" of the meningocele at the time of surgery in two patients, and one additional patient had an associated myelographic abnormality, the exact nature of which was not detailed further.[7] In another study, Delashaw et al described finding lipomeningomyelocele, tethered cord, and diastematomyelia in a cohort of four patients with cervical meningoceles. Most of these lesions were caudal to the level of the meningocele.[8]

Preoperative somatosensory evoked potentials (SSEPs) are rarely utilized or reported in the literature. Decreases in amplitude and prolonged latencies[10,26] may be noted, although this may also occur in normal patients.[15] The value of this testing may be in its use as a baseline dataset that surgeons would refer to either intraoperatively or in postoperative follow-up. Given the anecdotal nature of obtaining electrophysiological studies preoperatively, there is no consensus on its use.

■ Treatment

Intraoperative Monitoring

Several authors have reported the use of intraoperative anal sphincter electromyography (EMG) and stimulation of the pudendal nerve[2,25,27] and found the technology useful for the determination of functioning neural elements and for operative management of caudal TCS. These studies did not detail the number of instances in which

the technique was utilized, nor the subset in which the technique made a difference in intraoperative decision making. Furthermore, they do not compare the outcomes of patients who underwent surgery with or without monitoring.

The use of motor evoked potentials during surgery for patients harboring intramedullary neoplastic lesions, including lipomas, has been reported with 100% sensitivity and 91% specificity of the technique predictive of postoperative motor deficits.[28,29] However, this technique has not yet been reported as an adjunct in the surgical management of cervical tethered cord. Furthermore, there are technical limitations in the ability to perform intraoperative monitoring at the cervical level of certain functions, especially the bladder. Because the bladder is innervated from multiple levels and there are many supraspinal modulators, the accurate identification of bladder efferents remains technically challenging.[30]

Intraoperative SSEPs are also variably reported in the cervical TCS literature. The most dramatic result was demonstrated in the report by Eller et al, when the SSEPs were shown to have a significant and immediate improvement after releasing the tethering lesion intraoperatively.[10] It is the senior author's (DGM) experience, however, that SSEPs are not particularly useful in most situations because the act of untethering requires the surgeon to proceed with procedures that must be continued if the goals of the operation are to be realized, despite the monitoring results. Most importantly, there are no prospective studies reporting the use and comparative outcome of patients undergoing surgery for cervical TCS with intraoperative monitoring. Completion of such a study may be logistically difficult, owing to technical considerations and the rarity of the condition; however, it would be a valuable contribution to the field.

Surgical Technique

Almost all publications in the literature, regardless of etiology, report the use of microsurgical technique for untethering the spinal cord. Of utmost importance before embarking on this surgical procedure is the thorough understanding of the anatomy, the tethering lesions and their locations, and anticipation of any pitfalls. This includes the assimilation of all radiographic data, noting the epicenter of the lesion and presence of dysraphic laminae and prior postsurgical interventions, along with the characteristics of the spinal cord in relation to the lesion and whether the tethering is occurring in an eccentric fashion. A detailed discussion with the anesthesiologist is also mandatory to ensure proper handling of the patient at the time of anesthesia induction, intubation, positioning, and intraoperative course, especially if neurophysiological monitoring is utilized.

As with the surgical management of any dysraphic or traumatic lesion of the spine and spinal cord, we prefer to identify and delineate as much normal anatomy and landmarks as possible. It is not uncommon to lose tissue planes when dealing with tethering lesions, so a clear understanding of the local and regional anatomy is requisite before addressing the tethering pathology. Surgical loupe magnification is sufficient for the initial dissection and approach to the spine. At all times, the surgical team must be mindful not only of the responsible lesion that must be completely untethered but also of the exit strategy. By this, especially in patients with spinal dysraphism, it is necessary to assess the quality of the fascial layers and dura for an effective, watertight closure.

At this stage of surgery, in the posttraumatic cervical TCS literature, some authors utilize intraoperative ultrasonography to aid the localization of the tethered segment.[17] Once the normal anatomy is delineated and the surgical team is ready to address the tethering lesions, we feel the modern surgical microscope and microsurgical instruments are of paramount importance in the handling of these delicate surgical situations. Clearly, dissection is carried forth with great attention and care of the neural elements, utilizing sharp dissection techniques. Thorough inspection and lysis of all tethering lesions are required; otherwise there remains the risk of postoperative delayed recurrence of

symptomatic TCS, as reported by Pang et al with their experience in a cohort of patients with cervical myelomeningocele.[25] It is our experience that most congenital and acquired lesions causing TCS, upon close inspection, have a clear plane between the tethering segment and the normal neural tissue. The exception is the lipomyelomeningocele, where the lipoma occupies a juxtamedullary-subpial location with no discernable cleavage plane.[31] It is our practice that complete untethering with subtotal lipoma resection is the best surgical decision, so as not to jeopardize the patient's neurological function.

In the senior author's experience, the use of the handheld CO_2 laser substantially reduces the operative time for management of tethering lesions, with particular reference to lipomyelomeningoceles. Use of the laser also reduces the intraoperative blood loss because the lipoma is vaporized and small vessels are sealed simultaneously.[32] Only larger arteries require separate bipolar cauterization. The reduced blood loss is particularly important in infants, whose initial blood volume is small. In fact, these infants do not require intra- or postoperative transfusion. The laser also reduces the need to manipulate the tissues and thus prevents the consequent operative trauma. With $3\times$ loupe magnification, the handheld laser may be played over the exposed surface of the lipoma, reducing it layer by layer, down to the liponeural interface. Loupe magnification and manual laser manipulation are preferred by the senior author to the use of the operative microscope with coaxial laser resection because the surface area of the lipoma is large, and there is need for frequent changes in the angle of approach to the portion of lipoma exposed at any one time.

In the posttraumatic cervical TCS literature, after completion of the untethering procedure, many advocate duraplasty to expand the subarachnoid space. It is argued that this expanded space may result in decreased incidence of retethering by adhesive bands. It is possible that compared with primary closure of the dura, which will always lead to some loss of intrathecal volume, the expansile duraplasty will theoretically result in decreased retethering.[17] However, there are no prospective data on this practice, and the definition of retethering, on radiographic or clinical grounds, is also not uniform in the literature.

■ Outcomes

The most important feature of cervical TCS in common with the more prevalent caudal TCS is that patients derive clinical benefit, either improvement or stabilization in the majority of cases, from surgical intervention. Furthermore, the case reports and series in the literature are encouraging in the paucity of major morbidity and mortality associated with surgery. Therefore, the risk:benefit ratio is in favor of untethering.

In the cervical TCS literature, there are multiple case reports and small series relaying surgical successes[3,5–19]; one of the most thorough analyses of patient evaluation, treatment, and outcome was reported by Pang and Dias in 1993. In this cohort of nine patients with cervical myelomeningoceles, the first group of six patients had a simple subcutaneous resection of the sac and ligation of the dural fistula. No lysis of underlying tethering structures was performed. Five of these six patients deteriorated 13 months to 8 years after their initial surgery with worsening hand function and lower extremity spasticity. In contrast, the last three patients in this series underwent complete intradural lysis of tethering lesions at the initial surgery. At 3-year follow-up, two of three patients remained neurologically normal; one of the three patient required an additional surgical intervention due to return of symptoms 4 years after the initial surgery, and workup revealed a residual ventral tethering structure, which was addressed. Reoperations, which were performed in the five patients in the first group, were tolerated well and were successful in improving the patients' neurological function at 12 to 35 months of additional follow-up.[19]

Among the many publications of cervical region dermal sinus tracts,[5,6,11,15] in an interesting retrospective report on their cohort of patients with dermal sinus tracts in the cervical and thoracic spines, Ackerman et al found that all of their patients with dermal sinus tracts over the age of 12 months had a neurological deficit at presentation, whereas patients younger than 12 months were all neurologically normal. The patient ages ranged from 3 days to 55 years at presentation. Eighty percent of the patients presenting with neurological deficit "improved" after surgery, and the remaining patients had stabilization of symptoms.

In the acquired etiologies, the posttraumatic cervical TCS has several larger case series reporting the surgical outcome. In a cohort of 53 patients with PPCM and mean follow-up of 23.9 months, Lee et al report that 56% of patients improved when presenting with motor symptoms, 46% with spasticity, 45% with sensory loss, 47% with gait dysfunction, 36% with axial or radicular pain, and "minimal" relief in those who presented with paresthesias, sphincter dysfunction, or autonomic dysreflexia. Overall, 73% of patients had "satisfactory" results, 21% were clinically stabilized, and 7% were worse after surgery.[17]

In a cohort of 40 patients with PPMM, surgery resulted in 79% of patients improving when presenting with motor symptoms, 62% with pain, 50% with sphincter dysfunction, 43% with sensory level loss, and 75% with autonomic dysfunction. Overall, in this study, 83% of patients had "good" results and 17% were clinically stabilized.[18] Supporting these results, 95.8% of patients undergoing untethering felt that surgery was helpful in preventing further neurological deterioration.[12]

Taking the reported literature together with our own experience, the outcome from untethering cervical lesions is favorable, even among symptomatic patients. However, experience has also taught us that the natural history of untreated symptomatic tethered lesions is not favorable for a patient's good functional outcome, with improvement from surgical intervention dependent on the duration of symptoms. In fact, we believe that prophylactic surgery, when conducted at experienced centers with low associated procedural morbidity and mortality, portends the best outcome in these situations.

■ Conclusion

Cervical TCS is a distinct clinical entity that shares all of the protean features of caudal TCS. Cutaneous or structural abnormalities are often present at birth with congenital lesions, whereas the patients' past medical history and thorough physical exam are revealing in acquired cases. At a variable period of months to years, insidious neurological deterioration affects sensory and motor systems, as well as bladder and bowel function; unique to the cervical spine is the manifestation of TCS by autonomic dysregulation, hyperhydrosis, respiratory insufficiency, and Horner syndrome.

Surgical untethering stabilizes the clinical picture, and one can often anticipate significant improvement, especially if performed early in the course. Motor and sensory symptoms benefit the most from untethering, with the response to surgery unpredictable for preoperative bladder and bowel dysfunction. Similar to tethering at the caudal end of the spinal cord, retethering of the cervical spinal cord can occur after surgical untethering, and thus patients must be followed throughout life.

There are no prospective trials assessing the optimum technique and timing for intervention for the management of cervical TCS, owing largely to the diverse etiologies responsible for the tethering. For example, it is not known whether prophylactic surgical intervention is warranted in this situation, although extrapolation from the caudal TCS data would support this practice. Therefore, the literature contains many methodologies for patient management and operative intervention. Also, the long-term outcome of these patients is of interest, especially with the increasing recognition of retethering, whose surgical management has been successful. We recommend the creation of a multiinstitutional, prospective database of this unique disease entity that would facilitate the study of these important questions.

References

1. Hoffman HJ, Hendrick EB, Humphreys RP. The tethered spinal cord: its protean manifestations, diagnosis and surgical correction. Childs Brain 1976;2(3):145–155
2. Hendrick EB, Hoffman HJ, Humphreys RP. The tethered spinal cord. Clin Neurosurg 1983;30:457–463
3. Yamada S, Zinke DE, Sanders D. Pathophysiology of "tethered cord syndrome". J Neurosurg 1981;54(4):494–503
4. Yamada S, Knerium DS, Mandybur GM, Schultz RL, Yamada BS. Pathophysiology of tethered cord syndrome and other complex factors. Neurol Res 2004;26(7):722–726
5. Ackerman LL, Menezes AH, Follett KA. Cervical and thoracic dermal sinus tracts. A case series and review of the literature. Pediatr Neurosurg 2002;37(3):137–147
6. Beyerl BD, Ojemann RG, Davis KR, Hedley-Whyte ET, Mayberg MR. Cervical diastematomyelia presenting in adulthood. Case report. J Neurosurg 1985;62(3):449–453
7. Chaseling RW, Johnston IH, Besser M. Meningoceles and the tethered cord syndrome. Childs Nerv Syst 1985;1(2):105–108
8. Delashaw JB, Park TS, Cail WM, Vollmer DG. Cervical meningocele and associated spinal anomalies. Childs Nerv Syst 1987;3(3):165–169
9. Dogulu F, Onk A, Oztanir N, Ceviker N, Baykaner MK. Cervical dermal sinus with tethered cord and syringomyelia. Case illustration. J Neurosurg 2003;98(3, Suppl)297
10. Eller TW, Bernstein LP, Rosenberg RS, McLone DG. Tethered cervical spinal cord. Case report. J Neurosurg 1987;67(4):600–602
11. Erol FS, Topsakal C, Ozveren MF, Akdemir I, Cobanoglu B. Meningocele with cervical dermoid sinus tract presenting with congenital mirror movement and recurrent meningitis. Yonsei Med J 2004;45(3):568–572
12. Falci SP, Lammertse DP, Best L, et al. Surgical treatment of posttraumatic cystic and tethered spinal cords. J Spinal Cord Med 1999;22(3):173–181

13. Feltes CH, Fountas KN, Dimopoulos VG, et al. Cervical meningocele in association with spinal abnormalities. Childs Nerv Syst 2004;20(5):357–361

14. Hart DJ, Apfelbaum RI. Anterior cervical spinal cord tethering after anterior spinal surgery: case report. Neurosurgery 2005;56(2):E414, E414

15. Kuo MF, Wang HS, Yang CC, Chang YL. Cervical cord tethering mimicking focal muscular atrophy. Pediatr Neurosurg 1999;30(4):189–192

16. Lee TT, Alameda GJ, Gromelski EB, Green BA. Outcome after surgical treatment of progressive posttraumatic cystic myelopathy. J Neurosurg 2000; 92(2, Suppl)149–154

17. Lee TT, Alameda GJ, Camilo E, Green BA. Surgical treatment of post-traumatic myelopathy associated with syringomyelia. Spine 2001; 26(24, Suppl) S119–S127

18. Nishino A, Shirane R, So K, Arai H, Suzuki H, Sakurai Y. Cervical myelocystocele with Chiari II malformation: magnetic resonance imaging and surgical treatment. Surg Neurol 1998;49(3):269–273

19. Pang D, Dias MS. Cervical myelomeningoceles. Neurosurgery 1993;33(3):363–372, discussion 372–373

20. Harwood-Nash DCF, Fitz CR, Resjo IM, Chuang S. Congenital spinal and cord lesions in children and computed tomographic metrizamide myelography. Neuroradiology 1978;16.69–70

21. Bremer JL. Dorsal intestinal fistula; accessory neurenteric canal; diastematomyelia. AMA Arch Pathol 1952;54(2):132–138

22. Pang D, Dias MS, Ahab-Barmada M. Split cord malformation: Part I: A unified theory of embryogenesis for double spinal cord malformations. Neurosurgery 1992;31(3):451–480

23. Osborne DR, Vavoulis G, Nashold BS Jr, Dubois PJ, Drayer BP, Heinz ER. Late sequelae of spinal cord trauma. Myelographic and surgical correlation. J Neurosurg 1982;57(1):18–23

24. Shaw MDM, Russell JA, Grossart KW. The changing pattern of spinal arachnoiditis. J Neurol Neurosurg Psychiatry 1978;41(2):97–107

25. Pang D, Wilberger JE Jr. Tethered cord syndrome in adults. J Neurosurg 1982;57(1):32–47

26. Roy MW, Gilmore R, Walsh JW. Evaluation of children and young adults with tethered spinal cord syndrome. Utility of spinal and scalp recorded somatosensory evoked potentials. Surg Neurol 1986;26(3):241–248

27. Kothbauer KF, Novak K. Intraoperative monitoring for tethered cord surgery: an update. Neurosurg Focus 2004;16(2):E8

28. Kothbauer KF, Deletis V, Epstein FJ. Motor-evoked potential monitoring for intramedullary spinal cord tumor surgery: correlation of clinical and neurophysiological data in a series of 100 consecutive procedures. Neurosurg Focus 1998;4(5):e1

29. Morota N, Deletis V, Constantini S, Kofler M, Cohen H, Epstein FJ. The role of motor evoked potentials during surgery for intramedullary spinal cord tumors. Neurosurgery 1997;41(6):1327–1336

30. Schaan M, Boszczyk B, Jaksche H, Kramer G, Günther M, Stöhrer M. Intraoperative urodynamics in spinal cord surgery: a study of feasibility. Eur Spine J 2004; 13(1):39–43

31. Rogers HM, Long DM, Chou SN, French LA. Lipomas of the spinal cord and cauda equina. J Neurosurg 1971;34(3):349–354

32. McLone DG, Naidich TP. Laser resection of fifty spinal lipomas. Neurosurgery 1986;18(5):611–615

10 Indication and Treatment of Tethered Spinal Cord

James M. Drake and Harold J. Hoffman

Tethered spinal cord syndrome consists of a group of dysraphic conditions in which the conus medullaris is located in an abnormally low position and is fixed there in a relatively immobile state. Many of these conditions are seen in association with spina bifida occulta, whereas others are seen secondary to repair of a myelomeningocele or lipomyelomeningocele.

■ Embryology

During fetal life, the spinal cord grows much more slowly than the vertebral column. This leads to a progressive disparity between the termination of the spinal cord and that of the spine; in effect, there is a progressive ascent of the conus medullaris. The most distal part of the spinal cord forms through the process of secondary neurulation or canalization from day 28 to day 48 of the gestational period. Through this process, the caudal cell mass becomes canalized and forms the terminal neural tube, which eventually becomes the conus medullaris. Through the process of regression, the most caudal portion of the neural tube atrophies and forms a fibrous band (called the filum terminale). The band is initially identifiable at day 52. The conus medullaris then ascends within the spinal canal largely through the disproportionate growth of the vertebral column relative to that of the neural tube. At 20 weeks' gestation, the termination of the conus medullaris is at the level of the space between the L4 and L5 vertebrae. By 40 weeks' gestation or at term, the conus is at the L3 level and, by age 2 months, has reached the adult L1–2 level.[1]

■ Pathophysiology

Studies by Yamada et al[2] show that if stretch is placed on the conus medullaris, progressive ischemia can occur, leading inevitably to neurological sequelae. Anatomical studies by Breig[3] have shown that as the normal spine flexes, the spinal cord moves toward the C4 level. This upward movement during flexion is not possible in a conus medullaris that remains tethered. A sudden flexion movement of the spine in the patient with a tethered cord can produce further traction on the conus and lead to symptomatic onset of tethered cord syndrome, even after cessation of growth in adult life.

■ Historical Background

Johnson[4] first described the entity of lipomyelomeningocele in 1857. However, it was not until 1950 that Bassett[5] emphasized the progressive deterioration in function in patients with a lipomyelomeningocele and stressed the value of early prophylactic surgery. Despite this, management of these lesions remained controversial until relatively recent years. Matson[6] believed that surgical management should consist of a cosmetic repair. With the development of prophylactic surgery in cases of occult spinal dysraphism, lipomyelomeningoceles were excluded from consideration because of their complex anatomy and the difficulty of assessing the value of surgery. However, in recent years, the value of carrying out such early surgery has been stressed.[7]

In 1953 Garceau[8] described the filum terminale syndrome in three patients who had a thick filum terminale discovered at laminectomy and who improved following section of the filum terminale. Jones and Love[9] reported a further six patients in 1956. In 1976 the author and colleagues reviewed their experience with patients who had a thick filum or spinal cord tethering.[10]

■ Clinical Presentation

Cutaneous manifestations in patients with a tethered spinal cord are common. Patients with a lipomyelomeningocele will almost always have a fatty mass visible in the lumbosacral region, which can vary from a large expansive mass to a small lipoma to a caudal tail-like appendage (**Fig. 10.1A,B**). In addition, other cutaneous manifestations such as hemangioma or dimple may be present. Patients with a diastematomyelia typically have a large hairy patch in the region of the dysraphic spine (**Fig. 10.1C**). About one third of patients with simple tethering show some form of cutaneous lesion (such as a hairy patch, hemangioma, dimple, or area of thin atrophic skin) or a subcutaneous lipoma (**Fig.10.1D**). In patients who develop secondary tethering following repair of a myelomeningocele or lipomyelomeningocele, an obvious incision is visible on their backs.

Patients with a tethered spinal cord present with a progressive motor or sensory deficit in the lower limbs. Many are seen in the orthopedic surgeon's office because of a gait disturbance. They can display foot deformities such as pes cavus or an equines deformity (**Fig. 10.2**). The plastic surgeon may see these patients because of trophic ulceration of the foot due to sensory loss. Scoliosis alone or in combination with other problems is common in patients with a tethered spinal cord. If a spine-straightening procedure is performed with the cord still tethered, sudden and precipitous deterioration in neurological function can occur. Untethering the spinal cord in a patient with a mild scoliosis can frequently prevent progression of or even improve the scoliosis and thus avoid the need for instrumentation. A neurogenic bladder is a common event in patients with a tethered spinal cord, and in many of these patients, signs of a neurogenic bladder are their major manifestation. Back pain and root pain may occur in patients with a tethered cord. The pain is typically intractable and aggravated by movement. It is rarely seen in patients with diastematomyelia or lipomyelomeningocele; however, it may be seen in patients with secondary tethering after repair of a lipomyelomeningocele or myelomeningocele. The pain may radiate along dermatomes and may mimic pain due to other causes. Patients with a tethered spinal cord tend to deteriorate in their function with growth spurts during childhood but also in adult life as a result of trauma and flexion movements of the spine. Sudden and irreversible deterioration in neurological function is possible. Although treatment at first diagnosis has been recommended, recent reports question the effectiveness of prophylactic surgery in lipomyelomeningocele in preventing subsequent deterioration.[11,12]

■ Patient Evaluation

All patients with a tethered spinal cord should undergo careful evaluation and documentation of motor and sensory function. Plain x-rays of the spine may show evidence of spina bifida occulta in patients with a tethered spinal cord. The bifid spine is usually below L3 and frequently involves several segments. Ultrasonography helps delineate the level of the conus in the infant.

Magnetic resonance imaging (MRI) is currently the investigative tool of choice. It shows the low-lying cord and the conus fixed

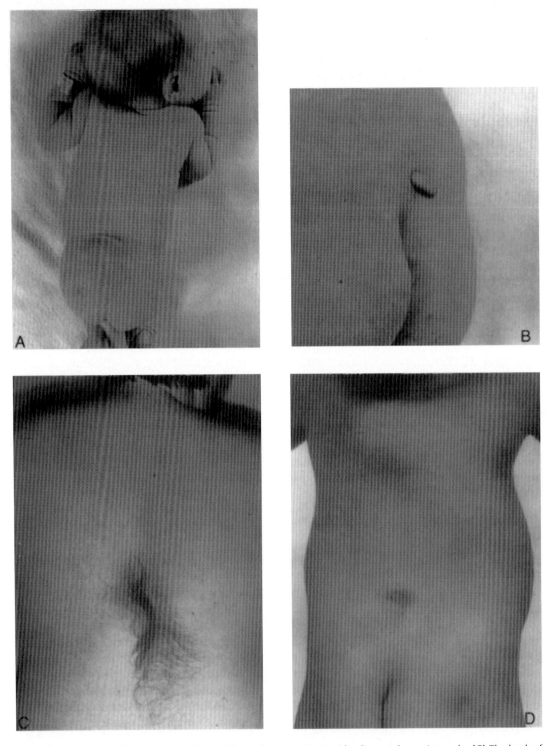

Fig. 10.1 Clinical manifestations in patients with a tethered spinal cord. **(A)** The back of an infant with a lipomyelomeningocele. Note the hemangioma in association with the lesion. **(B)** A caudal tail-like appendage in a patient with a lipomyelomeningocele. **(C)** The back of a patient with a diastematomyelia showing a large hairy patch. **(D)** The back of a patient with simple tethered cord showing a hemangioma.

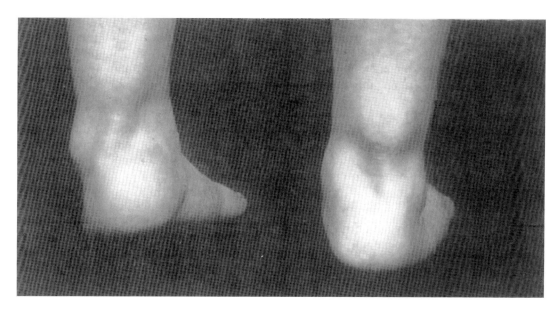

Fig. 10.2 A foot deformity in a patient with a tethered spinal cord.

posteriorly (if it is tethered at the site of a myelomeningocele repair) (**Fig. 10.3**). Several series of patients have been reported who had clinical features of a tethered spinal cord with normal imaging, or a normal level conus medullaris, and a portion of which improved following division of the filum terminale.[13-16]

Urodynamic testing is an important adjunct to the assessment of these patients, both before and after therapy, because it helps identify patients with a neurogenic bladder and records objective improvement after untethering. Urodynamic testing in infants is difficult, and the reproducibility of urodynamics may be imperfect.[17]

■ Treatment

Thick Filum Terminale

Patients with a thickened filum need a single-level laminectomy, usually at the level of the L5 and S1 vertebrae. Because the thickened filum is very different from the adjacent nerve roots in its size, tautness, and profusion of blood

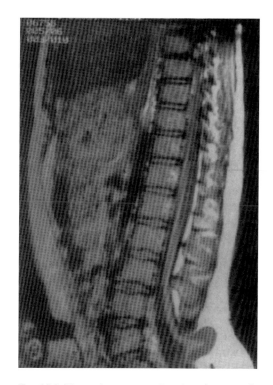

Fig. 10.3 Magnetic resonance imaging showing a low-lying spinal cord, tethered at the site of a myelomeningocele repair

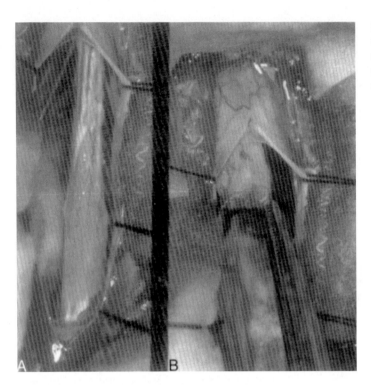

vessels, it is rarely necessary to stimulate the filum to differentiate it from the surrounding nerve roots. The thickened filum is divided after coagulation (**Fig. 10.4**).

Attached Spinal Cord

Patients with an attached spinal cord are treated similarly to patients with a thick filum terminale. However, the laminectomy is performed over the mid- to low sacral region. The cord is detached from the terminal dural sac and allowed to ride free. Frequently, the attached spinal cord is thinned out and stretched and may mimic a thick filum terminale on neuroimaging. During surgery, however, the nerve roots can readily be seen exiting the spinal cord and ascending to reach their exit foramina (**Fig. 10.5**).

Diastematomyelia

To correct diastematomyelia, the surgeon makes an incision over the abnormal vertebrae

extending downward to below the level of the diastematomyelia. The laminae are removed over the normal dural sac below the diastematomyelia. The bone removal continues in a cephalad direction over the split dural sacs until the normal dural sac is reached. Between the split dural sacs, there is usually a massive amount of bone and fat that, as it is removed, leaves a thin spike traveling in a cephalad direction between the split dural tubes and ending in a broad-based attachment to two vertebral bodies at the level of an absent disk space. The dura is then opened over the caudal single dural tube and extended in a cephalad direction over the split dural tube, exposing the split spinal cord. The spinal cord distal to the split is normally tight against the split in the dural tube and the bony spike (**Fig. 10.6**). A high-speed drill is used to drill the bony spike down to the vertebra anteriorly. Typically, an arterial blood vessel in the center of this bony spike bleeds profusely. Waxing the bone will control this bleeding. The anterior dura is then either left open or closed with one or two sutures. The

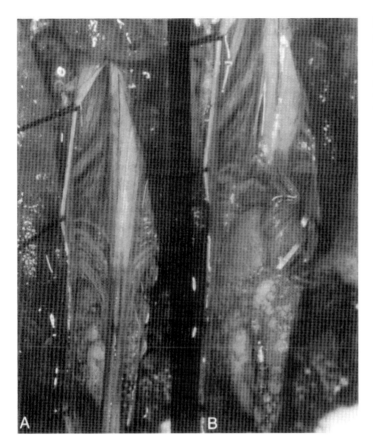

Fig. 10.5 (A) Operative photograph showing the spinal cord attached to the end of the dural sac, with the lower nerve ends ascending to their exit foramina. **(B)** After release of the tethering, the nerve roots take a horizontal course.

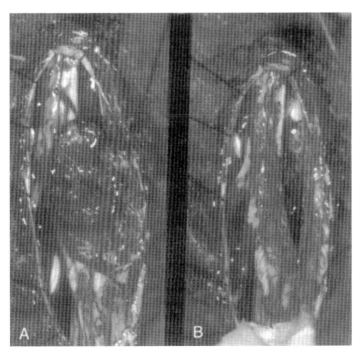

Fig. 10.6 (A) Operative photograph showing a diastematomyelia. Note the bony spike surrounded by dura and fat, with the spinal cord tight against the inferior portion of the spike. **(B)** After removal of the spike, the split in the spinal cord can be clearly seen.

posterior dura is reconstituted, either directly or with a dural graft. Because all patients with diastematomyelia have an associated thick filum, the dural opening is continued in a caudal direction to expose the conus and the filum terminale. The filum is then divided.

Lipomyelomeningocele

To repair a lipomyelomeningocele or myelocystocele, the surgeon makes an incision in the skin in the midline. The dissection is then performed at the cephalad extent to the last intact lamina. This lamina is removed, exposing the intact dural tube. The dura is opened at this level, and the dural opening is continued down to the region of the lipomyelomeningocele, where the dura is deficient. At the level of the lipomyelomeningocele, there are no posterior bony elements. A grooved director is used

to divide the dura laterally on either side of the lipomatous mass, just at its attachment to the lipoma. If the lipomyelomeningocele is dorsal, the dural tube is intact distally so the dural opening is continued down into the normal distal dural tube (**Fig. 10.7A**). If the lipomyelomeningocele is terminal or transitional, the distal dural tube will be abnormal because of dural schisis (**Fig. 10.7B**).

The dural incision is continued to the lowermost portion of the anterior dural tube. The massive proliferation of dorsal fat can now be identified and separated from the overlying mesodermal tissues. The fat is removed initially with scissors and gradually shaved down. A laser is an effective tool for melting and removing the fat. Complete removal of all of the fat, however, may jeopardize normal conus function; therefore, some fat is usually left. Intraoperative monitoring may help to identify nerve roots imbedded

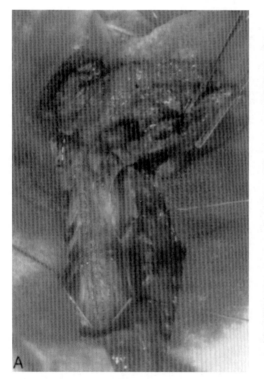
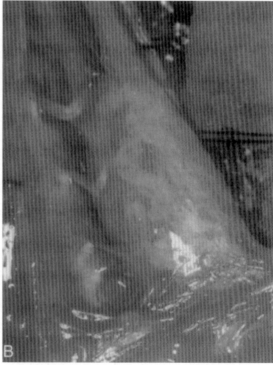

Fig. 10.7 (A) Operative photograph of a dorsal lipomyelomeningocele. Note that the spinal cord below the lipoma is tethered caudally by a thick filum terminale. **(B)** Operative photograph of a terminal lipomyelomeningocele.

in the fat, particularly in lipomas that extend through the intravertebral foramina.

In those patients with a dorsal lipomyelomeningocele, the thickened filum terminale must be divided to untether the spinal cord effectively. In patients with a terminal syrinx, as seen particularly in patients with a myelocystocele, the syrinx is effectively drained as the fat is removed. Patients with a repaired lipomyelomeningocele are always left with a large dural defect. A variety of dural substitutes can be used for reconstitution of the dural tube.

magnification, freeing the cord from mesodermal tissue. In these cases, the dural repair is often inadequate. Fat can frequently be seen extending from subcutaneous tissue into the spinal cord, mimicking the appearance of a lipomyelomeningocele.

Occasionally, in addition to tethering, other conditions such as diastematomyelia or dermoid tumor may be found. These conditions should be treated when the cord is untethered. Once the spinal cord is free, the dural closure must be secure to prevent neural tissue from adhering to mesodermal tissue.

■ Tethering at the Site of Myelomeningocele Repair

Frequently, the diagnosis of tethering at the site of repair is a diagnosis of exclusion. The child with a repaired myelomeningocele who shows evidence of secondary deterioration may have some condition other than tethering, such as shunt malfunction, Chiari malformation, hydrosyringomyelia, spinal dermoid cysts, diastematomyelia, or intracranial midline cysts. Only when these conditions are excluded should tethering at the site of repair be considered as the cause of the patient's symptoms. This is particularly important because all patients with a repaired myelomeningocele have a low-lying spinal cord.

Untethering at the site of the myelomeningocele repair must be performed with care under

■ Conclusion

A diagnosis of tethered spinal cord should be considered for any patient with spina bifida occulta in the lumbosacral region who presents with back or leg pain, scoliosis, neurogenic foot deformity, trophic foot ulceration, or a sphincter disturbance. This is particularly the case when there is an overlying cutaneous manifestation of spina bifida occulta, such as a hairy patch, a lipoma, a hemangioma, atrophic skin, or a dimple. Intensive investigation of these patients is warranted.

If the presence of a tethered cord is confirmed, early treatment is advocated, particularly in the presence of clinical deterioration. Prophylactic untethering in asymptomatic patients has also been advocated, but the risks and benefits of this surgery are being evaluated.

References

1. Barson AJ. The vertebral level of termination of the spinal cord during normal and abnormal development. J Anat 1970;106(Pt 3):489–497
2. Yamada S, Zinke DE, Sanders D. Pathophysiology of "tethered cord syndrome." J Neurosurg 1981;54:494–503
3. Breig A. Overstretching of and circumscribed pathological tension in the spinal cord: a basic cause of symptoms in cord disorders. J Biomech 1970;3:7–9
4. Johnson A. Fatty tumour from the sacrum of a child, connected with the spinal membranes. Trans Pathol Soc London 1857;8:16–18
5. Bassett RC. The neurologic deficit associated with lipomas of the cauda equina. Ann Surg 1950; 131:109–116, illust
6. Matson DD. Neurosurgery of Infancy and Childhood. Springfield, IL: Charles C Thomas; 1969
7. Hoffman HJ, Taecholarn C, Hendrick EB, Humphreys RP. Management of lipomyelomeningoceles: experience at the Hospital for Sick Children, Toronto. J Neurosurg 1985;62:1–8
8. Garceau GJ. The filum terminale syndrome (the cord-traction syndrome). J Bone Joint Surg Am 1953;35-A:711–716

9. Jones PH, Love JG. Tight filum terminale. AMA Arch Surg 1956;73:556–566

10. Hoffman HJ, Hendrick EB, Humphreys RP. The tethered spinal cord: its protean manifestations, diagnosis and surgical correction. Childs Brain 1976;2:145–155

11. Kulkarni AV, Pierre-Kahn A, Zerah M. Conservative management of asymptomatic spinal lipomas of the conus. Neurosurgery 2004;54:868–873, discussion 873–875

12. Pierre-Kahn A, Zerah M, Renier D, et al. Congenital lumbosacral lipomas. Childs Nerv Syst 1997; 13:298–334, discussion 335

13. Khoury AE, Hendrick EB, McLorie GA, Kulkarni A, Churchill BM. Occult spinal dysraphism: clinical and urodynamic outcome after division of the filum terminale. J Urol 1990;144(2, Pt 2):426–428, discussion 428–429, 443–444

14. Warder DE, Oakes WJ. Tethered cord syndrome and the conus in a normal position. Neurosurgery 1993; 33:374–378

15. Warder DE, Oakes WJ. Tethered cord syndrome: the low-lying and normally positioned conus. Neurosurgery 1994;34:597–600, discussion 600

16. Wehby MC, O'Hollaren PS, Abtin K, Hume JL, Richards BJ. Occult tight filum terminale syndrome: results of surgical untethering. Pediatr Neurosurg 2004;40: 51–57, discussion 58

17. Gupta A, Defreitas G, Lemack GE. The reproducibility of urodynamic findings in healthy female volunteers: results of repeated studies in the same setting and after short-term follow-up. Neurourol Urodyn 2004;23:311–316

11 Tethered Cord Syndrome Associated with Myelomeningoceles and Lipomyelomeningoceles

Shokei Yamada, Daniel J. Won, Alexander Zouros, and Shoko M. Yamada

This chapter concentrates on tethered cord syndrome (TCS) associated with two pathological categories: (1) myelomeningoceles (MMCs) and (2) lipomas or lipomyelomeningoceles (LMMCs). Earlier the goal of surgical treatment for MMCs, spina bifida aperta, was considered to be protection of the neural elements and prevention of infection to the exposed spinal cord and intradural-subarachnoid space,[1,2] and the consequent scar formation. It became apparent, however, that repair of MMCs in some patients, and of lipoma and LMMCs in the majority of patients, was followed by neurological improvement.

Such experiences were supported by research work with the following evidence. The impaired oxidative metabolism was associated with increased tension in the lumbosacral cord, and further, metabolic improvement occurred after release of tension by the repair of these anomalies.[3] It is a reasonable assumption that these clinically or radiologically demonstrable anomalies must be eliminated surgically if the signs and symptoms suggest the presence of TCS. Furthermore, untethering procedures should be performed on symptomatic patients at an early stage if operative risks are estimated as minimal. This chapter focuses on the symptomatology, prevention, and treatment of TCS.

■ Tethered Cord Syndrome Associated with Myelomeningoceles

MMCs in the lower lumbar and sacral regions are often associated with TCS. Until recently, it was believed that neurological deficits associated with MMCs were neither reversible nor progressive.[4,5] Thus it was assumed that the repair of such lesions was purely for better nursing care and cosmetic reasons. Understanding of the pathophysiology of TCS and the delayed neurological deterioration observed in children with spinal cord tethering has brought to light the importance of early correction and avoidance of retethering through proper surgical repair.[6,7]

Anatomical Considerations

In general, MMCs are the result of defective neurulation. The normal tubular formations of the dura mater and pia arachnoid remain cephalic and caudal to the dysraphic level. The dura is usually open and everted over the articular facets and often extends farther laterally to cover the paraspinal fascia. The arachnoid membrane is frequently everted and covers the inner side of the dura. However, when the normal skin covers the major portion of the MMC, the arachnoid usually underlies the skin and extends over the membranous sac. The arachnoid membrane can be clearly isolated and closed over the neural tissue. The pia mater is widely open lateral to the neural plaque, and the central canal terminates at the cephalic end of the neural placode and continues as a midline groove of the placode.

The MMC sac itself is composed of an aberrant membrane or an extension of the intermediate arachnoid,[8] which is interposed between the pia arachnoid and pia mater in the normal spinal canal. Hereafter, the MMC sac is referred to as the meningocele or meningeal sac. Nerve roots often pass through a layer of the meningocele sac or internal to the membrane. Cerebrospinal fluid (CSF) contained in the MMC communicates with the normal subarachnoid space at the junction of the meningocele sac and normal spinal canal. CSF probably circulates through the numerous small channels between the arachnoid trabeculations or the penetrations of the intermediate arachnoid formed at the base of the MMC.

Treatment

Objectives of Repair

The dispute has been long-standing as to whether early surgical intervention is beneficial in cases of MMC. Previously, no neurological improvement was expected after the repair of MMCs.[4,5] However, an increasing number of cases with postoperative neurological improvement have recently been reported,[6,7,9] and these results have encouraged early surgical intervention. It is now generally accepted that repair and closure of MMCs should be performed within 48 hours of birth.[4-6] It is believed that the repair of MMCs associated with untethering of the spinal cord may ameliorate neurological deficits,[6,7] particularly motor and sensory function.[6]

The repair and closure of MMCs have the following objectives: (1) to protect the externally exposed neural elements; (2) to prevent infection caused by the invasion of organisms; (3) to prevent and reverse neurological deficits by untethering the spinal cord[6,7]; (4) to prevent retethering after surgery[6,7,10]; (5) to improve nursing and, later, self-care; and (6) to facilitate cosmetic reconstruction.

Preoperative Considerations

Prior to surgery, consider the following two points to prevent central nervous system infection: (1) prophylactic use of antibiotics should be started within 24 hours of birth, and (2) an immunological factor for control of infection must be considered. Maternally acquired antibodies are typically present for up to 2 months after birth. If the infant is breast-fed, immunoglobulin M antibodies will remain during the course of breast-feeding. If the repair of the MMC is delayed beyond 2 months postpartum, then serum gamma globulin levels should be obtained, and if the level is decreased, intravenous immunoglobulin can be given prior to surgery (Nielsen-Canarella S, personal communication, 1998).

Surgical Anatomy

The authors, for surgical purposes, divide MMCs into three types based on anatomical differences. In the first type, the spinal cord, often buckled, travels inside the meningocele sac, and its neural placode surfaces along the dome of the sac. The placode is covered by a thin layer of poorly developed epithelial tissue but not by meningeal lining. The farther caudal part of the spinal cord often enters the spinal canal with defective laminae. The caudal end of the spinal cord or filum is either loosely or densely adhesive to the surrounding tissue. It is important to release the spinal cord from adhesion because a later occurrence of TCS is expected when the bucked spinal cord straightens as the vertebral column rapidly grows.

The second type of MMC is characterized by a spoon-shaped neural placode exposed to the surface without meningeal lining. The spinal cord terminates at the caudal extremity of the placode. Postoperative cord tethering may occur from adhesion of the spinal cord to the surrounding meninges or extradural fibrous tissue if meningeal closure is not complete.

In the third type, the spinal cord terminates abruptly inside the meningocele sac and the central canal is open to the CSF space. The nerve roots exiting near the caudal extremity surround the cord and are distributed to the meningocele sac. An incomplete form of the terminal ventricle may be present. Meningeal closure of the caudal end is essential for preventing development of TCS.

Surgical Technique

Type 1 Myelomeningocele

Under general endotracheal anesthesia intubation, the patient is placed prone and padded with a roll on each side of the trunk. An incision is made immediately outside the junction of the skin and membranous sac in a circumferential manner (**Fig. 11.1 A,B**). Careful microscopic dissection of the sac from the overlying skin allows for isolation of the neural plaque along its edges.

The neural plaque is an embryological dorsal cleft and has no meningeal lining in this type of MMC. The very thin, disorganized epithelial membrane covering the plaque is washed with saline irrigation and trimmed with microscissors. This prevents the enclosure of contaminated devitalized squamous elements under the skin coverage for the repair. Prior to dissection of the sac, it is often necessary to incise the dura longitudinally 0.5 to 1.0 cm cephalad or caudad to its base (**Fig. 11.1C**). The arachnoid membrane can now be easily identified where its dorsal aspect ends, cephalic and occasionally caudal to the neural plaque. The lateral extension of the arachnoid membrane can be seen everted on each side beyond its fusion with the pia, dorsolateral to the exit of the posterior nerve roots. When the skin covers the major portion of the meningo-

cele sac, the arachnoid extends to underlie the subcutaneous tissue (**Fig. 11.1D,E**). As soon as the meningocele sac is ruptured, CSF is drained out of the sac causing it to collapse immediately. The spinal cord sinks in the collapsed subarachnoid space and relaxes (**Fig. 11.1C**). The superficial edge of the meningocele sac is carefully dissected from the lateral end of the neural placode. The arachnoid membrane, which can be found everted lateral to the spinal canal, is then freed from the underlying dura. The dura that is everted over the lateral mass of the vertebrae is also isolated from the facet and fascia. Fibrous tissue around the caudal end of the spinal cord is then dissected free. Next, several 8–0 nylon sutures are passed through both pial edges and tied (**Fig. 11.1C**). This procedure allows formation of a nearly normal spinal cord and central canal contour (**Fig. 11.1C**). Both edges of the arachnoid flaps are then approximated over the reformed cord using 8–0 nylon sutures (**Fig. 11.1C**). Repair of the arachnoid membrane in this fashion establishes postoperative CSF circulation in the subarachnoid space and prevents adhesions from forming between the underlying neural tissue and dura or extrameningeal structures. Dural flaps are then freed from the underlying fascia bilaterally and closed with interrupted 6–0 nylon sutures. In some cases where the arachnoid membrane is not well formed around the meningocele sac, the dural flaps may be used directly to cover the spinal cord. At times, it may be difficult to form an adequate dural flap if the lateral mass of the vertebra is wide and protrudes posteriorly. If dural closure is defective (usually at the caudal end), then bilateral fascial flaps are developed to cover the entire meningocele sac for a watertight closure. However, if the arachnoid and dural layers are closed completely, fascial flap closure is not absolutely necessary. It is recommended that at least two of the three layers (the arachnoid, dura, and fascia) should be closed. Finally, the subcutaneous tissue and skin are closed in the standard fashion, with careful attention not to compress the underlying neural elements.

The closure of a large MMC that has skin coverage only to its base necessitates bilateral dissection of the skin anteriorly to the pararectal line of the abdominal wall for vertical closure, and to the scapulae and sacrum for horizontal closure. Before placing the sutures, skin color should be observed while the skin edges are approximated with the aid of skin hook traction.

If blanching occurs along the edges, further dissection is necessary. Relaxing incisions or Z-shaped skin flaps may have to be utilized, although these techniques are rarely required. Slightly bluish discoloration after closure is

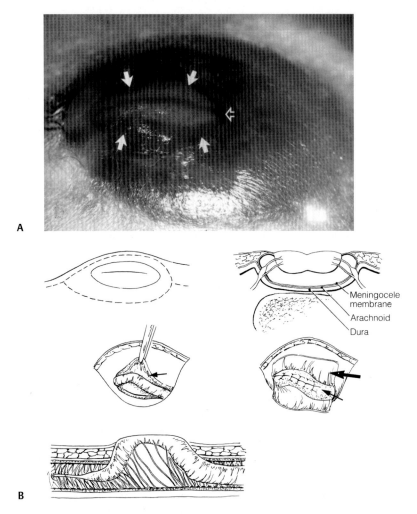

Fig. 11.1 (A) Photograph of a type 1 myelomeningocele (MMC) as viewed from the outside. The neural placode is exposed dorsally, with no meningeal covering (*solid arrows*). The midline groove is well identified, and a poorly developed translucent epithelial membrane covers the placode. The central canal (*open arrow*) is covered by a thin membrane. **(B)** An elliptical incision surrounds the myelomeningocele. The buckled spinal cord reaches the dome of the MMC where the placode is exposed. The spinal cord ends in the sacral canal with either loose or dense adhesion to the surrounding connective tissue. It is important to release the tethering of the cord.

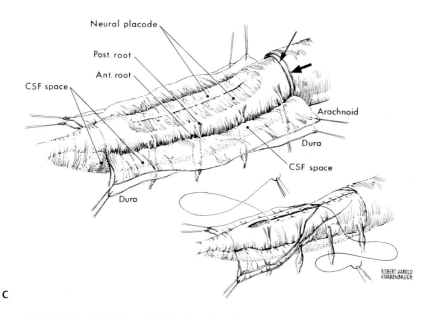

C

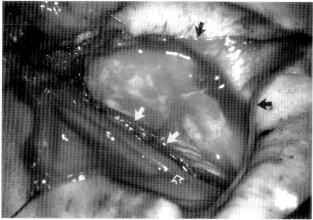

D

Fig. 11.1 *(Continued)* **(C)** After laminectomy at one level above the spina bifida, a midline dural incision is made to expose the cephalic end of the neural placode. The midline groove of the neural placode is continuous to the central canal. The trimmed edge of the meningocele sac is shown underneath the arachnoid membrane at the cephalic end of the sac, which is assumed to be a continuation of the intermediate arachnoid in the normal spinal canal. The lateral edges of the sac are excluded in the drawing. The arachnoid and the dura are everted away from the placode. The pia mater has been closed with 8–0 nylon sutures. The second figure shows sutures being placed through the arachnoid (dura is indicated by *large arrows* and the arachnoid by *small arrows* in. **(D)** The central placode has sunk to the anterior spinal canal after cerebrospinal fluid (CSF) draining, and the trimmed edge of the meningocele sac borders the placode (*white arrows*). The everted arachnoid has a broad base and its lateral extension has been isolated from subcuticular tissue (*black arrows*). The opening of the central canal (*open arrow*) and the midline groove of the neural placode are clearly seen. CSF draining from the central canal percolates through the thin membrane over the placode, causing constant wetting of the placode surface. The nerve roots directing cephalad (to the right) and exiting through the arachnoid and dura are identified. *(Continued on page 124)*

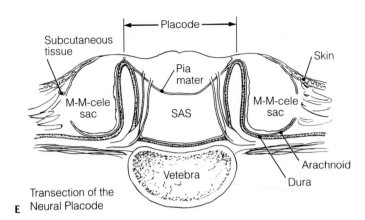

Fig. 11.1 *(Continued)* **(E)** Transection of the MMC shows the arachnoid membrane extending laterally to undermine the skin. The meningocele sac is fused with the arachnoid except for the area of the membrane directly attached to the placode edge (*arrows*). SAS, subarachnoid space.

tolerated, and sloughing skin or dehiscence rarely ensues. Kyphectomy has been advocated by Reigel[7] to prevent skin ischemia caused by the protruding lateral mass of the bifid vertebrae.

Type 2 Myelomeningocele

The repair of this type of MMC is similar to that of type 1. In this case, the skin is isolated from the meningocele sac, which is then incised around its junction to the neural placode. The spoon-shaped placode usually has no filum (**Fig. 11.2A**). The pia is closed with 9–0 nylon sutures, and formation of the spinal cord is completed (**Fig. 11.2B**). The arachnoid and the dura are closed in separate layers over the newly formed cord. Closure of the meninges is of utmost importance in preventing postoperative cord adhesion

Type 3 Myelomeningocele

The spinal cord in this type of MMC characteristically has an open central canal at its caudal end that forms the terminal ventricle (**Fig. 11.3A**). The caudal end of the spinal cord and the nerve roots are carefully dissected from the surrounding membrane and fibrous tissue for untethering (**Fig. 11.3B**). Next, the pia mater is closed around the end of the spinal cord to complete the closure of the central canal (**Fig. 11.3C**). The surrounding nerve roots are carefully dissected. The caudal end of the spinal cord is then closed with pial, arachnoid, and dural sutures. The arachnoid, dural, and fascial flaps are closed in a similar fashion as for type 1 MMC (**Fig. 11.3D,E**).

■ Postoperative Management and Complications

Postoperatively, the infant should be kept in the prone position with a protective covering over the repair site. Feedings may be started within 8 to 12 hours if bowel sounds are audible and the baby can be held by a nurse or parent for feedings.[7]

Complications subsequent to the initial MMC repair often necessitate a secondary surgery. The morbidities include the following: (1) dehiscence or CSF leakage[11]; (2) hydrocephalus[6,7,11]; (3) infection[6,7]; (4) new TCS or recurrence of TCS[1,6,12–14]; (5) local adhesive spinal cord dysfunction; and (6) hindbrain dysfunction[15] (which is outside the scope of this chapter).

Dehiscence, CSF leakage, and ulceration are almost inseparable problems. Further, incomplete meningeal closure healing results in scar formation around the spinal cord and nerve roots.

Hydrocephalus, which is frequently associated with MMCs (80%),[6] must be treated promptly by ventricular fluid shunting for protection of

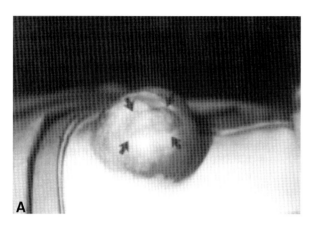

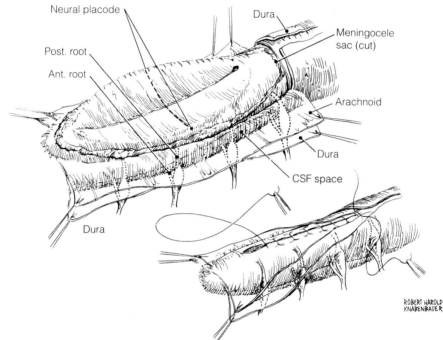

Fig. 11.2 (A) Photograph of a type 2 MMC with a placode covered by a thin epithelium (*black arrows*). **(B)** This type of myelomeningocele has a spoon-shaped placode. The caudal end has no filum terminale. The pial sutures reform the caudal spinal cord, and the arachnoid and dural sutures complete the covering of the reformed cord

cerebral function as well as prevention of CSF leakage through the MMC or repaired wound. The incidence of shunt infection after MMC repair is twice as high as for hydrocephalus from other causes.[16] Prophylactic antibiotic administration is useful for the prevention of shunt infection.[16–18] Shunt infection (with a 2 to 5% incidence rate[16,17]) almost always results in ventriculitis and can cause secondary infection of the repaired MMC.

The infection rates of MMC repair are variable (12% overall).[19] There are several reasons for postrepair infection. MMCs are contaminated soon after the patient's birth, and organisms

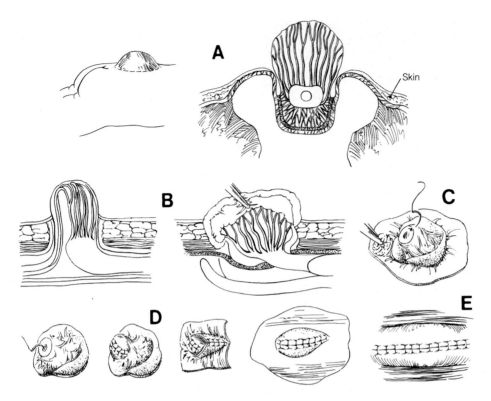

Fig. 11.3 (A) Drawings of a type 3 myelomeningocele (MMC). **(B)** Transection of the most cephalic part of the spinal cord shows a central canal. **(C)** The caudal end of the spinal cord is located in the MMC. The nerve roots arise from the spinal cord outside the central canal in the cerebrospinal fluid (CSF) space and terminate in the sac. **(D)** Pial sutures around the central canal close the spinal cord. Sutures through the arachnoid edges followed by **(E)** sutures through the dural and fascial flaps complete the watertight closure.

can invade the underlying structures through a thin membranous portion. Therefore, the infection is most likely related to the growth of organisms left in the membrane. When CSF leakage persists, organisms spread easily inside the subarachnoid space, resulting in meningitis. Meningitis can also occur secondary to shunt infection or septicemia from other serious infections in the newborn.

The infection rate has some bearing on the timing of MMC repair. Data reported by McLone and Naidich[6] show a significant difference in infection rates between early and late repair: 7% after repair within 48 hours of birth compared with 37% after repair later than 48 hours. The authors advised repair of the MMC within 48 hours, followed by prophylactic

antibiotic treatment. These data suggest that repeated contamination of the MMC contributes to postoperative infection, which also results in scar formation adjacent to neural elements.

The patient is more likely to develop postoperative cord adhesion if[10] (1) the spinal cord or nerve roots were not dissected completely from the surrounding scar and meningeal tissue, (2) dissection resulted in local ischemia, (3) the nerve structures are not covered by the meningeal structure or its inert substitute, or (4) dermal tissue is left under the skin closure.[20] Therefore, meticulous repair of neural tissue and meningeal structures cannot be overemphasized to minimize postoperative neurological complications.

■ Tethered Cord Syndrome Associated with Lipomas and Lipomyelomeningoceles

Due to their similarities in embryonic development, signs and symptoms, and surgical indications and procedures, both lumbosacral lipomas (leptomyelolipomas) and LMMCs are discussed together. Quite often these anomalies are considered to be the mechanical cause of cord tethering, and surgical untethering results in the alleviation of symptoms.[15,21-23] The authors' purpose in this part is to distinguish stretch-induced lesions associated with lipomas and LMMC from those due to spinal cord or nerve root compression and neuronal dysgenesis. Therefore, the discussion is limited to only those patients who underwent redox studies of cytochrome a,a$_3$ and who had proven impairment of oxidative metabolism in the cord segments proximal to the lipoma or LMMC that improved after untethering procedures, thus indicating that these patients had TCS

Classifications of Lipomas and Lipomyelomeningoceles

The definition of LMMCs[24] is often unclear because of the complexity of the anatomical arrangement of the spinal cord, nerve roots, and meninges. This is true particularly in the variation of the interface between the spinal cord and lipomatous (fibrolipomatous or fibroadipose) tissue and its relationship to meninges and subarachnoid space. Mainly, this complexity is derived from the disarray of the perineural tissue (mesodermal and ectodermal) in relation to the neurulation abnormality,[25,26] the timing of the caudal mass formation, and the arachnoid and dural development.[3,27]

Chapman[21] classified lipomas (leptomyelolipomas) into three types: caudal, dorsal, and transitional. In addition, he provided discrete diagrams to show that lipomas protrude outside the confinement of the arachnoid and dural canal (**Fig. 11.4A,B,D**). Others[28,29] added a filar type, which has been considered synony-

mous with the tethered spinal cord. French[30] defined lipomas as a fibroadipose mass located in the subarachnoid or intradural space (**Fig. 11.4C**), as opposed to LMMC in which a lipomatous mass protrudes external to the arachnoid and dura. Schut et al[22] have found that almost all LMMCs are fluctuant, indicating that CSF is contained in the mass.

The authors have modified Chapman's lipoma model[21] and classify LMMCs into three types, all of which have subarachnoid space extension into the lipomatous mass.

1. In the caudal type, the elongated spinal cord enters the meningeal sac through its narrow junction with the normal sacral CSF space. The lipoma–cord interface is located at the distal end of the sac (**Fig. 11.5A**). The fatty mass otherwise remains external to the meningeal lining (fused dura and arachnoid).[31,32]

2. In the dorsal type (**Fig. 11.5B**), the lipoma–cord interface is located in the dorsal surface of the incompletely neurulated spinal cord, consisting of intermingled fibroadipose and glial tissue. The lipomatous mass extends through the open meninges and laminae into the muscular layers and blends into the subcutaneous fat. The meningeal sac may extend into the lipomatous mass. The dura external to the junction is everted and covers the articular processes of the vertebrae. Apparently mesodermal (fibroadipose) tissue competed with neuroectodermal tissue to grow into the dorsal neural plate before the completion of neurulation. As in reconstruction of the neural plaque of the MMC, the closure of the pial edges of the dorsal spinal cord in the LMMC[33] assists in preventing future meningeal or muscular adhesion to the cord.

3. In the transitional type, the interface is located at the caudal extremity of the cord and extends farther to the dorsal aspect (**Fig. 11.5C**). The subarachnoid space extends around the filum that is the extension of the ventral half of the spinal cord.

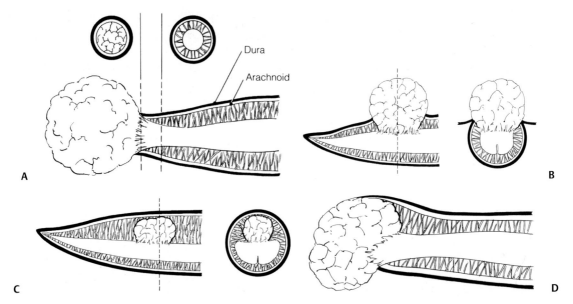

Fig. 11.4 Schematic drawings of the three types of lipomas. A lipoma is considered to result from the growth of fibroadipose tissue into the neural cleft before the closure of the neural crests.[18] **(A)** The caudal type. The interface of the cord and the lipoma is circumferentially united (fused) with the dura and pia arachnoid. The lipoma extends outside the subdural and subarachnoid space. **(B,C)** The dorsal type. The interface of the cord and the lipoma is located in the dorsal aspect of the cord, which corresponds to the neural placode of the myelomeningocele. The lipoma extends outside the dura in **(B)** and remains underneath the arachnoid in **(C)**. **(D)** The transitional type. The interface of the cord and the lipoma extends from the caudal extremity of cord to its dorsal aspect. (Modified from Chapman's model of leptomyelolipoma[21] with permission)

■ Clinical Presentation

Signs and symptoms of the tethered cord syndrome associated with LMMCs include motor and sensory dysfunction, incontinence, scoliosis, and various types of musculoskeletal deformities (including leg and foot deformities) and skin stigmata (Chapter 9, "Indication and Treatment of Tethered Spinal Cord"). The signs and symptoms are more severe in patients with multiple and very obvious congenital deformities. Tethering-induced symptomatology includes nonmyotomal and nondermatomal motor and sensory deficits in scattered or patchy patterns.[34] Associated with these signs are incontinence and hyporeflexia of a random fashion in any tendon. These signs are likely to occur in the caudal and transitional types of lumbosacral lipomas and LMMCs.

The compression of the spinal cord by a lipomatous mass may possibly result in neurological deficits manifested by motor and sensory dysfunction and hyporeflexia or hyperreflexia at and below the level of the lesion. In addition, manual pressure exerted on a large lipomatous mass can stretch the spinal cord and exacerbate stretch-induced neurological deficits. In contrast, total (congenital) paraplegia and incontinence may be the manifestations of neuronal agenesis of the entire lumbosacral cord.[23,35] The dense motor and sensory deficits in the distal lower limbs and incontinence are often related to lower lumbar and sacral agenesis. Involvement of all sensory modalities is likely to indicate neuronal agenesis, whereas the deficit only to pain and temperature sensation indicates the early TCS.

B   **Dorsal Type**

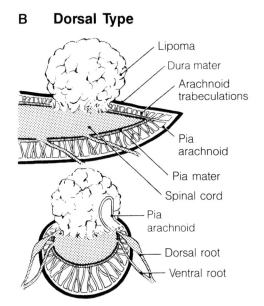

A   **Caudal Type**

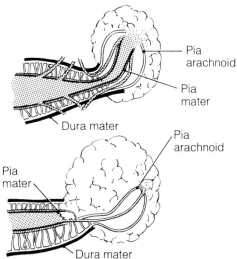

C   **Transitional**

Fig. 11.5 Schematic drawings of the three types of lipomyelomeningocele (LMMC). **(A)** The caudal (terminal) type. The interface of the spinal cord and the lipoma is located at the caudal extremity of the lower sacral or coccygeal cord. The fusion of the meninges (dura and arachnoid) with the spinal cord is located slightly caudal to the interface. **(B)** The dorsal type. The interface of the spinal cord with the lipoma is found at its dorsal aspect. A usually small subarachnoid space extends into or surrounds the fatty mass. **(C)** The transitional type. The interface of the cord and lipoma is located in the posterior part of the caudal extremity and extending to the dorsal aspect of the cord. The anterior part of the caudal extremity extends to the filum terminale that continues caudad and is surrounded by pia arachnoid and dura and ends at the fatty sac wall (see **Fig. 11.9C**).

Diagnosis

A swelling of the skin (elevated by the fat tissue), dimples, cutaneous hemangioma, tufts of hair, and sinus tracts are frequently associated with a lipoma or LMMC, but they are not necessarily pathognomonic for TCS. Soft fat tissue with fluctuation suggests the presence of CSF underneath the fat tissue. As the patient grows, progressive scoliosis and exaggerated lumbosacral lordosis are noticeable in the cases of TCS. Deep tendon reflexes of the lower extremities are usually hypoactive. Hyperactive reflexes associated with leg weakness with Babinski sign, which are found in ~10% of patients,[34] indicate higher lumbar or thoracic spinal cord lesions. In these cases, split spinal cord[29] or dermoid tumor in the thoracic cord concomitant with lumbosacral LMMC should be suspected.

Imaging

Plain films should be studied to find midline abnormalities such as spina bifida occulta, widely spread pedicles, and hemivertebrae with fused vertebral bodies, which suggest the presence of a lipomatous tumor or dermoid. Cystometrogram may reveal bladder distention for incontinent patients.

Magnetic resonance imaging (MRI) is a routine and valuable imaging tool for the diagnosis of LMMC or lipoma. The high signal in T1-weighted imaging and low density in T2-weighted imaging distinguish this disorder from fibromatous tumors (e.g., schwannomas and meningiomas), which show high signal in both imagings. A large mass with fat signal located posterior to the low lumbar and sacral cord suggests a transitional LMMC (see **Fig. 11.8**). Adjacent to the fat mass, a syrinx may be found in the lumbosacral canal.

One of the advantages of MRI studies is the demonstration of the posteriorly located conus or filum that touches the arachnoid membrane, that is, one of the signs of TCS.[35] Metrizamide-enhanced computed tomography is recommended for patients who have severe claustrophobia and therefore cannot undergo MRI.

Treatment

Surgical Indications

Opinions surrounding the prophylactic surgery in asymptomatic patients with a lipoma or LMMC vary depending on the experience of the neurosurgeon.

1. The first group[15,21–23] advocates that all children with a radiographically demonstrable lesion be operated on as soon as these lesions are discovered. McLone advocates surgical repair as early as 2 to 3 weeks of age, including repair of large lipomas or LMMCs, because lipomatous mass can be easily dissected from adjacent spinal cord and nerve roots (McLone DG, personal communication, 1995).
2. The second group emphasizes that the complex interrelationship between the lipomatous mass and neural and meningeal tissue does not warrant early surgery. This group advises to wait until a discrete separation of matured neural and meningeal structures can be executed at the later age.[32,34,36]
3. Hoffman et al[15] determined that 4 years of age was the maximum limit of the waiting period. Their opinion is based on their experience with LMMCs, which indicates that incontinence or motor deficit is usually discovered by this age in the patient with LMMC.

The authors believe that surgical risks must be weighted against the progressive symptomatology that may develop in association with these lesions. A small lesion in an asymptomatic patient may be removed completely or subtotally to untether the spinal cord as a prophylactic procedure earlier. Surgical procedures for large lesions in asymptomatic patients may be delayed until 3 to 4 years of age, when the patients are likely to become symptomatic. Patients who have developed any subtle or mild signs and symptoms must promptly undergo surgery. The following are criteria for surgical indications: an increase in (1) motor or sensory deficits; (2) signs of incontinence; (3) scoliosis and lumbosacral lordosis; (4) deformities in the lower extremities, particularly in distal muscles, causing a high arch, hammertoes, or pes equines; and (5) back and leg pain. Functional tests such as somatosensory evoked potentials, electromyography, and cystometrogram are also valuable (see Chapter 3, "Pathophysiology of Tethered Cord Syndrome").

Our concern is that the TCS associated with LMMC may be overlooked by physicians because the patient's family may be unaware of incontinence until the patient passes the age of toilet training, and similarly of stumbling in infancy or early childhood. A high incidence of psychological and infection-induced incontinence obscures incontinence due to TCS. Even though the progression of the neurological symptoms and musculocutaneous deformities may be continuous, recognition of the progression on a daily basis is extremely difficult. These diagnostic difficulties may favor prophylactic surgery. Subtle signs and symptoms that are difficult to perceive include occasional urinary dribbling, thinning (atrophy) of leg muscles, weakness limited to the extensor hallucis longus muscle, painless sores on the feet, difficulty in bending to touch toes, increasingly high arched feet, or a slight difference in the size of lower limbs and feet. Careful observation of children by the family members with instructions from physicians is crucial to the detection of this syndrome.

Hoffman et al[28] determined three significant facts: (1) the asymptomatic patients with LMMC fare the best after surgical removal for cord untethering; (2) the less symptomatic the patient, the better the outcome of surgery; and (3) inappropriate surgical procedures aimed only at cosmetic improvement were followed by progression of TCS. Although no postoperative worsening occurred, the second surgical procedure to correct the tethering mechanism did not alleviate the signs and symptoms, except in patients with only mild signs. Their observations support the authors' results, including severe urinary dysfunction that is not alleviated after untethering.

Prolonged and repeated tractions can cause irreversible damage to the conus more easily than to the lumbar or S1 cord, as proven by metabolic and electrophysiological studies (see Chapter 3, "Pathophysiology of Tethered Cord Syndrome"). The balance between enthusiasm and skepticism toward an early surgical removal of LMMCs has been swaying from one to the other. It is quite clear that the risks involved in the repair of large LMMCs are much greater than those in the repair of small lesions. As long as the patient remains asymptomatic, the surgical procedure may be postponed until later (within 3 to 4 years of age). Overall, our awareness of TCS in these conditions and the potential reversibility of some symptoms and signs before metabolic stresses result in cord damage and in fixed deficits lends optimism to the surgical indications. In addition, early development of subtle neurological signs and symptoms and musculoskeletal abnormalities serve to alert physicians that patients with evidence of a lipoma or LMMC should be referred to a neurosurgeon.

From the authors' experience, a great majority of adults with an LMMC had undergone repair and closure of the lesion early in childhood. They have already experienced persistent but stable neurological deficits. It is imperative that patients undergo untethering procedures as soon as neurological signs or symptoms are manifested or preexisting deficits show progression.[29,37,38] The filar type of lipoma (tethered spinal cord[9]) may be handled similarly to TCS in a patient with a tight filum.[28,29,39]

Surgical Technique

Lipoma Resection and Untethering of the Spinal Cord

The surgical principles for TCS associated with lipoma or LMMC are to remove the mass to negate the tethering effect on the spinal cord,[15,22,40] to preserve neural tissue, and to prevent recurrence of TCS.[23,41] The surgical procedure for each type of LMMC is described in the following text. It must be remembered that even a mild retraction on the fat tissue can result in caudal traction of the spinal cord and accentuate the tethering effects.

Caudal Type

The fibroadipose tissue is transected through or immediately caudal to the lipoma–cord interface. The transection through the dura is, however, performed cephalad to the fusion of the dura and arachnoid to the fibroadipose tissue. This technique allows tight closure of the arachnoid dura.

Dorsal Type

The lipoma is removed away from the spinal cord tissue. The line of the lipoma dissection should be flush to the pial surface surrounding cord tissue.

Transitional Type

Transection through the lipoma–cord interface, or slightly caudal to it, is performed first. The lipoma extending to the dorsal surface of the spinal cord is then dissected away from the line of the lipoma–cord interface. The surgical technique for cord untethering from the lipomatous tissue is similar to that for cord untethering from the LMMC, and, therefore, its details are included in the description of the surgery for the latter.

Lipomyelomeningocele Repair and Untethering of the Spinal Cord

Caudal Type

The caudal type of LMMC (**Fig. 11.5A**) is different from the lipoma in the strict sense because the fibroadipose (lipomatous) tissue surrounds the meningeal lining that contains the CSF and the elongated spinal cord.[31] In other words, the myelomeningocele is attached and surrounded by the fibroadipose tissue that is connected to the cord only at its caudal extremity.

An elliptical incision in the bulging area allows removal of the redundant subcutaneous fat tissue continuous to the lipomatous tissue in the muscular layer and extradural space. The lipomatous tissue in the muscular layer is easily isolated from the surrounding fascia and paravertebral muscles. The midline incision is extended over one or two spinous processes and to one lamina above the spina bifida. After laminectomy at this level, the dura is cut in the midline to the cephalic end of the LMMC, where the dura and the arachnoid join the LMMC sac. The arachnoid membrane is separated away from the spinal cord, then the spinal cord may be followed caudad into the lipomatous meningeal sac. Upon opening the meningeal lining in the LMMC, the spinal cord and a short filum terminale are clearly identified in the CSF space (**Fig. 11.6E**). Usually, the nerve roots exiting this portion of the spinal cord travel cephalad through the neck of the meningeal sac into the sacral subarachnoid space. After entering the spinal canal they exit the dura at the corresponding intervertebral foramina. The meningeal sac and fibroadipose tissue are totally resected except for a narrow strip of meninges that can be closed completely around the spinal cord. The aforementioned nerve roots can be kept untouched during the removal of the lipomatous mass. This mass may be reduced in size by electrocautery (Corrdies, CO)[23] or CO_2 laser aspirator (Cooper Medical, Stamford, Connecticut).[15,42,43] Functional neural elements may be identified by rectal sphincter contraction, elicited by electrical stimulation of nerve fibers in the operative site.[2,44]

Illustrative Case

A 4-year-old girl presented with a 6-month history of dribbling of urine after successful toilet training. At birth, a fluctuant mass was noted in her left gluteal area (**Fig. 11.6A**). A lumbosacral spine film demonstrated a spina bifida (**Fig. 11.6B**). A cystic extension of the lumbosacral subarachnoid space into the left gluteal region was seen on myelography (**Fig. 11.6C**). The LMMC was repaired as described earlier (**Fig. 11.6D,E**). Within 2 weeks of the untethering procedure, she regained bladder control.

Dorsal Type

This type of LMMC (**Fig. 11.5B**) requires laminectomy at one or two levels above and below the lipomatous protrusion from the spinal cord. The dura is incised in the midline, cephalad and caudad to the LMMC. The dura is separated from the arachnoid membrane to ensure that the spinal cord is not looped into the meningocele sac (**Fig. 11.7**). The fibroadipose mass is separated from the dura and arachnoid to its junction with the pia mater and resected flush to the pial surface. Both pial edges may be closed with 8–0 nylon sutures, if possible, to prevent postoperative adhesion.[34] The adipose tissue must be removed flush with the posterior surface of the spinal cord, not necessarily into the lipoma–cord interface. Untethering of the spinal cord is accomplished in the patients who show signs and symptoms for the lesion above the level. The dura is closed, then the dural defect formed after removal of the lipomatous mass is covered by a dural substitute: lyophilized dura,[15] Gore-Tex (W. L. Gore and Associates, Inc., Flagstaff, AZ),[45] Silastic (Dow Corning, Midland, MI),[3,46] or fascial graft. A Gel-Film (Gel-Pak, Hayward, CA) piece placed on the spinal cord and nerve roots prevents their adhesion to the dura. The Gel-Film edges are approximated to the surrounding arachnoid with a few 8–0 nylon sutures to be kept in place without slipping. The dural substitute is sutured circumferentially to the remaining dura with 6–0 nylon sutures.

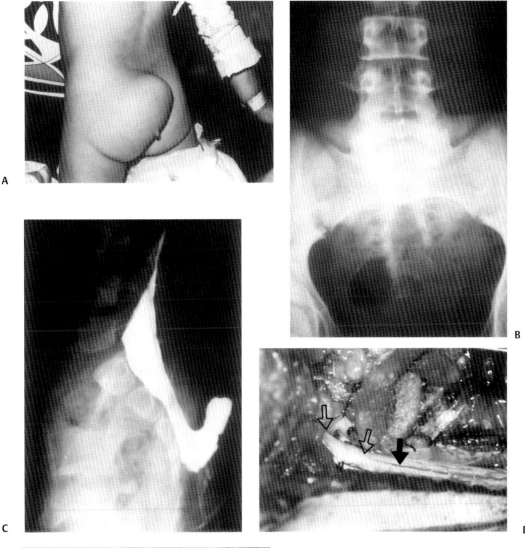

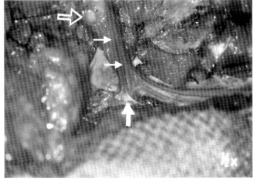

Fig. 11.6 (A) Photograph of a caudal-type lipomye-lomeningocele (LMMC). The left gluteal swelling is fluctu-ant. **(B)** A plain film shows spina bifida of the sacral spine. **(C)** The extension of the lumbosacral subarachnoid space into the LMMC sac is shown by myelogram (also demon-strated by T2-weighted magnetic resonance imaging (MRI). **(D)** Inraoperative photograhps of a cauldal-type LMMC show the spherical lipomatous mass being isolated from the surrounding fascia and muscles to the neck of the meningeal sac (an empty arrow on the left), and opening of the dura reveals thick arachnoid covering the spinal cord (two empty arrows). **(E)** An incision through the dorsal side of the fatty mass and an arachnoid-dural extension that contained cerebrospinal fluid exposed an elongated conus medullaris. The conus terminates at its interface with the lipoma.

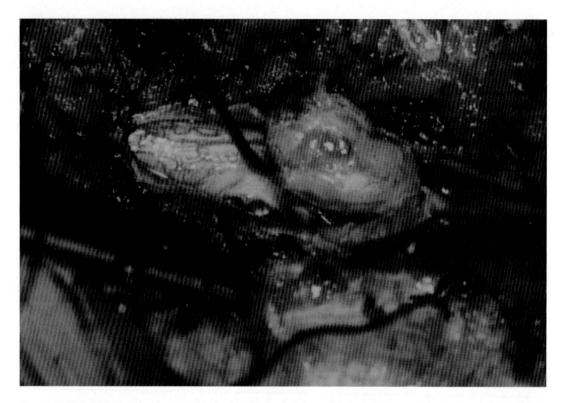

Fig. 11.7 Intraoperative photograph of a dorsal-type lipomyelomeningocele with an extension through the arachnoid and dura.

Transitional Type

The removal of the tumor needs special attention to prevent damage to the conus medullaris and sacral nerve roots because these nerve elements often pass through the fat tissue. The only ventral aspect of the conus tip extends into the meningeal sac covered by a lipomatous mass (**Figs. 11.5C, 11.8A**). This portion of the filum is transected with similar techniques as for caudal LMMCs. The dorsal portion of the transitional LMMC is dissected around the cord tissue as in the dorsal LMMC (**Fig. 11.7**). It is important to avoid even slight retraction on the lipomatous mass in any direction, which easily causes spinal cord stretching. The dural closure after removal of transitional LMMC is also the difficult part of the surgery requiring tight closure, particularly for the anterior-lateral dural defect (**Fig. 11.8B**).[47,48] The dural substitute must be conformed as sutures are placed to the edge of the defect. Watertight closure using 1.5 mm 6–0 nylon sutures with swathed round needles prevents CSF leakage that could easily occur through stitch holes created with larger needles.

Illustrative Case

In 1975, a 14-year-old girl noticed urinary incontinence while laughing, following a 7-year history of intermittent urinary tract infections. Marked pes equinus deformity necessitated the use of high-heeled shoes (**Fig. 11.9A**; compare with the postoperative dorsiflexion of the ankle joint to 90 degrees. **Fig. 11.9D**). Two dimples were noted in the sacrococcygeal region (**Fig. 11.9B**). Myelography showed a mass lesion in the caudal end of the spinal cord in the bifid lumbosacral canal. After S1–3 laminectomy, the fibroadipose mass was totally removed, including extradural and intradural portions, except for the intramedullary extension to the S2 and S3 cord segments (S2 vertebral body level).

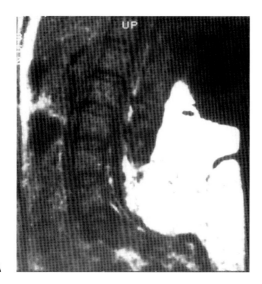
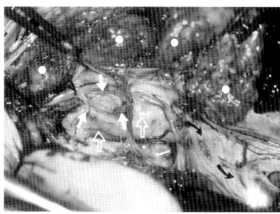

Fig. 11.8 (A) Magnetic resonance imaging shows a large transitional-type lipomyelomeningocele (LMMC) with adipose tissue extending to the extraspinal space and blending into subcutaneous fat. **(B)** Intraoperative photograph of a transitional-type LMMC extending from the caudal extremity to the anterolateral aspect of the cord. The flattened, wide lower conus (two empty arrow) is roated clockwise (to the left) in the middle is rotated clockwise (viewed from cephalad (i.e., from the right in the photograph), and the right posterior nerve roots (*curved arrows*) pass behind the conus, exiting the dura on the right. The intradural adipose tissue (*surrounded by three small arrows*) is continuous to the extradural lipomatous mass underneath the everted dural edge on the left.

Subpial resection reached the glial tissue of the lipoma–cord interface (**Fig. 11.9C**). Bladder control returned, and the pes equinus deformity lessened. She became able to walk in flat shoes within 3 years (**Fig. 11.9D**).

The filar type or fibroadipose filum. In this anomaly fibroadipose tissue is confined interior to Pia meter of filum, different from the lipoma, which extends outside the pia. A group of patients older than 16 years of age in this category is discussed in the chapter "Tethered Cord Syndrome in Adults and late teenage patients without dysraphism."

Outcomes

This series included 28 patients, 13 male and 15 female, with ages ranging from infancy to 72 years (average 9.5 years), who had a lumbosacral lipoma or LMMC during the period of 17 years from 1977. The caudal type of LMMC was found in nine patients, the dorsal type in seven, and the transitional type in 12. Patients were evaluated neurologically before and after surgery and were subjected to redox studies of cytochrome a,a_3. All patients showed oxidative shifts of cytochrome a,a_3 after untethering, as compared with the reduced state while the cord was tethered. These oxidative changes were correlated with neurological findings. The patients with a lumbosacral lipoma or LMMC who presented with neurological and musculoskeletal abnormalities were classified into three Categories, as described in Chapter 3, "Pathophysiology of Tethered Cord Syndrome).

Type 1

The chief complaint of the three patients in this group was intermittent urinary dribbling while bending over. All three regained bladder control within 2 weeks of untethering. Weakness in both legs found in one patient subsided within 1 month. One patient (a 21-year-old) with moderately high-arched feet also complained of low back and leg pain preoperatively

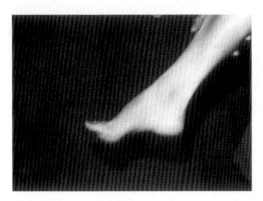

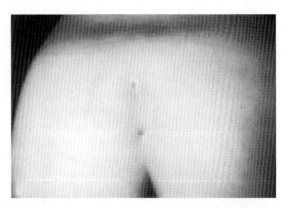

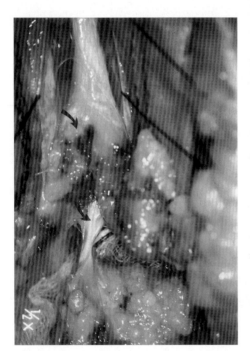

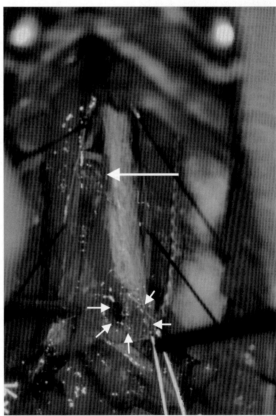

Fig. 11.9 Photographs for the patients with transitional lipomyelomeningocele (LMMC) are shown: **(A)** Presenting with prominent pes equines deformity, which necessitated the use of high-heeled shoes for walking, **(B)** two dimples in sacrococcygeal region, with no contour of subcutaneous LLMC faat noted from the outside. **Figs. 11.9C,D,E** show the sequence of surgical stages for the repair of a typical transitional LMMC (see Fig. 11.5). **(C)** Subcutaneous fibroadipose tissue was already removed to the dorsal attachment LMMC located in the spinal canal, and the posterior surface of the conus tip (*arrow at the top*) is ready to be dissected. The caudal part of LMMC formed a meningeal sac, which was anteriorly located and opened to show the conus-filum junction placed immediately above the neck of the meningocele sac. **(D)** Subpial resection of the lipomatous tissue was carried outil it blended to the glial tissue (five small arrows surrounding the transected conus end). The horizontal arrow points to the conus medullaris.

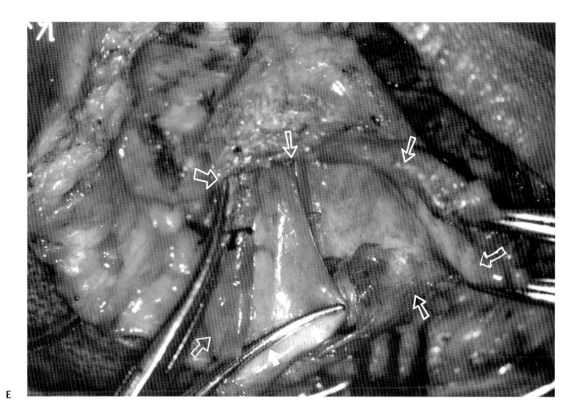

E

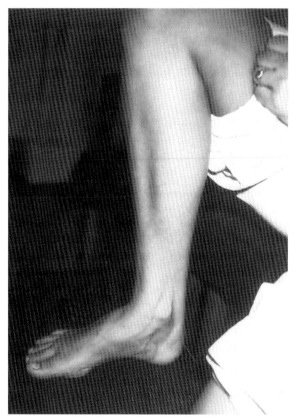

F

Fig. 11.9 *(Continued)* **(E)** The dura and arachnoid were sutured together around the conus medullaris while a clamp was placed on the caudal end of the dura *(two arrows)*, before its closure with dural sutures. The edge of the opened meningocele *(six empty arrows)* was closed later with sutures.

but was relieved of leg pain immediately after surgery and began to note lessening of the high arch of the feet within 6 weeks. The reductive shifts of cytochrome a,a_3 were only mild before untethering, and oxidative shifts after untethering indicated a normal redox state.

Type 2

Signs and symptoms in this group of 19 patients included 12 patients with incontinence (five subtle) and 17 patients with weakness, atrophy, or gait disturbance (weakness was mild in 14 patients and moderate in three), with 10 of these 17 having concomitant incontinence. Postoperative improvement in bladder or rectal function was striking: all the function returned to normal in the patients with subtle symptoms within 2 weeks and in the others within 2 to 3 months. Motor function returned to normal in the patients with mild preoperative weakness in 2 to 3 months and to normal or nearly normal within 3 to 24 months in patients with moderate weakness. Foot deformity in 14 patients lessened within 1 to 6 months. Redox studies showed a markedly reduced state before untethering, whereas the redox returned to the normal state after untethering.

Type 3

Moderate to severe weakness was noted in all six patients in this group, all of whom were ambulatory. Three were using crutches preoperatively but walked with only braces after the untethering procedure. Bladder control improved; one patient became continent and the others gained the ability to self-catheterize. Reductive shifts of cytochrome a,a_3 were pronounced before untethering, and the redox shifts after untethering were limited to subnormal levels.

In conclusion, the patients with type 1 LMMC made the fastest recovery from neurological dysfunction and musculoskeletal deformities, which were apparently caused by true TCS. The patients with type 2 LMMC also had good to excellent recovery but with varying recovery patterns among them. The patients with type 3 LMMC tend to have more serious neurological disabilities and made less recovery. We postulate that preoperative signs and symptoms in some of those patients may have been related to TCS and cord compression and other factors previously mentioned. Several authors reported surgical results on the patients with the mixture of occult spinal dysraphism, which included LMMCs and a combination of an elongated cord and a thick filum.[29,38,49–51] Although the number of our patients presented here is small, the prognosis of each patient was clearly predicted preoperatively and intraoperatively when the differences in neurological presentation and oxidative metabolic changes were correlated.

Complications

Three patients with transitional-type LMMC developed a CSF leak postoperatively. All three had developed a meningeal defect extending posteriorly or anterolaterally after LMMC repair. Two patients required resuturing of the dura, with an additional patch of the dural substitute to cover the stitch holes. The third infant patient, who had an original repair with a Silastic sheet, developed a CSF leak. The wound was infected, and meningitis ensued. Debridement of the wound and additional sutures placed between the Silastic sheet and the surrounding dura were combined with systemic antibiotic treatment. The meningitis and local wound infection were both controlled within 2 weeks. Two patients with the transitional type of LMMC who had incontinence (dribbling) developed temporary urinary retention, presumably due to detrusor-sphincter dyssynergy. After several months of intermittent catheterization, they began having better control.

Late complications included the following: (1) one patient developed TCS due to new fibrous formation of the filum, which had been viscoelastic at the first LMMC repair 10 years earlier; the filum resection resulted in neurological improvement; and (2) another patient developed a lumbosacral syrinx 6 years after dorsal lipoma removal, which was treated with a syringosubarachnoid shunt. Various authors discussed complications and related prevention and treatment[23,34,39] (see Chapter 7, "Lower Urinary Tract Dysfunction in Tethered Cord Syndrome"),[23]

■ Conclusion

Guidelines for treating MMCs, lipomas, and LMMCs associated with TCS are summarized as follows:

1. MMCs must be treated surgically as early as possible after birth to prevent or correct cord tethering. Other aspects of early surgery pertain as discussed.
2. TCS with an inelastic fibroadipose filum (tethered spinal cord) requires careful neurological follow-up. Any subtle signs and symptoms that indicate TCS should lead to early surgical untethering.

3. Lipomas of the spinal cord and LMMCs should be removed or repaired early in life (before 4 years of age). Various factors influence the timing of surgery. The caudal and small transitional types of lipomas and LMMCs are likely to cause stretch-induced symptomatology. The dorsal type can also be the cause of TCS above the lesion. Other factors must be considered before the decision making for surgical repair and untethering.
4. Neuronal agenesis is often difficult to distinguish from the far-advanced stage of cord tethering. Repair of an LMMC in patients with total paraplegia and flaccid bladder will not benefit the patients neurologically. Reflectance spectrophotometry of the lumbosacral cord has shown no signal from cord mitochondria and no improvement after cord untethering during the repair procedure.[52]

References

1. Begeer JH, Meihuizen de Regt MJ, HogenEsch I, Ter Weeme CA, Mooij JJ, Vencken LM. Progressive neurological deficit in children with spina bifida aperta. Z Kinderchir 1986;41(Suppl 1):13–15
2. James HE, Mulcahy JJ, Walsh JW, Kaplan GW. Use of anal sphincter electromyography during operations on the conus medullaris and sacral nerve roots. Neurosurgery 1979;4:521–523
3. Yamada S, Zinke DE, Sanders D. Pathophysiology of "tethered cord syndrome." J Neurosurg 1981;54:494–503
4. Heimburger RF. Early repair of myelomeningocele (spina bifida cystica). J Neurosurg 1972;37:594–600
5. Matson DD. Neurosurgery of Infancy and Childhood. 2nd ed. Springfield, IL: Charles C Thomas; 1969
6. McLone DG, Naidich TP. Myelomeningocele: outcome and late complications. In: McLaurin RL, Schut L, Venes JL, et al, eds. Pediatric Neurosurgery. 2nd ed. Philadelphia: WB Saunders; 1989:53–70
7. Reigel DH. Spinal bifida. In: McLaurin RL, Schut L, Venes JL, et al, eds. Pediatric Neurosurgery. 2nd ed. Philadelphia: WB Saunders; 1989:35
8. Nicholas DS, Weller RO. The fine anatomy of the human spinal meninges: a light and scanning electron microscopy study. J Neurosurg 1988;69:276–282
9. Linder M, Rosenstein J, Sklar FH. Functional improvement after spinal surgery for the dysraphic malformations. Neurosurgery 1982;11:622–624
10. Scott RM. Delayed deterioration in patients with spinal tethering syndromes. In: Holtzman RNN, Stein BM, eds. The Tethered Spinal Cord. New York: Thieme-Stratton; 1985:116–120
11. Pang D. Surgical complications of open spinal dysraphism. Neurosurg Clin N Am 1995;6:243–257
12. Oi S, Yamada H, Matsumoto S. Tethered cord syndrome versus low-placed conus medullaris in an over-distended spinal cord following initial repair for myelodysplasia. Childs Nerv Syst 1990;6:264–269
13. Tamaki N, Shirataki K, Kojima N, Shouse Y, Matsumoto S. Tethered cord syndrome of delayed onset following repair of myelomeningocele. J Neurosurg 1988;69:393–398
14. Venes JL, Stevens EA. Surgical pathology in tethered cord secondary to myelomeningocele repair. Concepts Pediatr Neurosurg 1983;4:165–185
15. Hoffman HJ, Taecholarn C, Hendrick EB, Humphreys RP. Management of lipomyelomeningoceles: experience at the Hospital for Sick Children, Toronto. J Neurosurg 1985;62:1–8

16. McCullough DC, Kane JG, Presper JH, Wells M. Antibiotic prophylaxis in ventricular shunt surgery, I: Reduction of operative infection rates with methicillin. Childs Brain 1980;7:182–189

17. Choux M, Lena G, Genitori L, et al. Shunt implantation: toward zero infection [abstract]. Childs Nerv Syst 1988;4:181

18. Scott RM. Preventing and treating shunt complications. In: Scott RM, ed. Hydrocephalus: Concepts in Neurosurgery. Vol 3. Baltimore: Williams & Wilkins; 1990:115–121

19. Reigel DH, McLone DG. Myelomeningocele: operative treatment and results. In: Marlin AE, ed. Concepts in Pediatric Neurosurgery. Vol 8. Basel: S Karger; 1987:41–50

20. Scott RM, Wolpert SM, Bartoshesky LE, Zimbler S, Klauber GT. Dermoid tumors occurring at the site of previous myelomeningocele repair. J Neurosurg 1986;65:779–783

21. Chapman PH. Congenital intraspinal lipomas: anatomic considerations and surgical treatment. Childs Brain 1982;9:37–47

22. Schut L, Bruce DA, Sutton LN. The management of the child with a lipomyelomeningocele. Clin Neurosurg 1983;30:464–476

23. Sutton LN. Lipomyelomeningocele. Neurosurg Clin N Am 1995;6:325–338

24. Johnson A. Fatty tumor from the sacrum of a child, connected with the spinal membranes. Trans Pathol Soc London 1857;8:16–18

25. Marin-Padilla M. The tethered cord syndrome: developmental considerations. In: Holtzman RNN, Stein BM, eds. The Tethered Spinal Cord. New York: Thieme-Stratton; 1985:3–13

26. McLone DC, Naidich TP. The tethered spinal cord. In: McLaurin RL, Schut L, Venes JL, et al, eds. Pediatric Neurosurgery. 2nd ed. Philadelphia: WB Saunders; 1989:76–96

27. Kunitomo K. The development and reduction of the tail and of the caudal end of the spinal cord. Comp Embryol Carnegie Inst 1918;8:163–198

28. Hoffman HJ, Hendrick EB, Humphreys RP. The tethered spinal cord: its protean manifestations, diagnosis and surgical correction. Childs Brain 1976;2:145–155

29. Pang D. Spinal cord lipomas. In: Pang D, ed. Disorders of the Pediatric Spine. New York: Raven Press; 1995:175–201

30. French BN. Midline fusion defects and defects of formation. In: Youmans JR, ed. Neurological Surgery. Vol 3. 2nd ed. Philadelphia: WB Saunders; 1989:1236–1380

31. Naidich TP, McLone DC. Congenital pathology of the spine and spinal cord. In: Taveras JM, Ferrucci JT, eds. Radiology. Philadelphia: JB Lippincott; 1986:1–23

32. Naidich TP, McLone DG, Mutluer S. A new understanding of dorsal dysraphism with lipoma (lipomyeloschisis): radiologic evaluation and surgical correction. AJR Am J Roentgenol 1983;140:1065–1078

33. Sakamoto H, Hakuba A, Fujitani K, Nishimura S. Surgical treatment of the retethered spinal cord after repair of lipomyelomeningocele. J Neurosurg 1991;74:709–714

34. Yamada S, Iacono RP. Tethered cord syndrome. In: Pang D, ed. Disorders of the Pediatric Spine. New York: Raven Press; 1995:159–173

35. Yamada S, Lonser RR. Adult tethered cord syndrome. J Spinal Disord 2000;13:319–323

36. Till K. Occult spinal dysraphism: the value of prophylactic surgical treatment. In: Sano K, Ishii S, Levay D, eds. Recent Progress in Neurological Surgery. New York: Elsevier; 1973:61–66

37. Iskandar BJ, Fulmer BB, Hadley MN, Oakes WJ. Congenital tethered spinal cord syndrome in adults. J Neurosurg 1998;88:958–961

38. Zide BM, Epstein FJ, Wisoff J. Optimal wound closure after tethered cord correction: technical note. J Neurosurg 1991;74:673–676

39. Garceau GJ. The filum terminale syndrome (the cord-traction syndrome). J Bone Joint Surg Am 1953;35-A:711–716

40. Sutton LN, Duhaime AC, Schut L. Lipomyelomeningocele. In: Park TS, ed. Spinal Dysraphism. Boston: Blackwell; 1992:59–73

41. Barolat G, Schaefer D, Zeme S. Recurrent spinal cord tethering by sacral nerve root following lipomyelomeningocele surgery: case report. J Neurosurg 1991;75:143–145

42. James HE, Williams J, Brock W, Kaplan GW, U HS. Radical removal of lipomas of the conus and cauda equina with laser microneurosurgery. Neurosurgery 1984;15:340–343

43. McLone DG, Naidich TP. Laser resection of fifty spinal lipomas. Neurosurgery 1986;18:611–615

44. Pang D, Casey K. Use of an anal sphincter pressure monitor during operations on the sacral spinal cord and nerve roots. Neurosurgery 1983;13:562–568

45. Inoue HK, Kobayashi S, Ohbayashi K, Kohga H, Nakamura M. Treatment and prevention of tethered and retethered spinal cord using a Gore-Tex surgical membrane. J Neurosurg 1994;80:689–693

46. Epstein FJ. Tethered spinal cord: summary discussion. In: Holtzman RNN, Stein BM, eds. The Tethered Spinal Cord. New York: Thieme-Stratton; 1985:142–147

47. Pang D. Tethered cord syndrome. Adv Pediatr Neurosurg 1986;1:45–79
48. Wilkins RH, Rossitch E Jr. Anterior and lateral spinal meningoceles. In: Pang D, ed. Disorders of the Pediatric Spine. New York: Raven Press; 1995: 265–276
49. Hüttmann S, Krauss J, Collmann H, Sörensen N, Roosen K. Surgical management of tethered spinal cord in adults: report of 54 cases. J Neurosurg 2001;95 (2, Suppl):173–178
50. Lee GYF, Gong GWK, Paradiso G, Fehlings MG. Adult tethered cord syndrome: clinical considerations and surgical management. Neurosurg Q 2006;16:55–66
51. van Leeuwen R, Notermans NC, Vandertop WP. Surgery in adults with tethered cord syndrome: outcome study with independent clinical review. J Neurosurg 2001;94(2, Suppl):205–209
52. Yamada S, Won DJ, Yamada SM. Pathophysiology of tethered cord syndrome: correlation with symptomatology. Neurosurg Focus 2004;16:E6

12 The Role of Folate Supplementation in Spina Bifida Occulta

Elias Rizk and Bermans J. Iskandar

■ Epidemiology of Spina Bifida Occulta

The incidence of spina bifida occulta (SBO) in the general population is unknown. Unlike the open neural tube defects (NTDs), namely anencephaly and myelomeningocele (spina bifida aperta or SBA), which are clinically obvious, detecting the closed defects requires imaging studies, and only recently have we truly appreciated that the finding of a subtle cutaneous anomaly in the newborn may be crucial to its future neurological, urological, as well as musculoskeletal development.[1] The incidence of bony anomalies that can be seen on radiographs, such as nonfusion of the laminae, is well known, but it is clear that the majority of patients with such lesions do not have spinal involvement.[2–4] Although the incidence of open NTDs is declining, such conclusions cannot be made with regard to the closed spinal defects because of the higher detection rate seen in recent years as a result of improved imaging.[5]

■ Familial Relationship between Open and Closed Neural Tube Defects

Open spinal defects (OSDs) have been associated with multiple maternal risk factors, such as diabetes, anticonvulsant use, and family history.[6] However, there is only limited information available on risk factors associated with the closed dysraphic states. There is, however, some evidence that open and closed NTDs may be genetically related.[5] This suggests that these different abnormalities may share some of the same risk factors. And until studies of risk factors in spina bifida occulta are conducted, this presumption may help guide health care providers with regard to prenatal screening, genetic counseling, and the use of periconceptional medications. In a region of Britain endemic for NTDs (prevalence of 0.8% or 10-fold higher than the current prevalence in the United States), Carter et al studied 364 siblings of 207 patients with all forms of OSD and found that there was a 4.12% prevalence of myelomeningocele or anencephaly in the series. This ratio was found to be similar to that of siblings of patients with open tube defects (4.45% and 5.18% in two major studies), and is approximately fivefold higher than the general prevalence in that region.[5] Recently, in a study of 52 families with a lipomyelomeningocele proband, the NTD Collaborative Group showed that the estimated sibling recurrence risk for *open* NTDs is 4%, which is not inconsistent with the generally recognized open NTD recurrence risk of 2 to 5% in families with an open NTD proband.[7] Further, Myers et al showed that periconceptional folate supplementation does decrease the risk of imperforate anus in the offspring,[8] and it is well recognized that there is a strong association between imperforate anus (and other manifestations of caudal agenesis) and spina bifida occulta.[9]

■ Periconceptional Folic Acid Supplementation in Open Neural Tube Defects

Although Smithells et al[10] in the 1980s made the first observation that periconceptional folate supplementation may reduce the risk of NTD recurrence, the correlation between NTD and folate was first suspected by Hibbard in 1964; in the past 2 decades, a series of well-designed studies in multiple countries confirmed that periconceptional folic acid supplementation in women with 0.4 to 0.8 mg/day results in a reduction in the prevalence of open NTD by at least 70%[11–14]; furthermore, supplementing women with a previous NTD-affected pregnancy with 4 mg of folic acid per day causes a 72% reduction in the NTD recurrence rate.[12,15–17] This persuaded the Public Health Service to recommend that any woman of child-bearing age who is sexually active should take a daily dose of 0.4 mg folic acid per day; similarly, women in the high-risk group (i.e., those who fit the latter criteria but who have also had a previous NTD-affected pregnancy) should take 4 mg of folic acid per day.[18] Since then, many countries have instituted similar policies[19] while initiating a flour fortification system, the results of which remain controversial.[20]

■ Periconceptional Folic Acid Supplementation in Spina Bifida Occulta

Currently, there are no data to support or dispute the use of high-dose (4 mg) periconceptional folate in families that have a child with SBO. However, because of the observation already discussed that a genetic relationship may well exist between the open and closed spinal defects, it has been the practice of some centers to recommend the 4 mg dose in mothers of SBO-affected children. That said, three points of contention arise: First, it is equally well established that folate supplementation decreases the risk of other malformations, namely craniofacial, urological, and cardiac.[21] Does this mean that women with a prior pregnancy affected by a craniofacial disorder should also be on the high folate dose? Second, although the 4 mg dose has had a positive effect on NTD prevalence, there are no data to suggest that this is the optimal dose, and that 0.4 mg is insufficient. The problem is that running an NTD folate dose–response study at this time would require the inclusion of thousands of subjects, and the cost of such a trial would be prohibitive (Berry RJ, CDC, personal communication). Third, although no folate toxicity has ever been reported, it is well established that folate supplementation, when not accompanied by B12, may mask pernicious anemia,[22] and there have been discussions in the recent literature about the possibility that overmethylation caused by high doses of folate may shut down the activity of certain genes[23]; however, this epigenetic phenomenon is still not well understood, and to this day, no negative consequences have been demonstrated in the dose ranges currently used in NTD prevention. *Thus the folic acid dose (0.4 mg vs 4 mg) to be recommended in women with a previous SBO-affected pregnancy remains controversial and hinges on individual preferences.*

References

1. Iskandar BJ, Oakes WJ. Occult spinal dysraphism. In: Albright AL, Pollack IF, Adelson PD, eds. Principles and Practice of Pediatric Neurosurgery. New York: Thieme; 1999
2. Boone D, Parsons D, Lachmann SM, Sherwood T. Spina bifida occulta: lesion or anomaly? Clin Radiol 1985;36:159–161
3. Fidas A, MacDonald HL, Elton RA, McInnes A, Wild SR, Chisholm GD. Prevalence of spina bifida occulta in patients with functional disorders of the lower urinary tract and its relation to urodynamic and neurophysiological measurements. BMJ 1989;298:357–359
4. Sutow WW, Pryde AW. Incidence of spina bifida occulta in relation to age. AMA J Dis Child 1956;91:211–217

5. Carter CO, Evans KA, Till K. Spinal dysraphism: genetic relation to neural tube malformations. J Med Genet 1976;13:343–350

6. Mitchell LE, Adzick NS, Melchionne J, Pasquariello PS, Sutton LN, Whitehead AS. Spina bifida. Lancet 2004; 364:1885–1895

7. Sebold CD, Melvin EC, Siegel D, et al; NTD Collaborative Group. Recurrence risks for neural tube defects in siblings of patients with lipomyelomeningocele. Genet Med 2005;7:64–67

8. Myers MF, Li S, Correa-Villaseñor A, et al; China-US Collaborative Project for Neural Tube Defect Prevention. Folic acid supplementation and risk for imperforate anus in China. Am J Epidemiol 2001;154:1051–1056

9. Davidoff AM, Thompson CV, Grimm JM, Shorter NA, Filston HC, Oakes WJ. Occult spinal dysraphism in patients with anal agenesis. J Pediatr Surg 1991;26: 1001–1005

10. Smithells RW, Sheppard S, Schorah CJ, et al. Possible prevention of neural-tube defects by periconceptional vitamin supplementation. Lancet 1980;1:339–340

11. Berry RJ, Li Z, Erickson JD, et al; Collaborative Project for Neural Tube Defect Prevention. Prevention of neural-tube defects with folic acid in China. China–U.S. N Engl J Med 1999;341:1485–1490

12. Czeizel AE, Dudás I. Prevention of the first occurrence of neural-tube defects by periconceptional vitamin supplementation. N Engl J Med 1992; 327: 1832–1835

13. Milunsky A, Jick H, Jick SS, et al. Multivitamin/folic acid supplementation in early pregnancy reduces the prevalence of neural tube defects. JAMA 1989;262: 2847–2852

14. Mulinare J, Cordero JF, Erickson JD, Berry RJ. Periconceptional use of multivitamins and the occurrence of neural tube defects. JAMA 1988;260: 3141–3145

15. Group MVSR; MRC Vitamin Study Research Group. Prevention of neural tube defects: results of the Medical Research Council Vitamin Study. Lancet 1991;338:131–137

16. Rosenberg IH. Folic acid and neural-tube defects: time for action? N Engl J Med 1992;327:1875–1877

17. Werler MM, Shapiro S, Mitchell AA. Periconceptional folic acid exposure and risk of occurrent neural tube defects. JAMA 1993;269:1257–1261

18. Recommendations for the use of folic acid to reduce the number of cases of spina bifida and other neural tube defects. MMWR Morb Mortal Wkly Rep 1992; 41(RR-14):1–7

19. Cornel MC, Erickson JD. Comparison of national policies on periconceptional use of folic acid to prevent spina bifida and anencephaly (SBA). Teratology 1997;55:134–137

20. Berry RJ, Carter HK, Yang Q. Cognitive impairment in older Americans in the age of folic acid fortification. Am J Clin Nutr 2007;86:265–267, author reply 267–269

21. Bailey LB, Berry RJ. Folic acid supplementation and the occurrence of congenital heart defects, orofacial clefts, multiple births, and miscarriage. Am J Clin Nutr 2005;81:1213S–1217S

22. Ellison AB. Pernicious anemia masked by multivitamins containing folic acid. JAMA 1960;173:240–243

23. Siegfried Z, Eden S, Mendelsohn M, Feng X, Tsuberi BZ, Cedar H. DNA methylation represses transcription in vivo. Nat Genet 1999;22:203–206

13 In Utero Repair of Myelomeningoceles

Nalin Gupta

Several diseases can be treated by surgical procedures performed directly on the fetus prior to the anticipated delivery date.[1] Most of these diseases, such as congenital diaphragmatic hernia and sacrococcygeal teratoma, are usually fatal if untreated. An open neural tube defect, or myelomeningocele, is different in that fetuses with this condition will usually complete a normal gestation and, if treated after birth, can live for many decades.[2] For this reason, the maternal and fetal risk factors of prenatal intervention must be balanced with the potential benefits. Currently, the reported benefits of fetal surgery include a reduction in shunt insertion rates and improvement in hindbrain abnormality.[3–5] Published reports of results from fetal myelomeningocele procedures are mostly retrospective case series compared with historical controls. To obtain more conclusive data, the potential benefit of fetal surgery for myelomeningoceles is being examined in a clinical trial directly comparing patients randomized into prenatal and postnatal treatment groups.

■ Rationale for Surgery

The neurological deficits caused by a myelomeningocele can be separated into two groups: primary and secondary. The primary neurological deficits are caused by the arrested development of the unclosed neural tube, known as the neural placode, which usually occurs in the lumbosacral region.[6] Because neural tube closure occurs during the third and fourth weeks of gestation, the spinal cord in this region is very immature at the stage when a myelomeningocele develops. It is unknown whether the neural placode is capable of further development. It is clear that the normal anatomy of the spinal cord is severely disrupted at the level of the placode.[7] The functional neurological level is either at the same level as the vertebral anomaly or actually higher than the vertebral level, resulting in worse neurological function in more than 80% of patients with spina bifida aperta but not with spina bifida occulta.[8] There is little that can be done in the postnatal setting to reverse the primary developmental abnormality of the affected spinal cord. Augmenting spinal cord function with tissue grafts or growth factors is speculative at this time.

The secondary neurological deficits in patients with spina bifida include delayed loss of motor function, worsening bowel and bladder control, and scoliosis. These symptoms and signs are typically attributed to a symptomatic tethered spinal cord. Magnetic resonance imaging (MRI) studies of most myelomeningocele lesions following repair show a dysplastic spinal cord terminating in the overlying soft tissues at the site of the repaired defect. The presence of the conus at the level of the repair site means that virtually all patients with spina bifida have a tethered spinal cord by radiological criteria. Fortunately, not all patients with spina bifida aperta, or a specific type of spina bifida occulta

145

(e.g., lipomyelomeningocele), will develop true tethered spinal cord syndrome, which consists of the development of clinical signs and symptoms above the area of repair. It is not clear why some patients with a myelomeningocele have either minor or no symptoms of a tethered spinal cord. One possibility is that those patients are likely to maintain normal viscoelasticity of the filum terminale, preventing the lumbosacral cord from unnecessary stretching.[9]

The theoretical advantage of fetal repair of myelomeningoceles is that the neural tube is covered and protected many months before the expected delivery date. The basis for expecting improved neurological function is that restoration of the dysplastic neural placode within the spinal canal isolates it from the amniotic fluid and prevents ongoing injury.[10,11] Additional experimental evidence is derived from experiments performed on fetal sheep. Meuli and others surgically created a spinal cord lesion in fetal sheep at 75 days of gestation that simulated a spontaneous spina bifida lesion.[12] After delivery at term, these animals were incontinent and had loss of sensation and motor function below the lesion level. The gross and microscopic appearance of the exposed spinal cord resembled a human spina bifida lesion. Animals with surgically created spina bifida lesions were then treated using a myocutaneous flap at 100 days of gestation. These animals were then carried to full-term gestation and had near-normal motor function and normal bowel and bladder control. The results of these experiments suggest that early repair of an exposed spinal cord may preserve neurological function and may allow improvement through plasticity.[13] Although provocative and interesting, these large-animal experiments clearly rely on a model system that does not have all the features of the human disease.

■ Timing for Surgery

Performing fetal surgery for myelomeningoceles would be expected to have the best results if performed as early as possible. However, this is limited by the timing of diagnosis and technical limitations of the actual surgical procedure. Most myelomeningoceles are detected during the second trimester, either to investigate a positive maternal screening test or during a routine ultrasound study. The quality of current ultrasonography allows detection of most fetuses with myelomeningoceles by the midportion of the second trimester.[14] From a practical viewpoint, this means that a diagnosis is made between 18 and 22 weeks of gestation. Taking into consideration current obstetrical practice, it is unlikely that detection of fetuses with spina bifida will occur any earlier unless new, more sensitive screening tests are discovered.

■ Surgical Technique

Fetal surgery cannot be performed without the participation of a well-trained team. Successful completion of a procedure requires specialized maternal and fetal anesthesia, the ability to perform uterine opening (hysterotomy) and closure with control of uterine contractions, and continuous intraoperative fetal monitoring. These techniques are described elsewhere and will not be addressed further in this chapter.[15]

The goals of the fetal procedure are similar to the standard postnatal procedure. They include identification of the neural placode, separation of the placode from the surrounding epithelium, closure of the dura and overlying soft tissues, and closure of the skin. These goals must be modified during a fetal procedure by several limitations. The first limitation is the tenuous nature of the fetal tissues. The neural placode is extremely fragile, and even limited manipulation leads to loss of tissue integrity. Although the nerve roots are able to withstand some handling, excessive tension causes avulsion. The dura is often insubstantial, is transparent when mobilized, and has the characteristics of arachnoid in older children. The skin is able to handle surgical dissection, but excessive tension leads to tearing.

A second limitation is the inability to properly place the fetus in a neutral position at all times during the procedure. The location of the hysterotomy is determined in part by the position of the fetus but also the location of the placenta. The orientation of the fetus can be confirmed prior to hysterotomy with intraoperative ultrasound, but at times it is difficult to maintain the lumbar spine in a horizontal position, which interferes with the closure of the lesion.

The neural placode is more visible in the fetus than in the term infant. The edges of the placode are continuous with the arachnoid, which is extremely thin and translucent. If the myelomeningocele sac is intact, the placode will be lifted upward away from the surface of the back (**Fig. 13.1A**). The epithelium of the skin does not usually reach the edge of the placode. The clear identification of the intervening arachnoid usually allows the placode to be divided from its attachments with sharp dissection. Depending upon the consistency of the placode, the neural tube can be retubularized; however, if the placode is particularly fragile, this step may not be possible. The dura is loosely attached to the underlying subcutaneous tissues just lateral to the spinal canal. After

incising the dura at its lateral junction with the dermis, gentle instillation of saline into the epidural plane lifts the dura away from the underlying tissues, which minimizes the manipulation of the dura. Between 18 and 20 weeks of gestation, the dura can be very thin and difficult to handle. After 22 weeks of gestation, the dura becomes more substantial and can be handled more easily.

Once the dura is detached from the dermis and separated from the underlying lumbar fascia, it can be closed using a running suture. If the amount of dura is insufficient, then a patch is used to close the opening. The use of acellular human dermis to repair the dura may contribute to the formation of intracellular dermoid cysts.[16] For this reason, a synthetic collagen matrix (DuraGen, Integra LifeSciences, Plainsboro, NJ) can be used to create a dural barrier. Following dural closure, the skin is closed as a single layer incorporating the superficial and deeper tissues (**Fig. 13.1B**). In general, dissection of the underlying muscle and fascia is not attempted because excessive fetal blood loss must be avoided and the duration of the procedure minimized. Elevation of the skin and separation from the

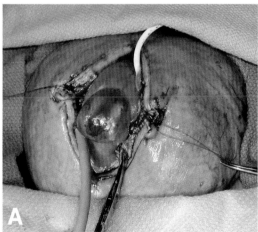
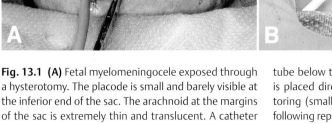
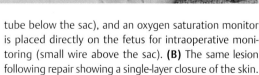

Fig. 13.1 **(A)** Fetal myelomeningocele exposed through a hysterotomy. The placode is small and barely visible at the inferior end of the sac. The arachnoid at the margins of the sac is extremely thin and translucent. A catheter is used to maintain the volume of amniotic fluid (large tube below the sac), and an oxygen saturation monitor is placed directly on the fetus for intraoperative monitoring (small wire above the sac). **(B)** The same lesion following repair showing a single-layer closure of the skin.

underlying subcutaneous tissues is relatively easy, although increased tension on the skin inevitably leads to tearing. Small openings in the skin caused by handling with forceps or tension from suture points generally close rapidly. If the skin can be brought together, the final postnatal appearance is often excellent. For situations where insufficient skin is available to close the lesion, either skin flaps, relaxing incisions, or synthetic material can be used.

There are substantial complications associated with open hysterotomy. These include placental separation, blood loss, premature labor, and delayed uterine rupture.[17,18] All of these reasons have led to most fetal procedures evolving toward endoscopic techniques. The treatment goals for myelomeningocele can be achieved by using endoscopic or open procedures, but the quality of the repair is substantially better with an open procedure.[19,20] Because endoscopic procedures are associated with fewer complications, new techniques may allow this approach to be reevaluated in the future.

■ Prenatal Imaging Studies Prior to Surgery

For postnatal treatment of myelomeningoceles, detailed imaging studies are often not obtained prior to surgery. A cranial ultrasound may be done to obtain a baseline assessment of the ventricular size. In contrast, preoperative fetal imaging studies begin with a detailed ultrasound examination. The specific goals of the ultrasound examination are to identify anomalies in ventricular shape and size, the position of the cerebellar tonsils, the level of the spinal defect, and the presence of lower-extremity deformities. In many cases, the dimensions of the anatomical defect can be accurately measured by ultrasound examination, although there can be difficulty determining the exact dysraphic level.[14]

Most patients being considered for fetal surgery will undergo a fetal MRI study (**Fig. 13.2A**). The preferred MRI technique performed at the University of California, San Francisco, is a single-shot, fast spin-echo T2-weighted sequence. The parameters of this sequence are repetition time (TR), 4000 millisecond; echo time (TE), 90 millisecond; field of view (FOV), 24 cm; slice thickness, 3 mm; no skip; bandwidth, 25 kHz; matrix, 192 × 160; and number of excitations, 0.5. These images are acquired in the axial, sagittal, and coronal planes, although adequate image quality is sometimes difficult to obtain because of fetal motion.[21] Images in sagittal, axial, and coronal planes are obtained randomly by repeatedly imaging the fetus over time. There is some evidence that MRI may improve the ability to detect coexisting spinal and brain anomalies that may not be apparent on ultrasound studies.[22,23]

■ Results

Experimental evidence suggested that early closure of myelomeningoceles should improve neurological function by preventing the secondary injury to the exposed nervous tissue.[10,12] Early clinical results, however, from fetal repair of human myelomeningoceles have been disappointing. Tubbs and others examined a cohort of patients ($n = 37$) who had undergone fetal repair between 20 and 28 weeks of gestation and compared their neurological function to a cohort ($n = 40$) of patients who underwent postnatal procedures.[24] No statistical difference was observed in lower-extremity function between the two groups. This study, along with others, has limitations inherent with any retrospective analysis, such as an unmatched control group, lack of standardization of surgical technique, and lack of randomization to treatment arms. Nevertheless, the lack of clear improvement in neurological function with fetal surgery suggests that the animal models used to study this disorder do not recapitulate the human disease.

The incidence of delayed signs and symptoms such as lower-extremity weakness, worsening of bladder and bowel control, and/or pain in patients who have had fetal surgery is unknown. Based on a few cases, reexploration

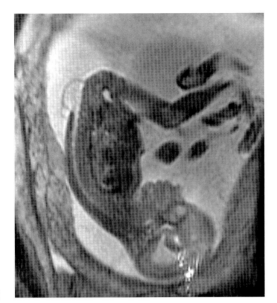

A

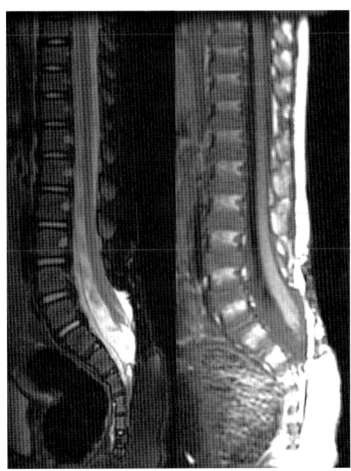

B

Fig. 13.2 (A) A fetal magnetic resonance imaging (MRI) scan (T2-weighted image) of the lumbar spine in a patient who subsequently had fetal surgery. The resolution of the image is low, but the spinal cord can be seen terminating in the placode. The myelomeningocele sac is clearly visible above the defect in the soft tissue. **(B)** A postnatal MRI (T1- and T2-weighted images) of the lumbar spine obtained in a patient at 1 year of age who had undergone fetal repair. The overall appearance is similar to patients who have had postnatal repair in that the end of the cord is low and appears to be adherent to the overlying soft tissues.

in patients who have had previous fetal repair appears to be more difficult because tissue planes in the area of the placode are poorly defined. Postnatal imaging studies of the distal spinal cord in patients who have had fetal repair, however, do not show an obvious anatomical difference compared with patients who have had postnatal repair (**Fig. 13.2B**). Urodynamics performed on a small group of children who had undergone fetal surgery showed clear abnormalities such as vesicoureteral reflux and a significant postvoid residual urine volume. These results were indistinguishable from those of patients who had undergone postnatal repair.[25] This is not unexpected given that urological function should be strongly related to sacral spinal cord function.

Data from centers performing fetal surgery for myelomeningocele have indicated that the benefits of surgery are a reduction in the rate of cerebrospinal fluid (CSF) shunt insertion, and improvement in the appearance of the Chiari II malformation on imaging studies.[3,26] The shunt rate in a cohort of 116 children treated with fetal surgery and followed in the postnatal period for at least 12 months was 54%.[27] The strongest predictor for postnatal shunt placement was the upper level of the spinal lesion, with those above L3 showing the highest rates of shunt insertion. This trend is similar to a historical series where lesion level affected shunt rates.[8] The overall percentage of patients requiring shunt placement, based on retrospective series, is usually in the range of 80 to 95%. By this measure, the reduction in shunt insertion rates reported in the fetal surgery group is encouraging. However, it is possible that selection bias alone may account for this benefit. To measure this presumed reduction in shunt insertion rates and to accurately assess maternal and fetal risks, a randomized, prospective clinical trial sponsored by the National Institutes of Health is under way. The Management of Myelomeningoceles Study (MOMS) will compare patients who will be randomly assigned to either postnatal or fetal surgery (**Table 13.1**). In addition to shunt insertion rates, other measures such as the Bayley Scale of Infant Development and neurological functional level will be used to assess the effect of fetal surgery.

Table 13.1 Inclusion and Exclusion Criteria for the Management of Myelomeningoceles Study

Inclusion criteria	1. Myelomeningocele must start at level T1 through S1 (may extend below S1) with hindbrain herniation. Lesion level will be confirmed by ultrasound, and hindbrain herniation will be confirmed by MRI at the fetal surgery unit.
	2. Maternal age ≥ 18 years
	3. Gestation age at randomization of 19 0/7 to 25 6/7 weeks gestation as determined by clinical information and evaluation of first ultrasound. If the patient's last menstrual period is deemed sure and her cycle is 26 to 32 days, and if the biometric measurements from the patient's first ultrasound confirm this last menstrual period (LMP) within ± 10 days, the LMP will be used to determine gestational age. In all other cases (i.e., if the LMP is unsure, if she has an irregular cycle or her cycle is outside the 26 to 32 day window, or if the measurements from her first ultrasound are more than 10 days discrepant from the ultrasound), the ultrasound determination will be used. Once the estimated date of confinement (EDC) has been determined for the purposes of the trial, no further revision is made.
	4. Normal karyotype with written confirmation of culture results. Results by fluorescent in situ hybridization (FISH) will be acceptable if the patient is 24 or more weeks pregnant.
Exclusion criteria	1. Multifetal pregnancy
	2. Abnormal fetal echocardiogram

Table 13.1 *(Continued)*

3. Fetal anomaly other than myelomeningocele or an anomaly related to myelomeningocele
4. Documented history of incompetent cervix
5. Short cervix < 20 mm measured by ultrasound
6. Preterm labor in the current pregnancy
7. History of spontaneous delivery < 37 weeks
8. Maternal-fetal Rh isoimmunization, Kell sensitization, or a history of neonatal alloimmune thrombocytopenia
9. Maternal HIV or hepatitis-B status positive or unknown because of the increased risk of transmission to the fetus during fetal surgery
10. Uterine anomaly such as large or multiple fibroids or mullerian duct abnormality
11. Other maternal medical condition that is a contraindication to surgery or general anesthesia
12. Patient does not have a support person (e.g., husband, partner, parent)
13. Inability to comply with the travel and follow-up requirements of the trial
14. Patient does not meet other psychosocial criteria (as determined by the case social worker) to handle the implications of surgery
15. Insulin-dependent pregestational diabetes
16. Obesity with a body mass index ≥ 35
17. Kyphosis in the fetus of ≥ 30 degrees
18. Placenta previa or placental abruption
19. Nonresident of the United States

■ Conclusion

Fetal surgery for myelomeningocele can be performed safely with acceptable maternal and fetal risks. Whether these risks are balanced by a benefit to the child over many years of follow-up is unknown. Initial reports do not indicate that fetal surgery improves neurological or urological function, although it may reduce the need for shunt insertion. The impact on other long-term disabilities such as tethered cord syndrome remains unknown and will only be determined as groups of patients are followed over time.

References

1. Harrison MR. Surgically correctable fetal disease. Am J Surg 2000;180:335–342
2. Mitchell LE, Adzick NS, Melchionne J, Pasquariello PS, Sutton LN, Whitehead AS. Spina bifida. Lancet 2004;364:1885–1895
3. Bruner JP, Tulipan N, Paschall RL, et al. Fetal surgery for myelomeningocele and the incidence of shunt-dependent hydrocephalus. JAMA 1999;282:1819–1825
4. Johnson MP, Sutton LN, Rintoul N, et al. Fetal myelomeningocele repair: short-term clinical outcomes. Am J Obstet Gynecol 2003;189:482–487
5. Tulipan N, Hernanz-Schulman M, Lowe LH, Bruner JP. Intrauterine myelomeningocele repair reverses preexisting hindbrain herniation. Pediatr Neurosurg 1999;31:137–142
6. Copp AJ, Greene ND, Murdoch JN. The genetic basis of mammalian neurulation. Nat Rev Genet 2003;4: 784–793
7. Hutchins GM, Meuli M, Meuli-Simmen C, Jordan MA, Heffez DS, Blakemore KJ. Acquired spinal cord injury in human fetuses with myelomeningocele. Pediatr Pathol Lab Med 1996;16:701–712
8. Rintoul NE, Sutton LN, Hubbard AM, et al. A new look at myelomeningoceles: functional level, vertebral level, shunting, and the implications for fetal intervention. Pediatrics 2002;109:409–413
9. Yamada S, Knerium DS, Mandybur GM, Schultz RL, Yamada BS. Pathophysiology of tethered cord syndrome and other complex factors. Neurol Res 2004; 26:722–726

10. Heffez DS, Aryanpur J, Hutchins GM, Freeman JM. The paralysis associated with myelomeningocele: clinical and experimental data implicating a preventable spinal cord injury. Neurosurgery 1990;26:987–992

11. Heffez DS, Aryanpur J, Rotellini NA, Hutchins GM, Freeman JM. Intrauterine repair of experimental surgically created dysraphism. Neurosurgery 1993;32:1005–1010

12. Meuli M, Meuli-Simmen C, Hutchins GM, et al. In utero surgery rescues neurological function at birth in sheep with spina bifida. Nat Med 1995;1:342–347

13. Walsh DS, Adzick NS, Sutton LN, Johnson MP. The rationale for in utero repair of myelomeningocele. Fetal Diagn Ther 2001;16:312–322

14. Patel TR, Bannister CM, Thorne J. A study of prenatal ultrasound and postnatal magnetic imaging in the diagnosis of central nervous system abnormalities. Eur J Pediatr Surg 2003;13(Suppl 1):S18–S22

15. Harrison MR, Evans MI, Adzick NS, eds. The Unborn Patient: The Art and Science of Prenatal Diagnosis. 3rd ed. Philadelphia: Saunders; 2000

16. Mazzola CA, Albright AL, Sutton LN, Tuite GF, Hamilton RL, Pollack IF. Dermoid inclusion cysts and early spinal cord tethering after fetal surgery for myelomeningocele. N Engl J Med 2002;347:256–259

17. Wilson RD, Johnson MP, Flake AW, et al. Reproductive outcomes after pregnancy complicated by maternal-fetal surgery. Am J Obstet Gynecol 2004;191:1430–1436

18. Wilson RD, Johnson MP, Crombleholme TM, et al. Chorioamniotic membrane separation following open fetal surgery: pregnancy outcome. Fetal Diagn Ther 2003;18:314–320

19. Bruner JP, Tulipan NB, Richards WO, Walsh WF, Boehm FH, Vrabcak EK. In utero repair of myelomeningocele: a comparison of endoscopy and hysterotomy. Fetal Diagn Ther 2000;15:83–88

20. Farmer DL, von Koch CS, Peacock WJ, et al. In utero repair of myelomeningocele: experimental pathophysiology, initial clinical experience, and outcomes. Arch Surg 2003;138:872–878

21. Coakley FV, Glenn OA, Qayyum A, Barkovich AJ, Goldstein R, Filly RA. Fetal MRI: a developing technique for the developing patient. AJR Am J Roentgenol 2004;182:243–252

22. Glenn OA, Goldstein RB, Li KC, et al. Fetal magnetic resonance imaging in the evaluation of fetuses referred for sonographically suspected abnormalities of the corpus callosum. J Ultrasound Med 2005;24:791–804

23. von Koch CS, Glenn OA, Goldstein RB, Barkovich AJ. Fetal magnetic resonance imaging enhances detection of spinal cord anomalies in patients with sonographically detected bony anomalies of the spine. J Ultrasound Med 2005;24:781–789

24. Tubbs RS, Chambers MR, Smyth MD, et al. Late gestational intrauterine myelomeningocele repair does not improve lower extremity function. Pediatr Neurosurg 2003;38:128–132

25. Holmes NM, Nguyen HT, Harrison MR, Farmer DL, Baskin LS. Fetal intervention for myelomeningocele: effect on postnatal bladder function. J Urol 2001;166:2383–2386

26. Tulipan N, Hernanz-Schulman M, Bruner JP. Reduced hindbrain herniation after intrauterine myelomeningocele repair: a report of four cases. Pediatr Neurosurg 1998;29(5):274–278

27. Bruner JP, Tulipan N, Reed G, et al. Intrauterine repair of spina bifida: preoperative predictors of shunt-dependent hydrocephalus. Am J Obstet Gynecol 2004;190:1305–1312

14 Epidermoid and Dermoid Tumors Associated with Tethered Cord Syndrome

David S. Knierim, Daniel J. Won, and Shokei Yamada

Epidermoid and dermoid tumors are usually thought of as developmental tumors. They may also be inclusions from previous surgery when elements of dermis or epidermis are retained with the neural placode at the time of myelomeningocele repair in spina bifida.[1] On rare occasions, these benign tumors can be caused by skin fragments that were implanted in the spine as a result of invasive procedure such as lumbar puncture.[2,3] They usually occur at or near the midline and can be associated with tubular dermal sinus tracts. They can be encountered in the nasofrontal region, the occipital region, and along the spine. The dermal sinus tracts that often connect to dural reflections or stalks are of greater potential for development of symptoms. Further tract communications with the central nervous system (CNS) are the potential source of three major complications: (1) CNS infection through the tract as a conduit for bacteria, (2) CNS compression by mass effect, and (3) tethered cord syndrome related to inelastic structures that anchor the caudal spinal cord, such as sinus tracts themselves, dural stalks, and inclusion cysts.

The incidence of dermal sinus tract is ~1 in 2500 live births.[4–6] Dermal sinus tracts have been reported all along the midline neuraxis from the nasion and occiput down to the lumbar and sacral region. The majority occur in the lumbar and lumbosacral region.[7,8] Often there is an associated cutaneous lesion overlying the midline anomaly or dermoid tumor, such as a cutaneous angioma, hypertrichosis, or a dimple at the surface of a dermal sinus.[9,10] The dermoid or epidermoid cysts may be extradural, intradural, and extramedullary. In the spinal form, the bony deformity of spinal dysraphism can be seen near the tumor on plain x-rays in adults. In children younger than 5 years of age, plain x-rays fail to show spinal dysraphism because the lamina and spinous processes have not yet fully ossified. There may be an increase in interpedicular space on plain films. A tumor located in a more rostral position may be in an intramedullary position, causing a concentric expansion of the spinal cord. Ultrasonography can sometimes be used as a screening study. Magnetic resonance imaging (MRI) has replaced myelography and computed tomography (CT) as the diagnostic study of choice. MRI, although noninvasive, provides great anatomical detail to help make a diagnosis and plan treatment.

The dermal tumor is often associated with spinal dysraphism and functionally with tethered cord syndrome. In addition, separate from the dermal sinus, an inelastic filum terminale continuous to the distal spinal cord is typically found attached to the caudally located area of dural schisis. The dermal sinus tract at this region alone can be another factor to cause tethered cord syndrome. Simply removing a dermoid cyst by itself might not be enough to reverse neurological impairment unless other mechanical tethering factors are eliminated. These lesions tend to have anomalous anatomical structures, and at times the true tethering point must be determined among multiple areas of suspected tethering.

■ Case Reports

Case 1

A 1-year, 11-month-old female presented with pain in the back. She had a past history of fevers treated with antibiotics but had never been diagnosed as having had meningitis. She would scream when she sat down hard. She could not tolerate sitting on a carpeted floor. She would not ever sit with her legs crossed or akimbo. She was unable to sleep through the night for 1 week prior to her admission because of low back pain. She exhibited a positive Gower sign where she would not bend over at the waist or hips to pick up objects from the floor.

A lumbosacral angioma and tandem spinal dimples were noted. Otherwise she was neurologically intact. At surgery tandem dermoid cysts were resected. The dural sinus stalk was excised, and the filum terminale was divided cephalic to the dural schisis, which was contiguous with the dural sinus (**Fig. 14.1A,B**). She was pain free after the surgery.

Case 2

An 11-year-old male had complained of bilateral foot pain at the age of 6 years. He had been seen in the orthopedic surgery clinic at age 9. He was unable to catch up with his friends when they were running. He was noted to have slightly high arches of both feet and was given a prescription for custom-molded inserts for his shoes. Purulent material was noted to be coming out of a dimple in his back 2 years later and

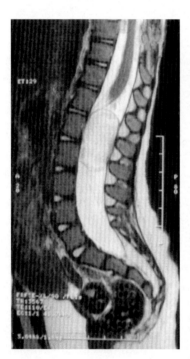 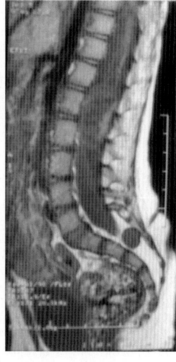

A   **B**

Fig. 14.1 Case 1. **(A)** Magnetic resonance imaging (MRI) showing a dermoid tumor just caudal to the conus medullaris causing some distortion of the nerve roots at the cauda equina. **(B)** MRI in the same patient showing a small caudally located tandem dermoid cyst associated with a dermal sinus. The rostral dermoid tumor is faintly outlined, and the conus medullaris is not seen as well as in **(A)**.

he was referred to the pediatric neurosurgery clinic. There was no history of meningitis and he had no complaint of back pain. A lumbar dimple was noted overlying the midline (**Fig. 14.2A**). MRI showed a sacral dermal sinus tract as well as a low-lying conus medullaris at the L3–4 region (**Fig. 14.2B,C**). At surgery (10/14/04) there was a dermal sinus tract extending from the cutaneous dimple into the spinal canal in the sacral region. The dermal sinus was resected,

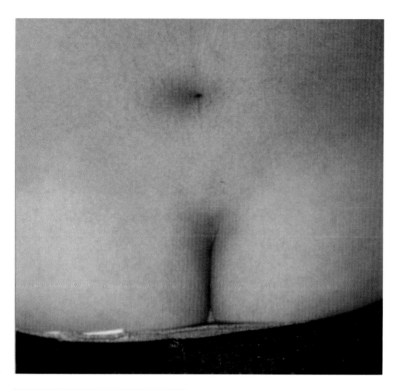

A

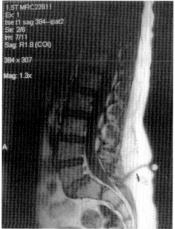

B

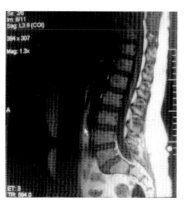

C

Fig. 14.2 Case 2. **(A)** Dermal sinus at lumbar region with subtle cutaneous angioma. **(B)** Magnetic resonance imaging (MRI) showing the cutaneous dimple, a dermal sinus connecting with a dural reflection or stalk. **(C)** MRI showing the low-lying conus in the same patient.

and the filum terminale was divided cephalic to its attachments in the fibrous region of the dural schisis. He remains neurologically intact without pain.

Case 3

A 7-month-old male presented with diarrhea and urinary retention requiring catheterization. During his hospitalization he developed fevers to 103°F and was noted to have stopped being as vigorous with his legs. He was noted to have a flaccid paraplegia. Lumbar puncture was attempted but yielded two dry taps. During the attempted lumbar punctures the patient was noted to have a small (1.5 cm diameter) cutaneous angioma in the midline at the lumbar spine. Close examination revealed a dimple in the center of the cutaneous angioma. MRI showed a dermal sinus at the sacral level with abnormal densities in the region of the cauda equina with a swollen appearing cord more superiorly (**Fig. 14.3**). On 7/3/04 a T9 through S3 multilevel laminotomy was conducted. Pus was drained from the gluteal, the paraspinous

regions, extradural, intradural and from the intramedullary regions via myelotomy. A dermal sinus was identified and resected, and the inelastic filum terminale was divided. Postoperatively the patient was noted to have an ascending paralysis that involved his arms. Another MRI scan revealed extension of intramedullary fluid to the cervical region. A multilevel laminotomy was performed from C7 through T3 on 7/8/04. Pus was again obtained via a myelotomy, and the region was irrigated with saline. Anaerobic *Bacteroides thetaiotaomicron* and *Peptostreptococcus magnus* were isolated from the spinal cultures. Diphtheroids were isolated from a transrectal drainage of a presacral abscess. Gradually he regained the use of his arms and legs.

Case 4

An 11-month-old female was noted to have a sacral dimple. She was referred to the pediatric neurosurgery clinic. A lumbar cutaneous angioma was noted to be associated with a midline dimple. Her legs were symmetrical and she walked without difficulty. MRI revealed a

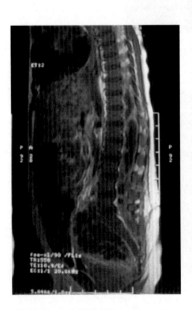 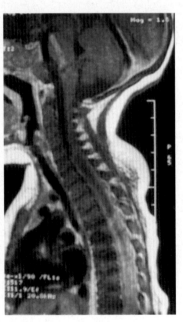

A B

Fig. 14.3 Case 3. **(A)** Magnetic resonance imaging (MRI) showing lumbar cystic fluid densities distorting normal cauda equina with a dermal sinus going toward the subcutaneous and cutaneous region dorsally. **(B)** Intramedullary abscess in the same patient extending to the upper cervical spine at the C5 level.

dural stalk associated with a dermal sinus tract (**Fig. 14.4**). On 4/16/04 she underwent L4, L5, and S1 laminotomy with resection of the dural stalk for untethering of the spinal cord. A laminoplasty was performed at L4–5. On her postoperative visit of 10/27/04 she was noted to be neurologically intact with no difficulty with voiding.

Case 5

A 7-year-old female experienced episodes of pain in her knees 3 years prior to her referral to pediatric neurosurgery. She was seen in the orthopedic surgery clinic and noted to have scoliosis with a 20 degree curvature from T10 through L4. Her exam was relatively unremarkable with the exception of a coccygeal dimple. Her history was complicated by the diagnosis of a liver abscess. MRI showed Chiari I malformation at the cervicomedullary junction with a conus at the L1 region. There was a fat signal in the filum and also a hint of hydromyelia. A dural stalk was noted at the dorsal midline at the termination of the thecal sac (**Figs. 14.5**). On 11/11/04 she underwent an S2 and S3 laminectomy and resection of the inelastic

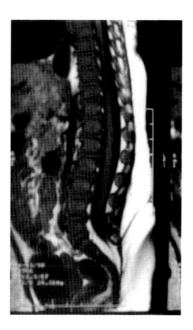

Fig. 14.4 Case 4. Magnetic resonance imaging (MRI) showing a dermal sinus communicating with a caudal dural stalk and a low-lying conus medullaris at the sacral region.

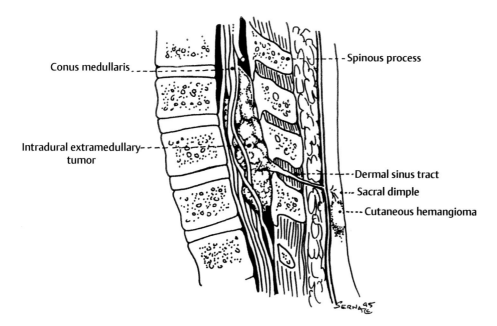

Fig. 14.5 Diagram of dural stalk with connecting dermal sinus and tumor in the region of the cauda equina.

fibroadipose filum and the dural stalk as a part of the dural schisis. Intraoperative sphincter monitoring showed normal responses.

■ Imaging Studies

Radiographic delineation of dermoid, epidermoid, and related abnormalities of the central nervous system can be challenging.[11,12] The radiographic density of the tumor can be very close to that of cerebrospinal fluid and unlike that of fat, neural tissue, bone, or other surrounding tissues. MRI is now the method of choice for the diagnosis of deep dermoid and epidermoid tumors and related sinus tracts, spina bifida, or craniorachischisis. However, extramedullary tumors may be misdiagnosed as an arachnoid cyst or a proteinaceous fluid pocket in what appears to be a generous thecal sac. In contrast, intramedullary tumors are easily identified on MRI because of the distortion of the surrounding spinal cord. Myelography is now largely of historical interest.

■ Embryological Aspects

The etiology of dermoid and epidermoid cysts or tumors is considered to be secondary to a rest or inclusion of either one or both layers of cutaneous dermis and epidermis. The sebaceous glands of the dermis are capable of secreting an excretion similar or identical to the sebum of a sebaceous cyst. Hair from the follicles originating in the dermis layer is often present, hence the name *dermoid tumor*. The dermis comes from the outer layer of mesoderm, whereas the epidermis comes from ectoderm.[13] The hair encountered in dermoid cysts seems to be relatively free from pigment. Neural tube defects and epidermoid and dermoid cysts are frequently associated with tethered spinal cord. About 60% of dermal sinuses either incorporate or end in a dermoid or epidermoid tumor, whereas ~30% of dermoid and epidermoid tumors are associated with dermal sinus tracts.[8,14,15] When occurring in the lumbosacral region, the defects are often associated with an inelastic, often thick

filum terminale. Embryologically, the neural tube closes by the twenty-fifth day of gestation at the cephalic neuropore and by the twenty-seventh day at the caudal neuropore.[16] It is believed that there is an aberration in the process prior to this time that could lead to formation of dermal inclusions and formation of sinus tract. Padget theorized that delamination or blistering of tissue occurs after the twenty-eighth day of gestation where a neuroschistic bleb formed, thus explaining the dysraphic state of spina bifida aperta.[6,17,18] This could result in dermal inclusions and sinus tracts communicating with underlying neural ectoderm. Although these tumors are considered to be histologically benign, the complications described in the introduction must be considered. With mesodermal involvement, lipomyelomeningoceles or skeletal muscle with the cells of spinal rests can occur.[19]

■ Treatment

Rationale for Surgical Treatment

Although dermoid and epidermoid cysts are histologically benign, their compression effect or traction effect on neural tissue within the spinal canal can be serious enough to require surgical treatment. By the definition of tethered cord syndrome, stretching of the spinal cord between the tethering site and the counteracting site, usually at the attachment of the lowest pair of dentate ligament, causes neurological dysfunction that are reversible. The dysfunction is manifested by motor and sensory deficit, musculoskeletal deformities in the lower limbs, and incontinence. A failure of the filum terminale to develop a normal viscoelastic structure during the embryonic stage (ninth to eleventh week) can cause insidiously progressive neurological signs and symptoms. Their worsening occurs with the passage of time by rapid spinal column growth and the repetition of insults, mainly excessive flexion and extension. However, development of the symptoms depends on the balance between the vertebral growth and spinal cord growth. Traction-induced dysfunction of the lumbosacral cord becomes most pronounced at the caudal portion (the conus medullaris) proportionate to greater stretching.[20] Mainly due to circulatory impairment of microvasculature (Yamada et al[21,22]) the gray matter is affected to a greater degree in patients with tethered cord syndrome. The reduction-oxidation ratio (redox) of cytochrome oxidase within the mitochondria shifts to the reduced state under cord traction, indicating impaired oxidative metabolism. This metabolic effect in the conus is the underlying mechanism for the bowel and bladder incontinence. Musculoskeletal adjustment in response to the tension within the cord accentuates natural curves of the lumbosacral lordosis and develops scoliosis of the lumbar and compensatory thoracic spine. The accentuation of these curvatures is to minimize the cord tension in the lumbosacral canal. The additional neuromuscular imbalance is manifested by foot deformities, such as high arches of the feet, pes equinus, hammertoes, and the asymmetry of the muscular mass and development of the lower extremities.

When these findings have been observed in total or in part, it is time to advise cord untethering. In addition, a space-occupying lesion of a dermoid cyst or epidermoid tumor must be considered as the symptoms progress and the need of decompression. If there has been previous surgery in the affected area, meticulous lysis of scar tissue and the release of adhesions around the spinal cord are mandatory. Chiari malformations, syringomyelia, hydrocephalus, or shunt malfunction should be considered for differential diagnoses or as the source of symptomatic aggravations. Epidermoid tumors have also been reported at the cerebellopontine angle mimicking acoustic neuroma or meningioma affecting long tracts that extend to the spinal cord.[23,24]

Surgical Technique

Precaution

When any degrees of bifid processes are encountered, it is important to gain anatomical understanding of the lesion, distinctly separate from scar, sinus tracts, abnormal dural planes, and the sources of cerebrospinal fluid leaks and bleeding.

Exposure of the laminae, especially when they are bifid, is a key to understanding the anatomy in the depths of the surgical site. Meticulous hemostasis is essential for successful clean surgical procedures at each depth of surgery utilizing microscopic magnification.

Operative Procedure

1. A skin incision is made in the midline and, if necessary, around the sinus tract opening. Palpation of the bifid processes can often outline the lesion, assisting in preservation of a dural sinus tract in the center of the operative field.
2. Paraspinal muscles are separated subperiosteally from the spinous processes and laminae to minimize bleeding and tissue damage. It is often necessary to expose one level above and below the preexisting extensive laminectomy or bifid site.
3. Laminectomy is performed to expose the normal dura around the sinus tract to its connection. Single or multiple laminae can be elevated with a high-speed rotating saw with a protective foot plate, leaving the rostral interspinous ligament. Then the laminal flap is rotated cephalad and held out of the operative site with sutures or a retractor.
4. The dura is exposed by careful dissection with the aid of a dural separator, the ligamentum flavum is divided, and epidural fat is separated from the dura. At this stage, the sinus tract, if present, passing through the bony defect and the dura at the site of spinal schisis can be clearly identified. There is usually no need to extend the laminectomy far laterally into the facet joints. At times a considerable dissection can be performed extensively between bifid spinous processes. In the presence of a wide interpedicular distance, normal dural planes must be

demonstrated superiorly and inferiorly before dural opening.

5. The dura is opened with a sharp blade and a dural hook. Dural retraction sutures aid in the exposure of the contents of the thecal sac. Hemostasis is aided by the use of Gelfoam (Pfizer Inc., New York, NY) and thrombin. There is often a tendency for dermoid tumors to protrude through the opening of the thecal sac.

6. The tumor is located extradural, intradural extramedullary, or intramedullary in the spinal canal. It is usually removed piecemeal, but at times large portions can be lifted off of neural elements. Associated dural stalks can be identified and resected at the time of initial exploration of the dural surface, including the dermal sinus tract all the way to the skin. After satisfactory resection of the inelastic filum, if present, for cord untethering, the arachnoid membrane is closed whenever possible using 5–0 Prolene suture (Ethicon, Inc., Piscataway, NJ). The dura is closed in a watertight fashion with 4–0 Nurolon. A large dural defect may require duraplasty with dural substitute. The single or multiple laminae, which was elevated for the exposure, can be reapproximated by placing sutures through the laminae as a laminoplasty. Muscle and fascia layers are closed using absorbable sutures and superficial layer of skin is closed using nylon sutures.

Dermoid tumors, histologically benign, carry a good prognosis when completely resected. They can be problematic in that they may recur, and neurological deficits are not always reversed.

A peripheral nerve stimulation in conjunction with a balloon rectal sphincter monitor helps identify nerve roots of the cauda equina when used. In particular, the sacral nerves (S2–4) can be preserved to spare bladder and bowel control. Alternatively, the use of intraoperative electromyography (EMG) of the external anal sphincter muscle as well as striated muscles in the lower limbs is advocated for distinction from the filum.[25]

■ Results

The authors have encountered three cases associated with infection with documentation of meningitis prior to or at the time of initial surgery. Of three patients that were unable to walk preoperatively, all regained the ability to walk. One of the cases with infection continues to require intermittent catheterization for bladder dysfunction. One case of intramedullary dermoid cyst has required an additional surgery for recurrence. All other patients did well postoperatively with neurological improvement or stabilization.

It has been noted that dermoid tumors, epidermoid tumors, and teratomas as a group make up ~1 to 2% of all spinal cord tumors.[12] According to Hendrick, spinal cord dermoid tumors are one tenth as common as dermoid tumors of the brain.

■ Conclusion

The topic of tethered cord may involve rests of cells that can form tumors. Fibrous stalks and dermal sinuses can create conduits that allow infectious complications. Growth over time can cause traction injuries to the spinal cord with resulting neuromuscular imbalance, deformities of the lower extremities, scoliosis, and bowel and bladder difficulties when the dysraphism involves the spine. Diagnostic technique continues to improve in the pre- and postoperative assessment of these conditions. One must continue to be vigilant in detecting this type of tumor. They are often mistaken for other diagnoses, such as demyelinating disorder, cerebral palsy, Guillain-Barré syndrome, encephalopathy, muscle strain, and many other phenomena, prior to a definitive workup and diagnosis at surgery.[26] MRI is the most useful diagnostic study for evaluating these patients. The correct diagnosis is seldom known with surety until surgery is performed and histological identification is obtained. One must not give up the evaluation for a cluster of

symptoms simply because of a limited radiographic exam. There are times when the entire spine and cervicomedullary junction must be scrutinized.

References

1. Storrs BB. Are dermoid and epidermoid tumors preventable complications of myelomeningocele repair? Pediatr Neurosurg 1994;20:160–162
2. Halcrow SJ, Crawford PJ, Craft AW. Epidermoid spinal cord tumour after lumbar puncture. Arch Dis Child 1985;60:978–979
3. Jeong IH, Lee JK, Moon KS, et al. Iatrogenic intraspinal epidermoid tumor: case report. Pediatr Neurosurg 2006;42:395–398
4. Cheek W, Laurent J. Dermal sinus tracts. In: Chapman PH, ed. Concepts in Pediatric Neurosurgery. Vol 6. Basel: Karger; 1985;63–75
5. McIntosh R, Merritt KK, Richards MR, Samuels MH, Bellows MT. The incidence of congenital malformations: a study of 5,964 pregnancies. Pediatrics 1954; 14:505–522
6. Powell KR, Cherry JD, Hougen TJ, Blinderman EE, Dunn MC. A prospective search for congenital dermal abnormalities of the craniospinal axis. J Pediatr 1975;87:744–750
7. Ackerman LL, Menezes AH. Spinal congenital dermal sinuses: a 30-year experience. Pediatrics 2003;112 (3 Pt 1):641–647
8. Boldrey EB, Elvidge AR. Dermoid cysts of the vertebral canal. Ann Surg 1939;110:273–284
9. Matson D. Neurosurgery of Infancy and Childhood. 2nd ed. Springfield, IL: Charles C Thomas; 1969: 647–688
10. Selfeshog E. Pediatric intraspinal tumors. In: Bradford DS, Hensinger RM, eds. The Pediatric Spine. New York: Thieme; 1985:155–162
11. Barkovich AJ, Edwards M, Cogen PH. MR evaluation of spinal dermal sinus tracts in children. AJNR Am J Neuroradiol 1991;12:123–129
12. Connolly E. Spinal cord tumors in adults. In: Youmans J. ed. Neurological Surgery. 2nd ed. Philadelphia: WB Saunders; 1982:3196–3214
13. Langman J. Medical Embryology. 2nd ed. Baltimore: Williams & Wilkins; 1969:37–68
14. Guidetti B, Gagliardi FM. Epidermoid and dermoid cysts: clinical evaluation and late surgical results. J Neurosurg 1977;47:12–18
15. McLone D, Dias M. Normal and abnormal early development of the nervous system. In: Pediatric Neurosurgery. 3rd ed. Philadelphia: WB Saunders; 1994:3–39
16. Sadler T. Langman's Medical Embryology. 7th ed. Baltimore: Williams & Wilkins; 1995:374–412
17. French B. Midline fusion defects and defects of formation. In: Youmans J, ed. Neurological Surgery. 2nd ed. Philadelphia: WB Saunders; 1982:1236–1380
18. Padget DH. Neuroschisis and human embryonic maldevelopment: new evidence on anencephaly, spina bifida and diverse mammalian defects. J Neuropathol Exp Neurol 1970;29:192–216
19. Knierim DS, Wacker M, Peckham N, Bedros AA. Lumbosacral intramedullary myolipoma. Case report. J Neurosurg 1987;66:457–459
20. Tani S, Yamada S, Knighton RS. Extensibility of the lumbar and sacral cord: pathophysiology of the tethered spinal cord in cats. J Neurosurg 1987;66: 116–123
21. Yamada S, Schneider S, Ashwal S, et al. Pathophysiologic mechanisms in the tethered spinal cord syndrome. In: Holtzman R, Stein B. eds. The Tethered Spinal Cord. New York: Thieme-Stratton; 1985: 29–40
22. Yamada S, Zinke DE, Sanders D. Pathophysiology of "tethered cord syndrome." J Neurosurg 1981;54: 494–503
23. Bikmaz K. Management of cerebellopontine angle epidermoid tumors. Contemp Neurosurg. 2004;26:1–4
24. deSouza CE, deSouza R, da Costa S, et al. Cerebellopontine angle epidermoid cysts: a report on 30 cases. J Neurol Neurosurg Psychiatry 1989;52: 986–990
25. Yamada S. Commentary in Surg Neurol 2004;62: 133–134. For the article "Quinones-Hinojosa A, Garkary CA, Gulati M, et al. Clinical outcome of adults after neurophysiologically monitored tethered cord release surgery. Surg Neurol 2004;62:127–135)
26. Hendrick E. Spinal cord tumors in children. In: Youmans J, ed. Neurological Surgery. 2nd ed. Philadelphia: WB Saunders; 1982:3215–3221

15 Tethered Cord Syndrome in Adult and Late-teenage Patients without Neural Spinal Dysraphism

Shokei Yamada, Russell R. Lonser, Austin R. T. Colohan, and Cheryl T. Yamada

Hoffman et al should be credited with linking the term "tethered spinal cord" to patients with lumbosacral signs and symptoms associated with elongated cord and thickened filum terminale.[1] Since the subsequent publishing of our report "pathophysiology of tethered cord syndrome (TCS)" in 1981,[2] we have sought to crystallize TCS as a distinct syndrome which corresponds to the pathophysiology.[3] This chapter describes how this goal was achieved by reviewing information from patients similar to those selected by Hoffman in 1976.[1] With the exception that our patients include those with TCS caused by an inelastic filum terminale, with or without cord elongation or filum thickening.[3,4,5] These late teenage and adult patients have descirbed their complaints and reactions in detail, including back and leg pain, urinary or rectal incontinence and sensory changes, which allows us to clearly group their symptoms and systematically document their physical and neurological signs. Such symptoms have become important sources of information for TCS diagnosis.

Research into the pathophysiology of tethered cord syndrome (TCS) indicates that its signs and symptoms are associated with characteristic impairments in oxidative metabolic and electrophysiological activities within the spinal cord rather than with histological damage.[1–6] This distinction is important because it may explain why untethering of the spinal cord reverses the symptoms of TCS. However, reported results of untethering surgery are complicated when patients with neural spinal dysraphism are included in adult TCS patients.[7–14] To account for these variations, we grouped patients as group 1 patients with neural spinal dysraphism, such as myelomeningocele (MMC) and lipomyelomeningocele (LMMC), and group 2 patients with no evidence of these anomalies but an inelastic filum that is anchoring the spinal cord at its caudal end.[3,5] Group 1 patients were known to have a certain degree of stabilized neurological deficits that progressed in adulthood (see the discussion of cord tethering category 2B), and group 2 patients presented with characteristic symptomatology only in the late teenage years or adulthood. Group 2 is the subject of this chapter, and from now on is referred to as adult TCS.

In this chapter we report on symptomatic patients with strict surgical indications based on a review of their signs and symptoms and imaging studies. These patients are typical of those with TCS, and surgery was recommended regardless of the presence or absence of an elongated cord or thickened filum. Surgical procedures consisted of sectioning or resection of the inelastic filum to untether the spinal cord.

Although this group of patients are included in Category 1 (true TCS) with sacral myelomeningocele and caudal lipomyelomeningocele among the visually expressed "tethered cord (or cord tethering)" patients, (See Discussion, Tethered Cord Syndrome and Various Interpretation and Prognosis), the latter two were excluded in the current series to avoid their complexity of the terminology.

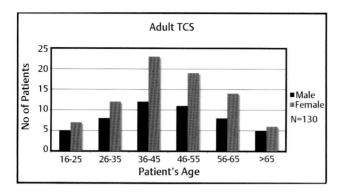

Fig. 15.1 The bar graph shows the distribution of the number of patients in age categories.

■ Signs and Symptoms

This report includes 130 patients (50 males; 80 females, ages ranging from 16 to 81 years as seen in the bar graph) (**Fig. 15.1**). Approximately 75% of these patients were originally referred for evaluation of "failed back"[15] or failed back surgery syndrome.[16] Each patient was subsequently diagnosed as having TCS and underwent untethering to alleviate the symptoms. Referral diagnoses included recurrent herniated disk, suspected herniated disk, osteoarthritic spondylosis, and back sprain. Twenty-three percent of these patients had a previous history of lumbar spine surgery without permanent pain relief and were categorized with failed back surgery syndrome.[17] Experiences in our group[5] and in others[12] have confirmed that detection of the reversible signs and symptoms for true TCS[18] is important for effective treatment of patients because accurate diagnosis and proper surgical untethering at an appropriate time have successfully reversed symptomatology. The following specific TCS symptoms should be identified in addition to routine physical and neurological examinations.

1. Pain pattern as characterized by the following:

   a. *Quality and location* TCS patients complain of constant aching in the back and legs or in one leg, localized deep in muscles.

   b. *Pain aggravation* Pain is worsened by flexing and extending the back. In particular, the following actions aggravated back pain immediately in all of our patients. Apparently, these actions straighten the lumbosacral lordosis and lengthen the canal, thus stretching the cord that is tethered by an inelastic filum.

      i. Sitting with legs crossed in a **B**uddha pose
      ii. **B**ending slightly over the sink, as for washing dishes or brushing teeth
      iii. Holding a **b**aby (or equivalent weight) at waist level (The three postures above are called 3B postures)
      iv. Lying supine
      v. Slouching as in a chair (95% of patients)

   c. When accentuated after forceful postural changes, the back and leg pain is expressed as a feeling of muscle cramping, pulling, or tearing. Occasionally, some patients complain of pain that extends to the thoracic back muscles, and rarely to the nuchal musculature. Presumably, such pain may be elicited by extensive reflex contractions of the longitudinal back muscle groups, such as erector spinae, longissimus thoracis, spinalis thoracis in the superficial layer and multifidus, semispinalis thoracis, cervicis and capitis in the deep layer, or by simultaneously isometric contraction through multisynaptic neuronal connections in the spinal cord.

2. Numbness in the lower limbs, often while walking

3. Bony pain in the legs and feet in the sclerotomal distribution.[19] For instance, one patient complained of severe pain in both calcanei and leg muscles. She wore a plaster of Paris cast to prevent bone irritation on standing and walking. After untethering surgery, her pain was rapidly relieved and she was able to walk barefoot. The pain in the calcaneus is likely to have corresponded to the sclerotome.

4. Difficulty in urination (80% of patients, $N = 130$) such as dribbling of urine, stress or urge incontinence, often barely reaching the bathroom, overflow incontinence, or retention[20] (see Chapters 7 and 8)

5. Rectal incontinence 30% ($N = 130$)

6. Decreases in tolerance of physical stresses often described as follows:

   a. Decrease in walking distance, giving up running

   b. Decrease in driving or riding distance in a car

   c. Difficulty in standing still, mainly due to aggravation of back and leg pain and back tightening

7. Negative symptoms are equally important for differential diagnosis, and include the following:

   a. No radiating pain in the lower limbs

   b. No aggravation of pain by coughing or sneezing, unlike the experience of patients with herniated lumbar disks

■ Imaging Studies

There are two noteworthy magnetic resonance imaging (MRI) findings in the group 2 patients: (1) cord elongation and filum thickening, and more significantly (2) posterior displacement of the filum, which is consistently found in these patients, signifying that the filum travels along the concave side of the lumbosacral lordosis, to minimize spinal cord tension.[5,21]

Due to limited resolution, MRI or computed tomographic (CT) myelographic visualization of the location of the conus tip in relation to the vertebral level and the thickness of the filum is less accurate than the determination at surgery. For example, the caudal end of the spinal cord can be determined by identifying the exit of the lowest coccygeal nerve (100 to 150 μm diameter) from the spinal cord, particularly for the conus tip located at the L3 vertebral level. From our experience, the caudal end of the spinal cord was found at the L2–3 intervertebral space or below in 64% of the patients, and the diameter of the filum was ≥ 2 mm in 42.3% ($N = 104$). These data clearly indicate that the preoperative diagnosis of adult TCS must rely primarily on the symptomatology and the specific imaging feature of posterior displacement of the conus and filum that attach to the posterior arachnoid membrane (see Chapter 18).

A capacious lumbosacral subarachnoid space is often associated with TCS. Cine-MRI motion pictures have been reported to show stiffness of an inelastic filum in contrast to a freely moveable cauda equina.[2] Although simulating the effects of ultrasonography in infants, this technology is not universally used.[22]

■ Diagnosis

Determination of the signs and symptoms characteristic of group 2 adult TCS patients is critical for accurate diagnosis and proper treatment. The specific features of TCS were previously described as a protocol for the diagnosis of adult TCS[23] and are listed in what follows. We have found that patients who show greater than 90% of these signs and symptoms are very likely to have TCS, and an urgent MRI study is recommended.

Protocol for symptoms associated with tethered cord syndrome

1. Maximum walking distance that has decreased over months to years

2. Walking that must be interrupted due to pain (and weakness)

3. Walking that causes leg numbness and urinary urgency
4. Aggravation of back and leg pain by spinal flexion and extension in general
5. Specifically, back pain that is aggravated by the following:

    a. Sitting in the Buddha pose with both legs crossed
    b. Bending slightly over the sink (**Fig. 15.2**)
    c. Holding a baby at waist level
    d. Lying supine (the patient prefers lying laterally in the fetal position)
    e. Slouching in a chair

6. Pain in the groin, genital, or anal area
7. Muscular pain, localized in different parts of the lower limbs, described as vague location by some patients

8. No radicular pain in legs and no accentuation by coughing, sneezing, or straight leg raising
9. Decreasing tolerance to driving because of back and leg pain, worse on a bumpy road
10. Pain extending to the buttocks on spinal extension or flexion
11. Intolerance to standing or sitting still

Protocol for signs associated with tethered cord syndrome

1. Absence of paravertebral back muscle spasms
2. Absence of local tenderness in the lumbosacral spine
3. Scoliosis and exaggerated lumbosacral lordosis (**Fig. 15.3**)
4. Foot or leg deformities: high-arched feet or hammertoes (the progression of these deformities is described by the patient's mother as he or she grows older to adulthood) (**Fig. 15.4**)

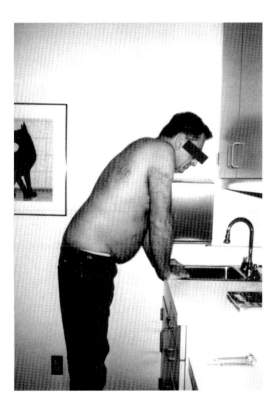

Fig. 15.2 Because his back and leg pain was aggravated while trying to bend over slightly to wash dishes, the patient had to hold onto the edge of the sink. After untethering surgery, the patient was able to wash dishes without developing pain.

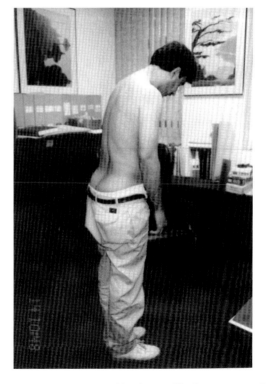

Fig. 15.3 Accentuated lumbosacral lordosis was noted in this tethered cord syndrome patient.

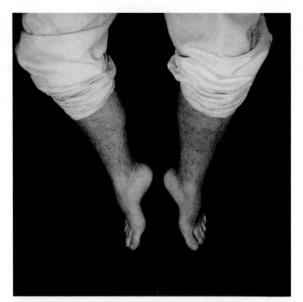

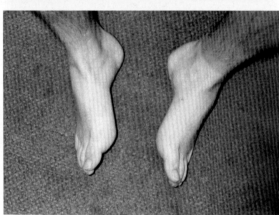

Fig. 15.4 (A,B) High-arched feet associated with mild bilateral hyperextension of the metatarsophalangeal joint and flexion of the phalangeal joint in the great toes (hammertoes) were found in these patients with early tethered cord syndrome. These deformities rapidly subsided after untethering. The patient in **(A)** shows more pronounced high arch than the patient in **(B)**. The tethered cord syndrome is more advanced in the former than in the latter patient.

5. Weakness of the extensor hallucis longus (**Fig. 15.5**)
6. Ankle joint instability on tiptoes or on heel standing, due to weakness of most often peroneus longus, less commonly, posterior tibialis, anterior tibialis, or gastrocnemius
7. Sensation to pinprick diminished
   a. in the dorsum of the foot
   b. in the perianal area and groin
   c. extensively in the lower limbs in patchy distributions
8. Diminished sphincter tone on digital insertion (reflex), on voluntary contraction, or anal wink reflex
9. Preoperative presence of postvoid residual urine, and postoperative marked decrease within 1 week
10. Flabby or atrophic muscles in lower limbs
11. Hypoactive deep tendon reflexes in lower limbs
12. No pain aggravation on straight leg-raising test
13. Patients with incontinence showed postvoid residual urine greater than 35 mL in all patients who complained of urinary incontinence.

Neurological signs and symptoms and musculoskeletal deformities are tabulated in

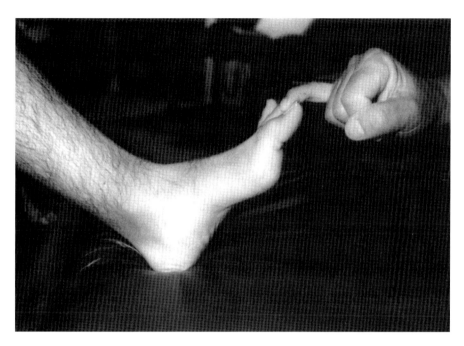

Fig. 15.5 At examination, mild but definite weakness of the extensor hallucis longus muscle was detected in this tethered cord syndrome patient, with the examiner using his little finger flexors to overcome dorsiflexion of the phalangeal joint in the patient's great toe. The patient regained normal strength of this muscle within a few days after untethering surgery.

Table 15.1. Negative findings are also important for diagnosis, such as the absence of a Babinski sign or straight leg-raising pain (except for one patient with concomitant herniated disk at L5–S1).

Table 15.1 Neurological Signs and Symptoms

Signs and Symptoms	%
Muscle weakness	94
Muscle atrophy	47
Gait difficulty	58
Sensory deficit	96
Bladder dysfunction	74
Anal sphincter dysfunction	90
Hyporeflexia of some of the knee and ankle jerks	95
Scoliosis	98
Exaggerated lumbosacral lordosis	74
Leg/foot deformity/high arches	76
Hammertoes	40
Leg or foot deformities/difference in length of legs or size of feet	3

Differential Diagnosis

To make a differential diagnosis of TCS, many other congenital or acquired diseases must be considered.

- Extradural lesions include acute herniated disk or recurrent herniated disk, inflammatory process of a disk, or painful disk degeneration, lateral recess syndrome or lumbar canal stenosis, epidural scar (pain due to irritation to the dura or spinal nerves) or pseudomeningocele-arachnoid cyst, and malignancy of the spine encroaching into the epidural space.
- Intradural-extramedullary lesions may produce symptoms similar to TCS, including meningiomas and schwannomas. A small schwannoma confined in the subarachnoid space needs to be considered in the differential diagnosis of TCS.
- Intramedullary lesions with symptoms overlapping or similar to those of TCS

include tumors, such as gliomas and ependymomas, which can be extraaxial, lumbosacral syringomyelia, multiple sclerosis, and exacerbation of poliomyelitis. Arachnoiditis or postoperative arachnoid adhesion that obliterates the subarachnoid space may result in spinal cord ischemia. For example, the authors found two cases that presented with TCS due to an encasement of the entire cauda equina with extensive arachnoid adhesion, causing lumbosacral cord tethering. After complete neurolysis of the entire cauda equina fibers, the lumbosacral cord was relaxed. Postoperatively both patients were completely free of back and leg pain and had subsidence of motor, sensory, and bladder dysfunction.

- Spine abnormalities, such as unstable lumbar and sacral spine or spondylolisthesis; lumbar facet syndrome or osteoarthritic spondylosis and ischiogluteal bursitis, trauma of vertebrae, fascia, muscle, and facet capsules also must be ruled out when seeking to diagnose TCS.
- Another complication in diagnosing TCS stems from lesions that originate outside the spinal canal. When back pain is the predominant symptom, for example, the pain may be due to TCS but it could also be due to (1) muscle spasms from physical overstress, (2) fibromyalgia, (3) peripheral nerve disorders, such as Guillain-Barré syndrome, (4) peripheral neuropathy due to diabetes mellitus, alcoholism, and heavy metal toxicity.

The most common area for confusion in the differential diagnosis of TCS is from a herniated lumbar or sacral herniated disk, and associated cauda equina syndrome. This diagnosis can easily be determined from the symptoms as shown in **Table 15.2**.

The diagnosis of TCS is clearly established with these characteristic signs and symptoms and with typical MRI findings. However, differential diagnosis of adult TCS requires special attention to three factors:

1. Signs and symptoms of TCS are subtle or their progression is insidious; in fact, patients are often referred to neurosurgeons as neurologically intact.
2. Acquired diseases in adults may obscure the typical signs and symptoms of TCS.
3. Imaging studies must be reviewed closely to find the characteristic features of TCS.

Table 15.2 Differential Diagnosis of Tethered Spinal Cord Syndrome

	Herniated Disk	Tethered Cord Syndrome
Radiating pain	+	−
Pain in inguinal and genitorectal area	−	+
Aggravated by coughing	+	−
Effects of 3B postures	−	+
Pain worse by slouching than by sitting straight	−	+
Pain worse on lying supine	−	+
Myotomal dysfunction	+	−
Dermatomal deficit	+	−
Perianal or distal hypalgesia	−	+
Extensive patchy hypalgesia	−	+
Incontinence	−	+
Paravertebral spasms	+	−
Pain on straight leg-raising test	+	−
Musculoskeletal deformities	−	+

■ Treatment

See Chapter 21 for a discussion of conservative treatment. Here we will discuss surgical treatment

Surgical Indications

Surgical indications for adult or pediatric TCS are determined by the combination of symptomatology and imaging studies. Symptomatology includes the following:

1. Aggravation of pain in the back and legs that is initiated or accentuated by repeated lumbosacral flexion and extension, particularly by special postural changes described in Signs and Symptoms
2. Physical exercises that accentuate spinal curvature
3. Progressive motor and sensory changes with skipped myotomal and dermatomal deficit, sometimes in sclerodermal distributions referred to bony or ligamentous structures[19]
4. Increasing difficulties with bladder or rectal control
5. Increasing lordosis or scoliosis or foot and toe deformities

The definite imaging signs of TCS are the posterior displacement of the conus medullaris and touching of the posterior arachnoid membrane by the filum;[5,21] however, there are other imaging signs that suggest TCS including the following:

1. A fibroadipose filum, although fat itself is not inelastic unless fibrous tissues grow together in large quantity
2. An elongated spinal cord[1,7–14]
3. A lipoma attached to the filum tip[24]
4. A thickened filum (Hoffman)
5. A capacious sacral sac, which is found in ~50% of our TCS patients[13] (**Fig. 15.6**)

Surgical Technique

If adult TCS is diagnosed, definitive treatment should be planned to reverse or prevent the

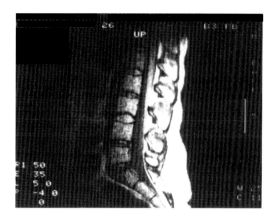

Fig. 15.6 T1-weighted magnetic resonance imaging shows a posteriorly displaced conus and a filum that is connected to high (fat) signal at the S2 vertebral canal and below. Note the capacious lumbosacral subarachnoid space.

progression of neurological deficits and spinal or foot deformities by releasing excessive tension within the spinal cord. The intraoperative stretch test is an important step to confirm lack of filum elasticity before the filum is sectioned.

Positioning

Under general endotracheal anesthesia, the patient is placed in the prone position, with the lumbosacral spine slightly flexed. Hyperflexion on the Wilson frame used for lumbar diskectomy should be avoided, or additional spinal cord stretching may precipitate spinal cord dysfunction.

Laminectomy

A laminectomy is performed at the level of the conus–filum junction, based on MRI or CT myelographic findings. If the junction is not clearly demonstrated by the imaging, laminectomy is done at the L2 or L3 level. Separation of the paraspinal muscles from the laminae should be limited medial to the facet to prevent avulsion of the mammillary branch, which could cause postoperative back muscle pain.

Intrathecal Endoscopy

Upon opening the dura, the tight filum is often found tenting the arachnoid membrane from underneath. A 2 to 3 mm long arachnoid incision is made in the midline with a Beaver blade, #59 knife, or microscissors. This tiny hole allows a curved endoscope to pass into the subarachnoid space. On the monitor, the posterior displacement of the filum is immediately identified. In each of two cases, a small extraaxial ependymoma was found at the caudal end of the conus, and in another case a small schwannoma was found arising from a sacral sensory nerve root.

Stretch Test

The dura and arachnoid are incised 1.5 cm long farther longitudinally. As soon as air enters the subarachnoid space, both the cauda equina and the filum sink anteriorly. However, the surgeon should be able to see the filum and isolate it from the surrounding cauda equina fibers, which are moving freely in the spinal fluid synchronous to pulsations, but the filum is seen tense, holding the conus tight. At this stage, a stretch test of the filum is performed by holding two points of the filum with two pairs of forceps and pulling them to the opposite direction (the cephalic forceps cephalad and the caudal forceps caudad). The fibrous or fibroadipose filum barely stretches (< 10%) with this maneuver in TCS patients, whereas the normal filum stretches at least 50% of the original length.

In addition, the following facts are to be remembered to enhance surgical efficiency. The conus is usually exposed medioposterior to the sensory nerve root attachments (**Figs. 15.7, 15.8**). The filum is sometimes found shifted laterally to the concave side of the scoliosis. (2) Under the microscope, the surgeon must determine the junction of the conus and filum before sectioning the filum by identifying the attachment of the lowest coccygeal nerve root as a landmark. This sensory nerve measures 100 to 150 μm in diameter. (3) The filum is often rotated as much as 90 degrees, and the anterior spinal vein is visible laterally on the anterior

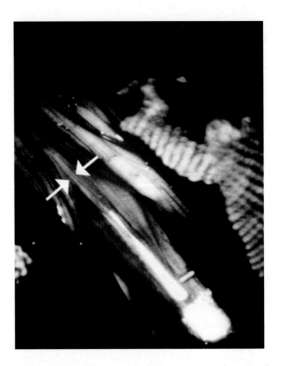

Fig. 15.7 The filum terminale (*arrows*) is inelastic and located posterior to the cauda equina fibers. The conus medullaris (*arrows*) is often found exposed between the cauda equina fibers. The filum is only 1.0 mm in diameter but inelastic and elongated less than 10% on the stretch test.

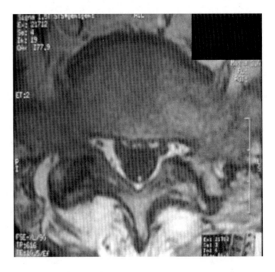

Fig. 15.8 The axial magnetic resonance imaging view for the same patient showed the filum pressing against the posterior arachnoid membrane.

surface of the filum. (4) The normal filum can be easily stretched and pulled freely into the open subarachnoid space and remains relaxed, even forming a coil like a noodle. Upon releasing the pull, however, the filum returns to its original shape and location within 15 minutes.

Partial Resection of the Filum

After the lack of filum viscoelasticity is confirmed, the filum is sectioned at two points with a Beaver blade knife or microscissors, 1 cm apart, at two points with the cephalic one 0.5 cm below the conus–filum junction. Two Wecke clips are placed at the sectioned ends. Postoperative CT scan demonstrates a gap between the two ends, 0.5 to 1.5 cm longer than the resected filum segment. The specimen is sent for histological studies.

Electrical stimulation of the nerve roots and filum is advocated to physiologically identify the filum,[13,25,26] whereas we determine the conus–filum junction anatomically with microscopic observation as described earlier.

■ Results

All surgical patients were relieved of leg pain on awakening from anesthesia. Neurological improvement followed, and postoperative back pain subsided within 2 weeks.

Motor power of patients with preoperative weakness improved after untethering procedures from the preoperative state 4/5 or 4+/5 to 5/5 in all patients, except one patient who had been involved in multiple motorcycle accidents since childhood. Accordingly, she had sustained leg fractures and peripheral nerve injuries, including the common peroneal nerve, yet showed improvement from preoperative $^3/_5$ to postoperative $^4/_5$ state. The sensory function improved to normal in patients who had hypalgesia in the distal legs and perianal area, or nearly normal.

Thirty-six of 50 patients with adult TCS (72%) complained of urinary control difficulties. Of these, 28 patients (77% of incontinent patients) who presented with stress or urge incontinence showed residual urine from 35 mL to more than 100 mL preoperatively, but 0 after surgery, and regained normal continence within 4 days. Of eight patients (23%) who presented with overflow incontinence with preoperative residual urine greater than 45 mL, six patients regained continence with postoperative residual urine less than 45 mL, and the other two patients who practiced intermittent catheterization for longer than 8 years still required catheterization after surgery. In all 50 patients, anal sphincter reflex was diminished preop but improved to normal or nearly normal after surgery.

An interesting finding is that as ambulation increased, postoperative patients complained of stress-induced muscle pain in their back and legs. This pain was described as similar to what paraparetic patients experience during muscle training. The duration of this pain depended on the preoperative pain severity and duration, with full disappearance after 3 to 18 months of muscle-strengthening therapy. Following surgery, 95% of patients had complete pain relief, and the others had marked pain reduction and resumed their jobs or daily work.

■ Case Reports

Case 1

A 38-year-old man complained of low back pain stemming from an automobile accident approximately 1 year earlier, although he did not actually notice the back pain until 2 days after the accident. He returned to work as a construction worker; however, the back pain persisted, necessitating that he work only 4 hours per day. After 3 weeks, he was laid off because he could not meet the contractual deadline required for his job. Bending slightly over the sink aggravated the low back pain, and tasks such as dishwashing could be tolerated for only a few minutes. He could not sit cross-legged (**Fig. 15.9A,B**) or pick up and hold his 2-year-old son while standing. The pain was partially alleviated by relaxed

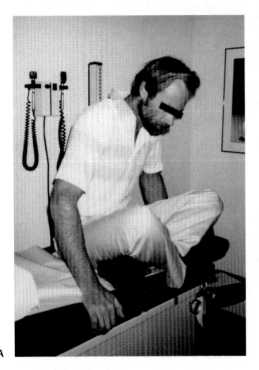
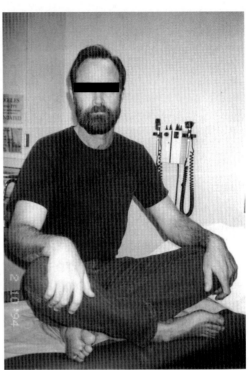
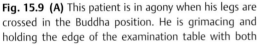

A

B

Fig. 15.9 (A) This patient is in agony when his legs are crossed in the Buddha position. He is grimacing and holding the edge of the examination table with both hands, trying to ease the back and leg pain. **(B)** The same patient is sitting comfortably in the Buddha position 3 weeks after surgery.

sitting or standing, but moving from one position to another caused it to worsen considerably. Physical therapy relieved his pain only slightly and temporarily. The patient reported "running to the bathroom" to avoid soiling his pants. Past medical history revealed seminoma of a testicle, which was resected successfully and irradiated. Physical examination showed an accentuated lordosis of the lumbar spine: ability to only touch his knees with the fingertips due to limited thoracolumbar flexibility and slightly high-arched feet. Neurological findings were mild weakness of the extensor hallucis longus muscles, diminished pinprick sensation in a patchy distribution in lower limbs, more so on the right than the left; no rectal tone found on digital insertion; decreased anal wink reflex to both right and left stimulation; and hypoactive right knee tendon reflex. MRI abnormalities were an elongated cord and slightly thick filum, and posterior displacement of the conus and filum.

After laminectomies at the L2 through L5 vertebrae, a fatty filum terminale was found, continuous to the conus at the level of the L5 vertebral body. The filum was sectioned below the attachment of the lowest coccygeal nerve to the spinal cord. The spinal cord immediately ascended and relaxed, resulting in a 1 cm gap between the two-sectioned ends.

One week after surgery, the patient began to ambulate and had complete relief from back and leg pain. By the 6-week clinical visit, motor, sensory, and rectal functions had returned to normal; he sat cross-legged, leaned over the sink without developing pain, and touched his toes. The high arch of his feet subsided within 2 years. The patient returned to his regular work 2 months after surgery.

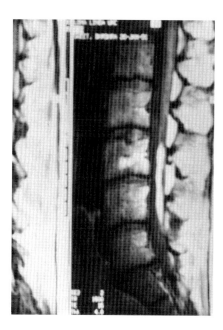

Fig. 15.10 T1-weighted magnetic resonance imaging, lateral view, demonstrates posterior displacement of the conus and filum, and high (fat) signal within the filum. At operation the filum was inelastic and found to be replaced by fibroadipose tissue, and adipose tissue extended into the conus.

Case 2

A 26-year-old woman fell during triathlon training and developed severe back and leg pain. Nine months of medical and physical treatment were of no effect. The referral diagnosis was a combination of herniated disk, back muscle sprain, and psychogenic factors. Pain was so severe that she could only walk a few yards at a time. She also complained of urinary incontinence (occasional dribbling), severe back stiffening, and patchy sensory changes in the thighs, legs, and genital area. Her leg muscles were flabby and thinner than they were prior to her fall but their motor power was within normal limits. Posterior displacement of the filum terminale was shown on MRI (**Fig. 15.10**). Urinary residual was 100 mL.

At surgery, the caudal tip of the conus was located at the L3 level (**Fig. 15.11A,B**), and the thick fibroadipose filum was sectioned. Her back and leg pain was relieved. As physical

therapy progressed, functional and occupational activities improved in both Prolos scores up to 5.[27] Four years after surgery, she graduated from college with a psychology degree and has returned to triathlon training. Her urinary control has returned to normal.

Case 3

A 36-year-old high school teacher, one of twin brothers, presented with a 10-year history of low back pain, some difficulty walking and urinary control. These symptoms worsened following a motor vehicle accident 1 year before presentation, when his car was hit from the side by another car. He complained of difficulty in continuing lectures because bending over the podium caused intolerable back pain. On examination, he showed difficulty sitting with legs crossed in a Buddha pose; weakness ($^4/_5$) in his left extensor hallucis longus and brevis and tibialis anterior; decreased sensation to pinprick in the dorsa of his feet, anterior thighs, gluteal regions, and the first and second toes bilaterally. His MRI of the lumbar spine reported that the conus tip was located opposite the L1 vertebra. An L1–2 laminectomy and division of a 1.3 mm thick inelastic filum terminale was performed, he was relieved of leg pain on awakening from anesthesia. Neurological improvement followed rapidly and he returned to teaching within 6 weeks. At his 2-month appointment, he brought his identical twin brother with a very similar symptomatology to our clinic. The second brother also underwent the same surgery and had an excellent recovery.

■ Discussion

Tethered Cord Syndrome and Various Interpretation and Prognosis

Pang extensively studied clinical cases of adult TCS, including those with a combination of elongated spinal cord and thickened filum, MMC, LMMC, occult MMC, fibrous adhesion, diastematomyelia,

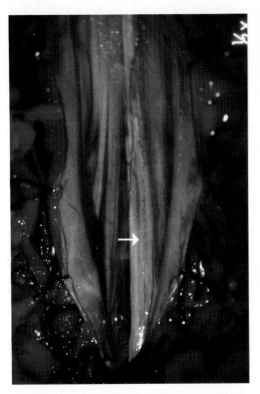
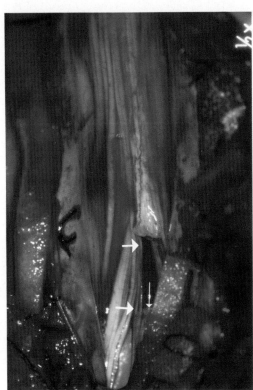

A

B

Fig. 15.11 Case 2. **(A)** The spinal cord is elongated, with its caudal end at the L3 vertebral level. The arrow indicates the lowest coccygeal nerve root. **(B)** A 1.2 cm gap developed after sectioning the filum, which was almost entirely replaced by fibroadipose tissue (*arrows*).

postmyelomeningocele repair, and dermal sinus tract.[13] Other publications on TCS followed with similar selection of anomalies.[10,12,14] Separately, Yamada et al selected adult TCS patients with only an inelastic filum, with or without thickening, and associated either with or without cord elongation.[5,21] Iskandar and colleagues described TCS patients with an elongated cord and thickened filum and those with LMMC.[11] Statistically and theoretically, surgical outcome is best in the cases with only inelastic filum, the least favorable is the postoperative repair cases. The surgical results of LMMC and MMC repair come between, with the former better than latter.[5,9,12,13,21,28–30]

The differences in the surgical outcome between various authors can be explained by the following analysis. The visual-impression-originated expression *cord tethering* was pathophysiologically grouped into three categories by Yamada and Won.[18]

Category 1 includes patients with the mechanical tethering site located at the caudal end of the spinal cord. The caudal LMMC and sacral MMC along with an inelastic filum are designated as category 1, the true TCS. These patients have excellent surgical outcome, although those with MMC and LMMC are not included in this series. Category 2 patients have variable surgical results and are divided into category 2A and 2B. Category 2A patients with a large dorsal or transitional LMMC and large plaque of MMC covering the lumbosacral cord often have no neurological improvement after surgical repair. Category 2B patients with a smaller LMMC and those with MMC that has a relatively small plaque have relatively better surgical outcome than the former group. Our group 1 adult TCS patients correspond to category-2B. Category 3 patients have no physiological function in the region of the lumbosacral cord (see Chapter 3 and Chapter 21).

Anatomical and Metabolic Implications in TCS

Since the publication of the "tethered spinal cord: its protean manifestations, diagnosis and Surgical Correction (please see reference 3)" by Hoffman et al[29], the combination of an elongated cord and a thickened filum has been emphasized as the structural characteristic abnormality of this disorder. We analyze the spinal cord length and filum diameter in normal individuals relative to TCS patients.

Spine and Spinal Cord Growth

Because the vertebral column grows faster than the spinal cord from the embryonic stage (ninth week of gestation) to early childhood, the spinal cord ascends in the spinal canal.[31,32] By 3 years of age (as in adults), the T12 and S1 cord segments lie between the T10 and L1 vertebrae,[33] and the caudal end of the cord is opposite the L1 or L2 vertebra.[24,33] Only 0.7%[34] or 7%[35] of unselected autopsy cases showed the caudal end of the spinal cord located opposite the L3 vertebra. The elongation of the spinal cord occurs primarily in the lumbosacral segments,[13] apparently secondary to stretching effect between the inelastic filum and the attachment of the lowest pair of dentate ligaments. This assumption can be made from the evidence that integrated fibers (not the growing axons) grow faster under stretching stress.[31,36] Therefore the cord elongation in TCS patients responds appropriately to stretch stress as compensation, and it is only under additional stretch stress, such as excessively rapid spinal growth and forceful flexion and extension that signs and symptoms of TCS would develop.

Filum Diameter

The normal filum diameter is reported as 1.1 or 1.2 mm.[37] The minimal filum diameter claimed to be diagnostic for TCS range from 1 mm[38] to 2 mm.[39,40] It seems that the filum thickness is not reliable for TCS diagnosis. Selden took an intermediate position in pediatric patients with TCS, where the filum thickness is crowded between 1.5 and 2.0 mm.[41]

Relevance of Abnormal Cord Length and Filum Thickness to TCS

Earlier, Warder and Oakes reported that 18% of the TCS patients showed the conus tip above the L1–2 interspace.[4] Our statistics showed 30% of our adult and later teenage patients failed to show either elongated cord (below L2–3 interspace) and thickened filum (equal to or greater than 2 mm), and > 50% of MRIs are negative for cord elongation and filum thickening. These data support that the cord elongation and filum thickening are of relative importance for TCS, and the essential mechanical cause for TCS is the traction effect of the inelastic filum. The subtle signs and symptoms reflect mild metabolic and physiological derangement in TCS without histological damage, and help explain the effectiveness of surgical untethering in reversing TCS symptomatology.

Delayed Manifestation of TCS in Adulthood

There are intrinsic and extrinsic mechanisms that explain the signs and symptoms that appear in late teenage years and adulthood.

1. Intrinsic factors

   a. Cumulative effects of oxidative metabolic impairment on neuronal function, similar to those in cats that were subjected to repeated cord traction, show prolonged cytochrome reduction.[42]

   b. Progressive fibrosis starting from the caudal end of the filum to involve its entire length, resulting in loss of filum viscoelasticity

2. Extrinsic factors

   a. Increasing physical activities due to repeated spinal cord stretching by increasing spinal mobility such as extreme flexion and extension (e.g., high leg-kicking for a dancer or in aerobic exercising, or leg stretching in yoga posturing, in contact sports, and running)

b. Single or multiple sudden blows to the back, often from rear-end automobile accidents or sitting down hard on the floor, thus causing a sudden straightening of the lumbosacral spine and stretching of the spinal cord

c. Osteophyte formation and thickening of the ligamentum flavum, which restricts cephalad movement of the spinal cord

Failed Back Syndrome and Tethered Spinal Cord Syndrome

A question is asked as to why the patients with TCS are undiagnosed and categorized as failed back syndrome.

First, many physicians are unaware of subtle signs and symptoms typical for TCS. In particular, aggravation of back pain by postural changes is the absolutely necessary symptom that must be documented to diagnose adult TCS. In our experience, no description of this symptom has been found in reports on patients who were referred as low back pain of unknown cause (failed back syndrome). Precise description of motor function (e.g., weakness of extensor hallucis longus, peroneus longus, perianal sensory loss) are often overlooked.

Second, the combination of an elongated cord and a thick filum was overemphasized, and MRI findings without these features are considered nondiagnostic for TCS. Whether the posterior displacement of the filum is present is not described.

Third, the negative findings such as no radiating pain in the legs and no leg pain aggravation by coughing or by straight leg-raising test are also diagnostically important.

Urinary and Rectal Incontinence

A high percentage of adult TCS patients suffer urinary or rectal incontinence (70%) similar to the statistics of others.[5,12,13] Considering the experimental model of tethered spinal cord, the conus is vulnerable to traction from the caudal end of the spinal cord (see Chapter 3). It is unfortunate that some patients were totally incontinent, requiring intermittent catheterization. These patients have clear memory of when they started to have intermittent dribbling or retention, and how soon afterward they became totally incontinent; usually constantly dribbling or intermittently pouring urine. They may have avoided such a serious state with untethering surgery performed during their early dribbling period. We believe that postvoid urinary residual measurement provides physicians with the warning sign for prompt and appropriate treatment. There is a high incidence of diminished reflex or voluntary sphincter contraction, which is similar to the urinary control through the conus. Constipation is listed as a frequent symptom for TCS,[12,13] but it is controlled by the balance between the vagus and sympathetic system control, and TCS itself may not be greatly contributing to its mechanism.

Mechanism of Back and Leg Pain

1. Based on clinical examinations, the pain that patients describe as vague and often dull in the low back and legs is directed to the musculature in the thighs or legs. Postoperatively, it becomes apparent that preoperative pain disappeared on awakening from anesthesia, but when physical therapy begins, patients begin to have pain in the back and leg muscles, and admit the location of the preoperative pain and postoperative pain is exactly the same. We postulate that mechanisms of pain in TCS patients is muscular in origin, caused by excitation of the sensory-motor synapses in the interneuron pool of the tethered spinal cord, similar to mildly ischemic neurons.[43,44]

2. Back and leg pain is expressed as muscle cramping, pulling, or tearing, after TCS patients sustain a sudden blow to the back at an automobile accident, particularly

rear-end collision, sit hard on the floor, misstep into a hole, fall downstairs, or perform repeated forceful flexion and extension of the lumbosacral spine.[13,42] Spinal cord stretching that occurs simultaneously to these spinal dynamic changes is likely to cause instant back and leg muscle contractions, followed by skeletal muscle spasms. The pain due to spasms is similar to an incapacitating muscle pain that highly trained athletes develop after an episode of strenuous muscle pull.

3. Pain sensation may be elicited by stretching of the dorsal root entry zone.

4. Stretching of the sensory sacral nerve roots that travel caudad from their spinal cord attachment to the fibrosed foraminal tissue may be the cause of leg pain in children because relaxation of these nerve roots after untethering is followed by pain relief. (McLone DG, personal communication, 2004). However, we have not observed such an occasion in adult cases.

5. Referred pain may be an important factor in the differential diagnosis of TCS. The lesion in the upper lumbar vertebrae or in the lower lumbar facets[45] may cause referred pain in the groin region. Pain in the buttock or greater trochanteric area may be referred from the facet lesions, due to innervation overlap with various sensory distributions of the spinal cord.[46]

Socioeconomic Considerations

Failed back syndrome or failed back surgery syndrome has been considered to be a serious socioeconomic problem, requiring prolonged multidisciplinary treatment by various specialists including neurosurgeons, neurologists, physiatrists, physiotherapists, orthopedic surgeons, rheumatologists, psychiatrists, psychologists, and other specialists.[47] An early diagnosis and proper treatment of TCS can significantly reduce the expenses inherent to this disorder.

■ Conclusion

Despite a clear-cut definition of TCS, there has been misunderstanding of this syndrome. Clinicians must clearly distinguish between category 1, 2, and 3 of visually oriented cord tethering, and further identify the basic differences between group 1 and group 2 adult TCS patients. Reliance upon the combination of an elongated cord and a thickened filum as a requirement for diagnosis overlooks TCS, especially in adult and late teenage patients. Keys to the proper diagnosis and treatment of TCS are the understanding of typical signs and symptoms and MRI findings. Complex ramification of diagnosis, treatment, and prognosis of TCS can be solved by understanding the pathophysiology.

References

1. Yamada S, Zinke DE, Sanders D. Pathophysiology of "tethered cord syndrome." J Neurosurg 1981;54:494–503

2. Yamada S, Iacono R, Morgese V, Douglas C. Tethered cord syndrome in adults. In: Menezes A, Sonntag VK, eds. Principles in Spinal Surgery. New York: McGraw-Hill; 1996:433–445

3. Hoffman HJ, Hendrick EB, Humphreys RP. The tethered spinal cord: its protean manifestations, diagnosis and surgical correction. Childs Brain 1976;2:145–155

4. Warder DE, Oakes WJ. Tethered cord syndrome and the conus in a normal position. Neurosurgery 1993;33:374–378

5. Yamada S, Lonser RR. Adult tethered cord syndrome. J Spinal Disord 2000;13:319–323

6. Yamada S, Clark L. Tethered cord syndrome. Contemporary Neurosurgery. 1990;12:1–6

7. Cochrane DD. Cord untethering for lipomyelomeningocele: expectation after surgery. Neurosurg Focus 2007;23:1–7

8. Gupta SK, Khosla VK, Sharma BS, Mathuriya SN, Pathak A, Tewari MK. Tethered cord syndrome in adults. Surg Neurol 1999;52:362–369, discussion 370

9. Finn M, Walker ML. Spinal lipomas: clinical spectrum, embryology, and treatment. Neurosurg Focus 2007;23:1–12

10. Hüttmann S, Krauss J, Collmann H, Sörensen N, Roosen K. Surgical management of tethered spinal cord in adults: report of 54 cases. J Neurosurg 2001;95 (2, Suppl):173–178

11. Iskandar BJ, Fulmer BB, Hadley MN, Oakes WJ. Congenital tethered spinal cord syndrome in adults. J Neurosurg 1998;88:958–961

12. Lee GYE, Paradiso G, Tator CH, Gentili F, Massicotte EM, Fehlings MG. Surgical management of tethered cord syndrome in adults: indications, techniques, and long-term outcomes in 60 patients. J Neurosurg Spine 2006;4:123–131

13. Pang D, Wilberger JE Jr. Tethered cord syndrome in adults. J Neurosurg 1982;57:32–47

14. van Leeuwen R, Notermans NC, Vandertop WP. Surgery in adults with tethered cord syndrome: outcome study with independent clinical review. J Neurosurg 2001;94 (2, Suppl):205–209

15. Wilkinson HA. The Failed Back Syndrome, Etiology and Therapy. 2nd ed. New York: Springer-Verlag; 1992

16. Zucherman J, Schofferman J. Pathology of the failed back surgery syndrome. In: White AH, ed. Failed Back Surgery Syndrome. Philadelphia: Hanley Belfus; 1996:159–175

17. Yamada S, Won DJ, Siddiqi J, Colohan ART. Tethered cord syndrome presented as failed back syndrome. Presented at: Annual Meeting of the American Association of Neurological Surgeons/Congress of Neurological Surgeons Pain; April 25, 2008; Chicago, IL

18. Yamada S, Won DJ. What is the true tethered cord syndrome? Childs Nerv Syst 2007;23:371–375

19. Austin GM. Dermatomes, sclerotomes and spinal cord relationship. In: Austin GM, ed. The Spinal Cord. 3rd ed. New York: Igaku-Shoin; 1983:727–750

20. Yamada S, Won DJ, Yamada BS, Colohan ATR, Siddiqi J. Post-void urinary residual for evaluation of tethered cord syndrome. Poster presented at: Annual Meeting of American Association of Neurological Surgeons; April 27–May 1, 2008; Chicago, IL

21. Yamada S, Won DJ, Kido DK. Adult tethered cord syndrome: new classification correlated with symptomatology, imaging and pathophysiology. Neurosurg Q 2001;11:260–275

22. Guo WY, Ono S, Oi S, et al. Dynamic motion analysis of fetuses with central nervous system disorders by cine magnetic resonance imaging using fast imaging employing steady-state acquisition and parallel imaging: a preliminary result. J Neurosurg 2006;105 (2, Suppl):94–100

23. Yamada S, Siddiqi J, Won DJ, et al. Symptomatic protocols for adult tethered cord syndrome. Neurol Res 2004;26:741–744

24. McLone DG, Naidich TP. The tethered spinal cord. In: McLaurin RL, Schut I, Venes JL, Epstein F, eds. Pediatric Neurosurgery. 2nd ed. Philadelphia: WB Saunders; 1989:76–96

25. James HE, Mulcahy JJ, Walsh JW, Kaplan GW. Use of anal sphincter electromyography during operations on the conus medullaris and sacral nerve roots. Neurosurgery 1979;4:521–523

26. Quinones-Hinojosa A, Garkary CA, Gulati M, et al. Clinical outcome of adults after neurophysiologically monitored tethered cord release surgery. Surg Neurol 2004;62:127–135

27. Prolo DJ, Oklund SA, Butcher M. Toward uniformity in evaluating results of lumbar spine operations: a paradigm applied to posterior lumbar interbody fusions. Spine 1986;11:601–606

28. Garceau GJ. The filum terminale syndrome (the cord-traction syndrome). J Bone Joint Surg Am 1953;35-A:711–716

29. Hoffmann GT, Hooks CA, Jackson IJ, Thompson IM. Urinary incontinence in myelomeningoceles due to a tethered spinal cord and its surgical treatment. Surg Gynecol Obstet 1956;103:618–624

30. James CCM, Lassman LP. Spinal dysraphism: the diagnosis and treatment of progressive lesions in spina bifida occulta. J Bone Joint Surg Br 1962;44:828–840

31. Barry A, Patten BM, Stewart BH. Possible factors in the development of the Arnold-Chiari malformation. J Neurosurg 1957;14:285–301

32. Kunitomo K. The development and reduction of the tail and of the caudal end of the spinal cord. Contrib Embryol Carnegie Inst 1978;8:161–198

33. Yamada S, Perot PL Jr, Ducker TB, Lockard I. Myelotomy for control of mass spasms in paraplegia. J Neurosurg 1976;45:683–691

34. Reimann AF, Anson BJ. Vertebral level of termination of the spinal cord with report of a case of sacral cord. Anat Rec 1944;88:127–138

35. Tubbs RS, Elton S, Bartolucci AA, Grabb PA, Oakes WJ. The position of the conus medullaris in children with a Chiari I malformation. Pediatr Neurosurg 2000;33:249–251

36. Pfister BJ, Iwata A, Meaney DF, Smith DH. Extreme stretch growth of integrated axons. J Neurosci 2004;24:7978–7983

37. Yundt KD, Park TS, Kaufman BA. Normal diameter of filum terminale in children: in vivo measurement. Pediatr Neurosurg 1997;27:257–259

38. Hochhauser L, Chaung S, Harwood-Nash DS, Armstrong D, Savoie J. The tethered cord syndrome revisited [abstract]. AJNR Am J Neuroradiol 1986; 7:543

39. Harwood-Nash D. Neuroradiology A: computed tomography. In: Holtzman RNN, Stein BM, eds. The Tethered Spinal Cord. New York: Thieme-Stratton; 1985:41–46

40. Pang D. Tethered cord syndrome. In: Hoffman HJ, ed. Advances in Neurosurgery. Vol 1, no 1. Philadelphia: Hanley and Belfus; 1986:45–79

41. Selden NR. Occult tethered cord syndrome: the case for surgery. J Neurosurg 2006;104(5, Suppl):302–304

42. Yamada S, Won DJ, Pezeshkpour G, et al. Pathophysiology of tethered cord syndrome and similar complex disorders. Neurosurg Focus 2007;23:1–10

43. Yamada S, Sanders DC, Haugen GE. Functional and metabolic responses of the spinal cord to anoxia and asphyxia. Proceedings of the 13th Annual Meeting of the Federation of Western Societies of Neurological Science. In: Austin GM, ed. Contemporary Aspects of Cerebrovascular Disease. Dallas: Professional Information Library; 1976:239–246

44. Yamada S, Sanders DC, Maeda G. Oxidative metabolism during and following ischemia of cat spinal cord. Neurol Res 1981;3:1–16

45. McCall IW, Park WM, O'Brien JP. Induced pain referral from posterior lumbar elements in normal subjects. Spine 1979;4:441–446

46. Descartes E. L'Homme. Paris: C Angot, 1664. Cited by Weinstein JN. The perception of pain. In: Kirkaldy-Willis WH, ed. Managing Low Back Pain. 2nd ed. New York: Churchill Livingstone; 1988:83–90

47. Yamada S, Siddiqi J, Yamada SM, Yamada VA. Tethered cod syndrome with new conceptual development. Arab J Neurosurgery 2009; In press

16 Tethered Cord Syndrome in Adults with Spina Bifida Occulta

Sharad Rajpal, Samir B. Lapsiwala, and Bermans J. Iskandar

Congenital tethered cord syndrome (TCS) presenting in adulthood is an uncommon entity that can potentially become symptomatic. The management of adult-onset TCS, however, remains controversial even though the necessity of early surgery in children with TCS is well established. The long-term surgical outcome after tethered cord release (TCR) in the adult population is generally favorable because most patients report improvement or stabilization of their symptoms. In addition, the overall postoperative complication rate is low. Although special consideration should be given to older patients with a poor general medical condition, it seems reasonable to recommend early surgical treatment in patients with TCS as well as asymptomatic patients with spina bifida occulta. This chapter reviews the major publications that discuss congenital tethered spinal cord (spina bifida occulta) presenting in adulthood. Data discussing acquired tethered cord from prior myelomeningocele repair will not be addressed.

Congenital anomalies of the spinal cord arise from incomplete formation of the dorsal midline structures and comprise a spectrum of malformations involving the neural tissue, meninges, bone, and skin. These malformations are divided into two broad categories: spina bifida aperta (SBA) and spina bifida occulta (SBO). SBO represents a set of "covered" spinal cord lesions that include lipomyelomeningocele (LMM), split cord malformation (SCM), meningocele manqué (MM), ectodermal inclusion tumor or cyst, neurenteric cyst, and tight filum terminale. SBO lesions are often concealed, or occult, even though coexisting cutaneous (hypertrichosis, capillary hemangioma, subcutaneous lipoma, dermal sinus, caudal appendage, atretic meningocele) or orthopedic (musculoskeletal) anomalies, including vertebrae or lower extremity manifestations are present in greater than half the cases. The absence of such external stigmata may delay diagnosis until later in life.

Tethering, or stretching of the spinal cord, results from fixation of the cord by inelastic structures. Most SBO lesions cause spinal cord tethering by their mere presence; such pathophysiology is similar to that caused by scar tissue following myelomeningocele repair[1] (refer to Chapters 3 and 11 on pathophysiology and on myelomeningocele and lipomyelomeningocele for details). In fact, some cases of postrepair myelomeningocele TCS may be caused by residual tandem lesions, such as a tight filum terminale or SCM, which is not recognized at the time of initial myelomeningocele closure.[2] Regardless of the cause of tethering, the physiological changes that occur within the spinal cord and the resultant clinical presentation seem to be consistent, but the age of presentation can be variable.

It is well established that all children with SBO require TCR to prevent neurourological deficits.[3] The situation is less clear, however, in adult-onset congenital TCS, mainly because of the lack of natural history studies.[4,5]

In this chapter, we review the clinical and radiographic characteristics of SBO presenting in adulthood using a broad literature search. Then, based on major relevant publications, we discuss the specific criteria for diagnosis and surgical management of this patient population, with special emphasis on the evidence for or against preventive surgery. Neither SBA (adult and pediatric) nor pediatric SBO is discussed, and publications that include such patients are not addressed.

■ Method and Materials

We systematically reviewed the literature on adult TCS using a Medline search. Most series reported mixed data that included either mixed SBO and SBA patients or mixed adult and pediatric populations. Fourteen series of adult TCS were found, but only five reported either adult SBO-only data or presented data in a fashion that allowed the exclusion of children and SBA patients.[6-9] The remaining nine series were excluded (**Table 16.1**). The largest SBO-only pediatric tethered cord series to date was used to compare adult and pediatric outcomes.[2] Because all patients with SBO are assumed tethered, the terms *SBO* and *TCS* are used interchangeably in this chapter. Because of the paucity of data in adults, we will not attempt to subclassify our discussion of the congenital TCS according to the various spinal anomalies.

■ Results

Classification of Adult-Onset Spina Bifida Occulta

Congenital TCS in adulthood presents more often in females (M:F ratio 1:1.3 to 1:2.8), and patient ages can range from 18 to 75 years (mean 37 years).[4,5,9,10] Although the majority of these patients present with symptoms of TCS, some are discovered incidentally (e.g., cutaneous or orthopedic anomalies that were previously unrecognized). Symptomatic patients are divided into three groups according to the classification by Pang and Wilberger[5]: (1) patients with no neurourological deficits, cutaneous, or skeletal anomalies in childhood, but with symptom development later in life; (2) patients with either cutaneous and skeletal deformities or stable neurological deficits in childhood but who suffer progressive neurological symptoms and signs starting in adulthood (some of these patients may have undergone corrective surgery for orthopedic, urological, or cosmetic cutaneous problems earlier in life); and (3) patients with progressive neurological symptoms and signs starting in childhood and continuing into adulthood.

Approximately 75% of adult patients remember precise circumstances leading to the acute onset of symptoms. Pang and Wilberger grouped these symptoms into three pathophysiological mechanisms.[5] The first mechanism

Table 16.1   Reasons for Exclusion of Large Reported Series from this Review

Authors	Reason for Exclusion
Begeer et al[28]	Mixed adult and pediatric populations
Huttmann et al[11]	Mixed SBO and SBA data
Kirollos et al[4]	Mixed SBO and SBA data; mixed adult and pediatric populations
Koyanagi et al[29]	Mixed adult and pediatric populations
Lee et al[30]	Mixed SBO and SBA data
Pang et al[5]	Mixed SBO and SBA data
Sharif et al[31]	Mixed SBO and SBA data; mixed adult and pediatric populations
Van Leeuwen et al[10]	Mixed SBO and SBA data
Yamada et al[16]	Mixed SBO and SBA data

Abbreviations: SBA, spina bifida aperta; SBO, spina bifida occulta.

(50% of cases) consists of momentary stretching of a tethered conus medullaris, as would occur after prolonged sitting, forward bending, straight leg-raising exercise, or being placed in the lithotomy position during childbirth.[5,11] The second mechanism (20% of precipitating events) consists of spinal canal narrowing from lumbar spondylosis and/or disk herniation with crowding of intraspinal contents in the presence of a TCS, and can be attributed to activities such as heavy lifting. The third mechanism involves trauma to the low back or buttocks as can occur with sudden forward and backward bending during a motor vehicle accident. There remains a 3- to 8-year delay between symptom onset and actual diagnosis.[5,8,11,12]

Approximately two thirds of SBO patients have cutaneous anomalies (**Fig. 16.1**).[6,8,9] These cutaneous anomalies are often ignored or surgically removed for cosmetic reasons without concomitant attention to the spinal abnormality (these patients fit into group 2 of Pang's classification scheme). Musculoskeletal deformities include lumbosacral lordosis; foot deformities such as high-arched feet and hammer toes; vertebral anomalies such as a bony septum or split vertebrae; and sacral agenesis. Mild scoliosis is present in up to 20% of patients,[9] and the incidence of foot deformities ranges from 11 to 33%.[6,8,9] The spinal cord is tethered by a variety

of spinal anomalies in 11 to 20% of patients with sacral agenesis or an imperforate anus; thus the classic recommendation is to obtain magnetic resonance imaging (MRI) on all patients with caudal regression syndrome of any severity.[3,13,14]

Presenting Signs and Symptoms

Pain

Low back and/or leg pain is the most common finding in adults with SBO-related TCS (**Fig. 16.2**).[2,6–9] Pain occurs in a nondermatomal pattern with a shocklike sensation and burning quality. In a series of 61 adult patients by Rajpal[15] et al, 34 (56%) and 30 (49%) patients presented with back and leg pain, respectively.[2] Pain is usually exacerbated by physical activity, particularly involving flexion and extension of the lumbosacral area. Yamada[12] et al described three postural changes that typically worsen pain in TCS patients. These were referred to as the "three B's": (1) the inability to sit with the legs crossed like Buddha, (2) difficulty with slight bending at the waist, and (3) holding a baby or light object (< 2.3 kg) at waist level while standing. These maneuvers straighten the lordotic lumbosacral spine and presumably stretch the tethered spinal cord. Tethered cord pain thus

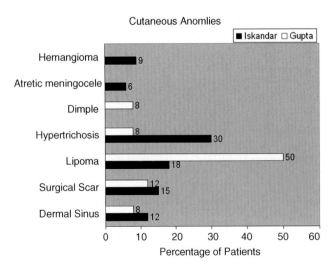

Fig. 16.1 Bar graph depicting the percentage of patients with cutaneous anomalies as reported in the Iskandar and Gupta series of adult patients with tethered cord syndrome.[8,9] The term *surgical scar* is used to describe several patients who underwent previous surgery to correct cutaneous deformities.

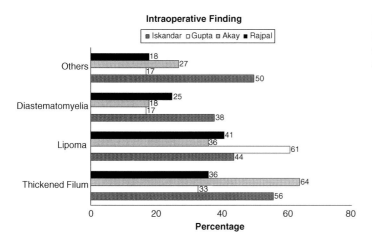

Fig. 16.2 Bar graph displaying the percentage of patients with the various spinal anomalies noted intraoperatively.[1,7,10,11]

often worsens with sitting, straining, and prolonged bed rest due to increased tension on the spinal cord caused by straightening of the lumbar curvature.

Sensorimotor Symptoms and Signs

Progressive leg weakness, paresthesias, and gait difficulty are common findings in SBO. Between 49 and 80% of adult patients with TCS present with motor or sensory signs or symptoms (**Fig. 16.2**).[2,6–9] Motor deficits are usually asymmetric and include atrophy of the lower limbs, whereas sensory changes affect the lower lumbar and sacral regions and typically do not follow a specific dermatomal distribution.

Genitourinary Dysfunction

A history of sexual dysfunction should alert physicians that further evaluation might be necessary. Approximately 35% of adult patients present with bowel or bladder dysfunction

(**Table 16.2**), and only 3% complained of sexual dysfunction (e.g., dyspareunia, retrograde ejaculation).[2] Bladder dysfunction includes spastic small-capacity bladders with uninhibited contractions, hypotonic large-capacity bladders, and frequent urinary tract infections. At our institution, we routinely obtain preoperative urodynamic studies on all patients. Urodynamic studies may reveal low bladder capacity, overflow incontinence, detrusor-sphincter dyssynergia, or a spastic bladder. Bowel incontinence in adult SBO is rare but has been reported to occur in ~10% of patients.[5,10]

Imaging Studies

In addition to high clinical suspicion, imaging studies are essential in diagnosing SBO, as well as for operative planning. MRI findings compatible with a tethered spinal cord include a tight filum terminale, characterized most commonly by a low-lying conus medullaris[10] or the presence of a thick (> 2 mm) and fatty

Table 16.2 Clinical Presentation of Adults with Congenital Tethered Cord Syndrome

Authors	Number of Patients	Pain	Sensorimotor Symptoms or Signs	Bowel or Bladder Dysfunction
Akay et al[6]	11	11(100%)	3(27%)	4(36%)
Filler et al[9]	12	6(50%)	8(67%)	8(67%)
Gupta et al[8]	18	9(50%)	15(83%)	6(33%)
Iskandar et al[9]	34	27(79%)	27(79%)	18(53%)
Rajpal et al[15]	61	45(74%)	30(49%)	21(35%)

filum terminale, LMM, SCM, MM, ectodermal inclusion tumor, or cyst with an associated dermal sinus tract.[3,16] The association between TCS and the presence of fat in the filum is discussed in detail elsewhere.[17] A preoperative cystometrogram may show a clinically subtle urodynamic deficit and may serve as a baseline for postoperative follow-up.

Surgical Treatment

After a complete workup including careful history, physical examination, MRI, and urodynamic studies, treatment consists of surgical release of the tethered cord. The operation involves a laminectomy followed by dural opening and release of all tethering structures. This may involve sectioning of a tight filum, split cord release from a midline septum, lipoma removal, and others. Arachnoidal adhesions and tethering bands, when present, should be lysed. Intraoperative electrophysiological monitoring with posterior tibial somatosensory evoked potentials (SSEPs), lower extremity and anal sphincter electromyography (EMG), and/or cystomanometry may be used at the discretion of the surgeon. It is recommended that the dura be closed using a synthetic or autologous dural graft to provide a capacious dural sac and minimize the chance of retethering. This is particularly helpful after LMM repair.

Intraoperative Findings

The most common congenital spinal anomalies that cause cord tethering are displayed in **Fig. 16.2**. In the series by Rajpal et al,[15] 41% of patients had an LMM, 36% had a thick/fatty filum, 25% had an SCM, 11% had a syringomyelia, 3% had a dermoid cyst/tumor, and 2% had MM.[2] More than one abnormality can be present simultaneously, but not all abnormalities are visible on MRI.

Outcomes

Surgical outcome after adult TCR is generally favorable; most patients report improvement or stabilization of their symptoms, not unlike the main pediatric series (**Table 16.3**). Of the five series reviewed, one series did not sort outcomes by signs and symptoms,[6] and another series may have underestimated its results by reporting only the percentage of patients whose symptoms improved, rather than including patients with symptom stabilization.[8] This latter group of patients is important because the surgical goal is often that of halting the progression of the symptoms rather than reversing the deficit.

Pain

In all four series (**Fig. 16.3A**), more than 65% of patients had improvement in their pain soon

Table 16.3 Surgical Outcomes of Adults and Children

Signs and Symptoms		Adult (%)*	Pediatric (%)†
Pain	Improved	65–89	100
	Stable	16	0
	Worse	4	0
Sensorimotor	Improved	42–80	43
	Stable	25–44	48
	Worse	8–12	9
Sphincter dysfunction	Improved	33–61	42
	Stable	33	45
	Worse	6	12

Representative papers from the adult and pediatric literature are compared with respect to outcome after tethered cord release in patients with spina bifida occulta. The overall surgical success rate seems to be equivalent between the two groups.

*Data taken from the Rajpal,[11] Iskandar,[9] Gupta,[8] and Filler[7] series.

†Data taken from the Anderson[21] series.

after surgery. Approximately 15% of patients had stabilization of their symptoms, and up to 4% of patients continued to have progression of their pain postoperatively.

Sensorimotor Symptoms and Signs

Approximately 42 to 63% of patients showed sensorimotor improvement postoperatively, 25 to 44% had symptom stabilization, and ~10%

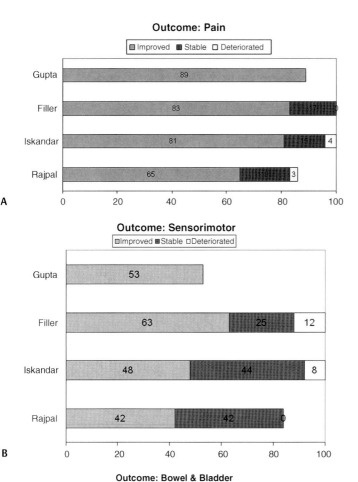

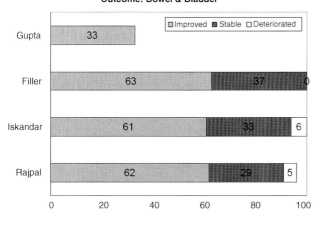

Fig. 16.3 Bar graph depicting the postoperative outcome of the various presenting symptoms and signs: **(A)** pain, **(B)** sensorimotor, and **(C)** bowel and bladder dysfunction, as reported in the Rajpal, Iskandar, Gupta, and Akay series.[1,7,10,11] Note: the Gupta series only reported the percentage of patients whose symptoms improved postoperatively, with no mention of the symptoms that stabilized or deteriorated; the Rajpal series outcomes do not necessarily total 100% because an additional category of "recurrence" was reported (not displayed).

worsened (**Fig. 16.3B**). In the pediatric TCS literature, TCR tends to stop the progression of symptoms and is less effective in reversing motor and sensory deficits. Improvement in spasticity and motor function also leads to gait improvement.

Outcome of Bladder Dysfunction

There is postoperative improvement of bowel/bladder dysfunction in 33 to 63% of patients, stabilization in 29 to 37% of patients, and ~10% of patients suffer from progressive bowel/bladder dysfunction long term despite TCR (**Fig. 16.3C**). Along those lines, it is important to note that distinguishing between progressive neural dysfunction and chronic bladder wall weakness remains subject to interpretation of the various bladder studies.

In mixed populations of SBA and SBO, Huttman[11] et al compared the duration of symptoms with outcome and concluded that pain and spasticity respond favorably to surgery regardless of the duration of symptoms, whereas improvement in the sensorimotor exam and bladder function is inversely related to the duration of symptoms.

Other Symptoms and Signs

Sixty-six percent of adult SBO patients presenting with trophic ulceration in the legs and feet had satisfactory healing of their lesions within 3 to 8 months of surgery.[5,8] Scoliosis typically stabilizes after TCR, even though severe scoliosis may still require surgical realignment and fusion.[18,19]

Work History and Subjective Assessment of Outcome by Patients

Long-term results collected by Iskandar et al on 28 patients showed that 22 patients (79%) considered the operation to be a "success."[9] Akay et al reported that 70% of patients thought the results of surgery were "good," whereas 30% thought they were "fair."[6] A review of the long-term work history of adult SBO patients who underwent TCR showed that of 22 patients who had worked preoperatively, 19 returned to their job after surgery. The remaining three patients stopped working within months of surgery due to circumstances unrelated to the surgery. Of six patients who did not work preoperatively, two had full-time jobs after TCR.

Surgical Morbidity

The complication rate of TCR in adulthood has been reasonably low in published series and compares favorably with the major pediatric series (**Table 16.4**). Main complications have included standard perioperative and anesthesia-related problems, as well as cerebrospinal fluid (CSF) leakage, pseudomeningocele formation, meningitis, neurological injury, and bladder dysfunction. The one reported mortality occurred in an adult patient who developed acute respiratory distress syndrome and sepsis postoperatively and died a few days following surgery.[2] Anecdotally, there is a correlation between the complexity of the tethering lesion and long-term results. For instance, there is a higher risk of bladder dysfunction after LMM repair, whereas postoperative deficits are rare after sectioning of the filum terminale. Similarly, the rate of retethering is

Table 16.4 Postoperative Complications

	Adult*	Pediatric†
Total Patients	107	73
Neurological	2	1
Nonneurological	14	NR
Death	1	0

Comparison of the rate of postoperative complications between the major adult (Iskandar et al,[10] Filler et al,[5] and Rajpal et al[11]) and pediatric (Anderson[2]) tethered cord series. Overall, there was one mortality but the rate of neurological complications was low. Nonneurological complications have included cerebrospinal fluid leakage, pseudomeningocele formation, and wound infection.

Abbreviation: NR, not reported.

*Data taken from the Iskandar,[10] Filler,[5] and Rajpal[17] series

†Data taken from the Anderson[21] series

high after LMM repair, and negligible after sectioning of the filum terminale. Although they tend to be more difficult and may present more risk of neurourological dysfunction, reoperations for symptomatic retethering usually yield good results.[20]

■ Discussion

Although the majority of SBO patients become symptomatic in childhood, some may remain asymptomatic until they reach adult age. TCR in children with SBO is believed strongly to be beneficial in preventing neurological deterioration.[3] The role of surgery in newly diagnosed adult patients, however, has been controversial. In this chapter, we conclude that TCR in adults is safe and likely to be beneficial to the long-term neurological outcome. In fact, the complication rate is not as high as previously assumed. It is important to realize, however, that most of the data presented are from institutions with significant experience in TCR surgery. It is conceivable that the low complication rate may not be replicated at low-volume institutions.

Pediatric versus Adult Tethered Cord

Pathophysiology and Risk Factors

The distribution of occult spinal dysraphic lesions between the adult and pediatric population is comparable with a few exceptions[5,21] (in the adult series there is a slightly lower frequency of dermal sinus tracts, and possibly a higher frequency of SCM). This leads us to presume that the pathophysiology of TCS is similar in children and adults. It has been postulated that the degree of traction on the conus determines the age of symptom onset.[5] Accordingly, a small change in the tension on the spinal cord may remain subclinical or cause only minor and nonprogressive deficits in childhood, until it is later aggravated by sudden or repetitive additional traction. Whereas in children the

onset of symptoms may often follow a growth spurt, the majority of patients with adult-onset symptoms report specific events that precipitated the neurological injury. It has been hypothesized that with each postural change, the tethered conus medullaris suffers episodes of minor injury that accumulate over time to lead to neurological deficit.[8] Yamada and colleagues have demonstrated that stretching of the lumbosacral cord in experimental animals and humans causes reductive shifts of cytochrome a, a_3 in mitochondria (i.e., impaired oxidative metabolism and subsequent neuronal dysfunction). Already dysfunctional spinal cord neurons are therefore vulnerable to additional stretching associated with the aforementioned injury, leading to neuronal damage.[22,23] In adult patients, bony spurs and herniated disks ventral to the spinal cord may accentuate the stretch, which would account for the observation that symptoms of TCS coincide with increasing lumbar spondylosis.[24] Nonetheless, there is no reason to believe that there is a significant difference in the actual cellular pathophysiology of childhood and adult-onset TCS.

Clinical Presentation

Children usually present with visible congenital anomalies such as cutaneous lesions and musculoskeletal deformities (described earlier). Neurological deficits, however, occur later in life as is evident from the natural history studies.[3] Foot deformities are the most common presenting features in children with congenital TCS, compared with only 21.7% of adults in Pang's series.[5] Such deformities do not progress over time. Limitations in function, such as gait, may only become noticeable once the patient reaches early childhood. Similarly, progressive scoliosis has been described in up to a third of pediatric TCS patients but is less common in adults.[25,26] Although pain is an uncommon presenting symptom in children, it is very common in adults. Childhood back pain is lumbosacral with variable radiation into both lower extremities. The anal and perianal pain often seen in adult patients is rarely noted in children, though very young children may not be able to express pain.

Diagnosis and Management

With advances in imaging techniques, delays in diagnosis have been reduced. Factors that contribute to late diagnoses include the lack of cutaneous or orthopedic (musculoskeletal) deformities at birth, the insidious onset or progression of the symptoms and signs,[27] and the concomitant presence of complicating factors such as a history of multiple back operations for degenerative or disk disease. The diagnostic and management problems become even more complicated in the presence of additional circumstances, especially prevalent in adult patients with back problems: a prior label of "failed back syndrome," the presence of pending lawsuits in cases of precipitating events such as falls or car accidents, and the involvement of workers' compensation issues.

■ Conclusion

Regardless of etiology, it seems fair to conclude that in the setting of low surgical complication rates and evidence that adult congenital TCS patients often present with progressive neurourological problems, TCR is a reasonable option in this group of patients to prevent neurological deterioration. The decision for surgery in adults, however, should be made on a case-by-case basis and should be weathered by other considerations such as nonneurological surgical risk, complexity of SBO lesion, patient age, and the extent to which there has been recent neurological deterioration.

References

1. Bowman RM, McLone DG, Grant JA, Tomita T, Ito JA. Spina bifida outcome: a 25-year prospective. Pediatr Neurosurg 2001;34:114–120
2. Iskandar BJ, McLaughlin C, Oakes WJ. Split cord malformations in myelomeningocele patients. Br J Neurosurg 2000;14:200–203
3. Iskandar BJ, Oakes WJ. Occult spinal dysraphism. In: Albright AL, Pollack IF, Adelson PD, eds. Principles and Practice of Pediatric Neurosurgery. New York: Thieme; 1999:321–352
4. Kirollos RW, Van Hille PT. Evaluation of surgery for the tethered cord syndrome using a new grading system. Br J Neurosurg 1996;10:253–260
5. Pang D, Wilberger JE Jr. Tethered cord syndrome in adults. J Neurosurg 1982;57:32–47
6. Akay KM, Erçahin Y, Cakir Y. Tethered cord syndrome in adults. Acta Neurochir (Wien) 2000;142:1111–1115
7. Filler AG, Britton JA, Uttley D, Marsh HT. Adult postrepair myelomeningocoele and tethered cord syndrome: good surgical outcome after abrupt neurological decline. Br J Neurosurg 1995;9:659–666
8. Gupta SK, Khosla VK, Sharma BS, Mathuriya SN, Pathak A, Tewari MK. Tethered cord syndrome in adults. Surg Neurol 1999;52:362–369, discussion 370
9. Iskandar BJ, Fulmer BB, Hadley MN, Oakes WJ. Congenital tethered spinal cord syndrome in adults. J Neurosurg 1998;88:958–961
10. van Leeuwen R, Notermans NC, Vandertop WP. Surgery in adults with tethered cord syndrome: outcome study with independent clinical review. J Neurosurg 2001;94(2, Suppl):205–209
11. Hüttmann S, Krauss J, Collmann H, Sörensen N, Roosen K. Surgical management of tethered spinal cord in adults: report of 54 cases. J Neurosurg 2001;95(2, Suppl):173–178
12. Yamada S, Won DJ, Kido DK. Adult tethered cord syndrome: new classification correlated with symptomatology, imaging and pathophysiology. Neurosurg Q 2001;11:260–275
13. Davidoff AM, Thompson CV, Grimm JM, Shorter NA, Filston HC, Oakes WJ. Occult spinal dysraphism in patients with anal agenesis. J Pediatr Surg 1991;26:1001–1005
14. Walton M, Bass J, Soucy P. Tethered cord with anorectal malformation, sacral anomalies and presacral masses: an under-recognized association. Eur J Pediatr Surg 1995;5:59–62
15. Rajpal S, Tubbs RS, George T, et al. Tethered cord due to spina bifida occulta presenting in adulthood: A tricenter review of 61 patients. J Neurol Spine 2007;6:210–215

16. Yamada S, Lonser RR. Adult tethered cord syndrome. J Spinal Disord 2000;13:319–323

17. Fitz CR, Harwood Nash DC. The tethered conus. Am J Roentgenol Radium Ther Nucl Med 1975;125: 515–523

18. McLone DG, Herman JM, Gabrieli AP, Dias L. Tethered cord as a cause of scoliosis in children with a myelomeningocele. Pediatr Neurosurg 1990-1991-1991;16:8–13

19. Reigel DH, Tchernoukha K, Bazmi B, Kortyna R, Rotenstein D. Change in spinal curvature following release of tethered spinal cord associated with spina bifida. Pediatr Neurosurg 1994;20:30–42

20. Jones PH, Love JG. Tight filum terminale. Arch Surg 1956;73:556–566

21. Anderson FM. Occult spinal dysraphism: a series of 73 cases. Pediatrics 1975;55:826–835

22. Yamada S, Iacono RP, Andrade T, Mandybur G, Yamada BS. Pathophysiology of tethered cord syndrome. Neurosurg Clin N Am 1995;6:311–323

23. Yamada S, Mandybur GT, Thompson JR. Dorsal midline proboscis associated with diastematomyelia and tethered cord syndrome: case report. J Neurosurg 1996;85:709–712

24. Sostrin RD, Thompson JR, Rouhe SA, Hasso AN. Occult spinal dysraphism in the geriatric patient. Radiology 1977;125:165–169

25. Hoffman HJ, Hendrick EB, Humphreys RP. The tethered spinal cord: its protean manifestations, diagnosis and surgical correction. Childs Brain 1976;2: 145–155

26. Yamada S. Tethered cord syndrome in adults and children. Neurol Res 2004;26:717–718

27. McLone DG. Spina bifida today: problems adults face. Semin Neurol 1989;9:169–175

28. Begeer JH, Wiertsema GP, Brakers SM, Mooy JJ, Wiemme CA. Tethered cord syndrom: Clinical signs and results of operation in 42 patients with spina bifida aperta and acculta. Z Kinderchin 1989;(44 Suppl 1): 5–7

29. Koyanagi I, Iwasaki Y, Hida K, et al. Surgical treatment supposed natural history of the tethered cord with occult spinal dysaphism. Childs Nerv Syst 1994; 13:268–274

30. Lee GY, Paradiso C, Tatar CH, et al: Surgical management of tethered cord syndrome in adults: Indications, techniques, and long-term outcomes in 60 patients. J Neurosurg Spine 2007;4:123–131

31. Sharif S, Allcutt, D, Marks C, Brennan P. "Tethered cord syndrome": Recent clinical experience. Br J Neurosurg 1997;11:49–51

17 The Normal Position of the Conus Medullaris Does Not Exclude a Tethered Spinal Cord

R. Shane Tubbs and W. Jerry Oakes

Since the inception of the term *tethered spinal cord* (TSC), most have intuitively accepted that the spinal cord must be located distal to its normal termination.[1] Many have declared coni located inferior to the L2 vertebral level and in patients with symptoms of lower spinal cord dysfunction as abnormally low and thus tethered. However, we have previously described a small series of patients in whom symptoms of a TSC were evident clinically yet radiologically their conus was found to lie at a widely acceptable normal anatomical level.[2,3] In fact, after a review of the extant literature prior to our publication in 1993, several authors had operated on patients for symptoms of a distally TSC in whom a conus was either retrospectively or prospectively found to terminate at a "normal" vertebral level.[4–10] Justifying surgical treatment for bona fide symptoms of a tethered cord seems appropriate in the fact that some authors advocate operative intervention for patients who are asymptomatic and are merely found to have fat within the filum terminale.[11] Of importance is where should the "normal" conus terminate? To some, below the L1–2 disk space is abnormally low, whereas to others, below the inferior border of L2 is abnormally displaced. From sonograms, one group concluded that a conus termination at the L3 level is indeterminate for abnormality.[12] This is confounded by the fact that the conus at times has no definite tip but gradually tapers to a very thick filum.[13,14] Operatively, however, the caudal end of the spinal cord is identified by the lowest coccygeal nerves as described by Yamada et al.[15,16]

■ Embryology of the Conus Medullaris and Filum Terminale

The human embryo has a distinct tail bud, which gradually regresses, and by 9 weeks gestation it is no longer seen externally.[13] The tip of the vertebral coccygeal segments contains an epidermal cell rest, the caudal cell mass. Secondary neurulation involving this cell rest apparently only gives rise to the filum and ventriculus terminalis, which may be identified from days 43 to 48, at which time it lies adjacent to the coccyx.[17] By 5 years of age, this "ventriculus terminalis" was found in only 2.6% of 418 children in a magnetic resonance imaging (MRI) study.[18] The filum terminale is composed of primarily pia mater, a neural crest derivative.[19] The filum terminale is created when the caudal neural tube regresses between the ventriculus terminalis and the caudal cell mass and is first seen on day 52.[17,20] The distal conus may also arise from the process of secondary neurulation.[21] In the term infant, the inferior tip of the conus has been described as being located at the L2–3 interspace in 98% of the cases and at the L3 level in 1.2% of the cases. Presumably, by 3 months of age, the tip of the conus achieves its adult position by "ascending" to the L1–2 interspace.[1] Robbin et al, with sonography, have refuted this idea of ascension during childhood and think that by ~19 weeks gestation the conus has achieved its adult position.[12] Therefore, with these data it is unlikely that significant additional ascent of the conus medullaris will occur after birth. Wilson and Prince have concluded that a conus positioned at L2–3 should be considered normal at any age.[22] DiPietro has shown that with sonography, children less than 2 months old had a mean conus termination at the lower third of the L1 vertebral body, children from 1 to 4 years of age had a mean conus termination at the upper third of the L1 vertebral body, and children greater than 4 years of age but less than 13 years also had a mean termination of the conus at the upper third of the L1 vertebral body.[23] Their study also concluded that as the conus ascends throughout childhood, the criteria for conus level should alter depending on the age of the patient. One study using sonography has found that in 92.1% of term babies the conus was above the L2 vertebral level and at the L2–3 disk level in only 6.3%.[24] Reimann and Anson reviewed 801 adult spinal cords and found that the conus medullaris is found above the L2–3 disk level in ~98%, whereas the mean conus lies at the lower third of the L1 vertebrae.[25] Saifuddin et al also found the mean termination of the conus at the lower third of the L1 vertebrae.[26] It is also said that the conus may tend to terminate differently in various races.[27]

The filum terminale is an elastic formation usually less than 2.0 mm wide,[13,28] which allows the conus medullaris to ascend during flexion of the spine. Distally, the filum travels to fuse with the dorsal dura mater then continues with this dural sheath as the coccygeal ligament.[19] If it is insufficiently elastic [e.g., abnormally thick, fat laden (decreased elasticity due to increased fibrous tissue)], this supposedly reduces the ability of the cord to move cephalad and thus places undue stress on the distal conus.[29] Incidental fat within the filum is seen in ~3.7 to 17% of the normal adult population.[17,30] In one of our series, fat was found in 91% of TSC patients.[30] Although the presence of fat may demonstrate possible pathology, it is

the amount of fibrous tissue within this fat that dictates the degree of viscoelasticity of the filum. In addition, the lack of denticulate ligaments along the caudal cord allows for more mobility if caudal forces are placed upon them.[31] We have found with cadaver studies that the denticulate ligaments, even cephalically, do little to abort either cranial or caudal traction on the spinal cord.[32] Supposed failure of involution of the terminal spinal cord and/or failure of the lengthening process of the filum terminale results in the TSC.[1,33]

■ Tethered Cord Syndrome with a Normally Positioned Conus

This entity, first described in 1953[34] with a normally positioned conus, is diagnosed on a clinician's ability to interpret the filum terminale on sagittal MRI as being taut. A more objective finding is a dorsally displaced conus and filum on MRI.[15,16,35] The term *tethered* has unfortunately been used both for cases in which the tip of the conus medullaris is at normal levels as well as for cases in which it is at abnormal vertebral levels.[1,4] In one series of tight fila, the tip of the conus resided at L2 or above.[13] Breig[36] has shown that the distal spinal cord becomes attenuated with flexion of the pelvis and that this biomechanical feature causes insult to the spinal cord during motion and increase in growth. However, these studies were performed in cadavers that had lost a great deal of their viscoelastic characteristics. We and others have found the distal cord to be hyperemic (indicating stress/tension) following sectioning of fila in patients with a normally or an abnormally positioned conus.[1,17,37] Yamada et al[38] have eloquently shown in a cat model that the TSC produces changes in the redox activity of cytochrome a,a_3 with a decrease in oxidation metabolism, presumably from mitochondrial anoxia.

The term *tethered* usually implies abnormally positioned.[13] Most definitions of normal cord termination levels are based on the anatomical measurements of Barson, who, quite intuitively, concluded that his findings in embryos were minimally inaccurate due to the hyperextension of the specimens during dissection.[39] Many series have suggested that incontinence in children who essentially have normal MRI scans of the lumbosacral region and usually have cystometrographic findings indicative of a neurogenic bladder can be successfully treated by simple sectioning of the filum terminale.[5–8,34,37] These series have had patients with both normal and fat-infiltrated fila.[5–8,30,34,40] Improvement of bladder function in these series showed improvements of 58%, 44%, 59%, and 67% at 1, 26, 13, and 20 months, respectively. Most patients in these series demonstrated little if any elements of occult spinal dysraphism. However, one should be clear that this is a diagnosis of exclusion and should be carefully considered.

In patients who present with symptoms indicative of TCS yet with imaging demonstrating a "normally" positioned conus medullaris, which can be visualized on sonography by the nineteenth week, the approximate same frequency of the following is observed (patients with normally positioned cord versus those with low-lying conus): cutaneous signatures of occult spinal dysraphism (46% vs 52%), abnormalities of the extremities (39% vs 32%), bony abnormalities (100% vs 95%), dysraphic abnormalities (62% vs 78%), and neurological abnormalities (77% vs 87%).[3] We stress that in our series none of the patients presented solely with urological dysfunction.[2,3] One criticism of the normally positioned conus in a patient with symptoms of a TSC is that these individuals may have additional vertebrae in the lumbar region thereby distorting this diagnosis if one does not number vertebrae from a cephalad to caudal direction. Often imaging of the lumbosacral region is only obtained in evaluation of these patients. The degree of potential error introduced into the aforementioned study by the possible occurrence of undetected transitional vertebrae or six lumbar vertebrae was found to be negligible.[22] In a review of 1614 lumbosacral spine radiographs the incidence of transitional vertebrae was found to be 8%.[22]

In support of biomechanical stress on the conus medullaris without alteration of its termination site at a normal level is the simple concept that a static midsagittal MRI of the lumbosacral region is all revealing in the absence of flexion or extension of the spine. Even with Barson's historic publication, he stated, "Our data represents the vertebral segments as though they were of constantly equal length both in respect of position and time. . . . This is obviously not so, although no adequate physical measurements exist of the precise size of the various vertebral segments at varying gestational ages and the normal ranges to be expected." Barson also makes an important query with regard to conus position by asking whether conus level is a result of an unusually short vertebral column or an abnormally long spinal cord, or whether both factors play a part.[39]

In our original report of patients with TCS and the conus in a normal position,[2] we reviewed our experience over 12 years with 73 patients with TCS. Of these, 13 (18%) had a cord termination at or above the L1–2 vertebral disk space. The mean age for this group was 11.3 years. These patients otherwise displayed characteristics usually associated with the patient with an abnormally low conus. The most common neurological complaints were lower extremity weakness and bladder dysfunction, each occurring in 40% of patients. Bowel dysfunction occurred in 30%. Six of these patients had cutaneous signatures indicative of occult spinal dysraphism; four had lumbosacral hemangiomas; one had a lumbosacral subcutaneous lipoma, and one had a midline lumbar skin tag. Five of these patients presented with extremity abnormalities, including three with leg-length discrepancy and two with foot deformities. Adipose tissue was found in 92% of patients either radiologically or histologically.

Radiologically and radiographically, several bony anomalies were identified in this population of patients. Ten of the 13 had bony abnormalities. These abnormalities included scoliosis (three patients), bifid vertebrae (10 patients), hemivertebrae, and segmentation errors. Other nonbony dysraphic anomalies included meningocele manqué in two patients, intradural lipoma in four patients, split cord anomaly (without median septa) in two patients, and terminal syringomyelia in two patients. Twelve of the 13 patients were operated. The average follow-up at that time was 2.2 years. Three patients presented neurologically normal. Seventy-five percent of patients with lower extremity weakness improved with surgery. For urinary complaints, at follow-up, two patients had normal urinary control, one patient had improved control, and one patient in whom there was a neurogenic bladder had no postoperative change. Of patients presenting with bowel complaints, all three had cessation of complaints at follow-up. Two patients presented with back pain that had resolved after their operation. The one patient that did not undergo surgery presented with low back pain and radicular leg pain that had improved at 6 months follow-up. Our follow-up publication on TCS and the normally positioned conus compared this subgroup to patients with TCS and a low-lying conus medullaris, which consisted of 60 patients.

Moufarrij et al have reported a series of patients with findings of TSC in which three patients had a cord termination at the L2 vertebral level.[9] Only one of these patients had a fatty filum terminale. Presenting symptoms in these three children were gait disturbance with lower-extremity weakness, leg cramps with foot inversion, and progressive kyphoscoliosis. These patients were noted at operation to have the cut ends of their fila retract 1 to 3 cm. Raghavan has reported 25 patients with TSC in which four had coni superior to the middle segment of the L2 vertebrae.[10] Two of the four presented with urinary incontinence, and fatty fila were found in three of the four, one of which did not present with urinary difficulties. Interestingly, tonsillar ectopia was found in five of nine patients with imaging of the craniocervical junction. Curiously, we have found previously that there is no significant difference in the level of cord termination between controls and children with a Chiari I malformation.[41]

Urinary Dysfunction

Although our description of TSC with a conus in the normal position did include patients who had urinary incontinence, this was only in four patients. In our report, three of the four patients had improved bladder function at postoperative follow-up.[2] Other sporadic reports in the literature have shown that urinary complaints, especially incontinence, are dealt with by sectioning the filum terminale in the face of a conus that is in a "normal" position.[7,8,34,40,42] Khoury et al have discussed sectioning of the filum for this scenario.[5,6] In their first publication, 23 children were operated on, all with normally positioned coni per myelography. Approximately 72% had resolution of their preoperative incontinence.[5] However, urinary incontinence unrelated to TSC must be considered. For example, some children may have persistent nocturnal enuresis secondary to developmental delay and not TSC.

■ Conclusion

There is a subset population of the patient with TSC in whom the tip of the conus lies at even liberally accepted normal levels. We would encourage clinicians treating patients with symptoms of TCS not to treat the patient based simply on imaging but imaging coupled with clinical symptoms and physical exam. It is important to point out that in lieu of the many publications of conus termination, one accept that there is no one single "normal" position of the terminal cord but rather a normal range. In addition, one may consider a patient with a supposedly normally positioned conus to actually have caudal descent of the cord in that, if not placed under stress it would have terminated superior to its current location. This would infer that earlier intervention might address an abnormally taut cord prior to its displacement. Perhaps a superior way of interpreting "tethered" cord is to view this as abnormal tension on the cord and not necessarily elongation of the distal cord. Finally, we stress that, with our experience, this group is the exception and not the rule with regard to TSC.

References

1. McLone DG. Occult dysraphism and the TSC. In: Choux M, De Rocco C, Hockley A, et al, eds. Pediatric Neurosurgery. Philadelphia: Churchill Livingstone; 1999:61–78
2. Warder DE, Oakes WJ. Tethered cord syndrome and the conus in a normal position. Neurosurgery 1993;33:374–378
3. Warder DE, Oakes WJ. Tethered cord syndrome: the low-lying and normally positioned conus. Neurosurgery 1994;34:597–600, discussion 600
4. Hendrick EB, Hoffman HJ, Humphreys RP. The tethered spinal cord. Clin Neurosurg 1983;30:457–463
5. Khoury AE, Hendrick EB, McLorie GA, Kulkarni A, Churchill BM. Occult spinal dysraphism: clinical and urodynamic outcome after division of the filum terminale. J Urol 1990;144(2 Pt 2):426–428, discussion 428–429, 443–444
6. Khoury AE, Balcom A, McLorie GA, Churchill BM. Clinical experience in urological involvement with tethered cord syndrome. In: Yamada S, ed. Tethered Cord Syndrome. Park Ridge, IL: American Association of Neurological Surgeons; 1996:89–98
7. Kondo A, Kato K, Kanai S, Sakakibara T. Bladder dysfunction secondary to tethered cord syndrome in adults: is it curable? J Urol 1986;135:313–316
8. Kondo A, Gotoh M, Kato K, Saito M, Sasakibara T, Yamada H. Treatment of persistent enuresis: results of severing a tight filum terminale. Br J Urol 1988;62:42–45
9. Moufarrij NA, Palmer JM, Hahn JF, Weinstein MA. Correlation between magnetic resonance imaging and surgical findings in the tethered spinal cord. Neurosurgery 1989;25:341–346
10. Raghavan N, Barkovich AJ, Edwards M, Norman D. MR imaging in the tethered spinal cord syndrome. AJR Am J Roentgenol 1989;152:843–852
11. Yundt KD, Park TS, Kaufman BA. Normal diameter of filum terminale in children: in vivo measurement. Pediatr Neurosurg 1997;27:257–259
12. Robbin ML, Filly RA, Goldstein RB. The normal location of the fetal conus medullaris. J Ultrasound Med 1994;13:541–546
13. Fitz CR, Harwood Nash DC. The tethered conus. Am J Roentgenol Radium Ther Nucl Med 1975;125:515–523
14. Grogan JP, Daniels DL, Williams AL, Rauschning W, Haughton VM. The normal conus medullaris: CT criteria for recognition. Radiology 1984;151:661–664
15. Yamada S, Iacono RP, Douglas C, Lonser RR, Shook JE. Tethered cord syndrome in adults. In: Yamada S, ed. Tethered Cord Syndrome. Park Ridge, IL: American Association of Neurological Surgeons; 1996:149–165
16. Yamada S, Iacono R, Morgese V, Douglas C. Tethered cord syndrome. In: Menezes AH, Sonntag VKH, eds. Principle of Spinal Surgery. Vol 1. New York: McGraw-Hill; 1996:433–445
17. Warder DE. Tethered cord syndrome and occult spinal dysraphism. Neurosurg Focus 2001;10:e1
18. Coleman LT, Zimmerman RA, Rorke LB. Ventriculus terminalis of the conus medullaris: MR findings in children. AJNR Am J Neuroradiol 1995;16:1421–1426
19. Hansasuta A, Tubbs RS, Oakes WJ. Filum terminale fusion and dural sac termination: study in 27 cadavers. Pediatr Neurosurg 1999;30:176–179
20. Kriss VM, Kriss TC, Babcock DS. The ventriculus terminalis of the spinal cord in the neonate: a normal variant on sonography. AJR Am J Roentgenol 1995;165:1491–1493
21. Nievelstein RAJ, Hartwig NG, Vermeij-Keers C, Valk J. Embryonic development of the mammalian caudal neural tube. Teratology 1993;48:21–31
22. Wilson DA, Prince JR. John Caffey award. MR imaging determination of the location of the normal conus medullaris throughout childhood. AJR Am J Roentgenol 1989;152:1029–1032
23. DiPietro MA. The conus medullaris: normal US findings throughout childhood. Radiology 1993;188:149–153
24. Şahin F, Selçuki M, Ecin N, et al. Level of conus medullaris in term and preterm neonates. Arch Dis Child Fetal Neonatal Ed 1997;77:F67–F69
25. Reimann AF, Anson BJ. Vertebral level of termination of the spinal cord with report of a case of sacral cord. Anat Rec 1944;88:127–138
26. Saifuddin A, Burnett SJD, White J. The variation of position of the conus medullaris in an adult population: a magnetic resonance imaging study. Spine 1998;23:1452–1456
27. Vettivel S. Vertebral level of the termination of the spinal cord in human fetuses. J Anat 1991;179:149–161
28. Zerah M, Pierre-Kahn A, Catala M. Lumbosacral lipomas. In: Choux M, Di Rocco C, Hockley A, et al, eds. Pediatric Neurosurgery. Philadelphia: Churchill Livingstone; 1999:79–100
29. Salbacak A, Büyükmumcu M, Malas MA, Karabulut AK, Seker M. An investigation of the conus medullaris and filum terminale variations in human fetuses. Surg Radiol Anat 2000;22:89–92

30. McLendon RE, Oakes WJ, Heinz ER, Yeates AE, Burger PC. Adipose tissue in the filum terminale: a computed tomographic finding that may indicate tethering of the spinal cord. Neurosurgery 1988;22:873–876

31. Tani S, Yamada S, Knighton RS. Extensibility of the lumbar and sacral cord: pathophysiology of the tethered spinal cord in cats. J Neurosurg 1987;66:116–123

32. Tubbs RS, Salter G, Grabb PA, Oakes WJ. The denticulate ligament: anatomy and functional significance. J Neurosurg 2001;94(2, Suppl):271–275

33. Selçuki M, Coşkun K. Management of tight filum terminale syndrome with special emphasis on normal level conus medullaris (NLCM). Surg Neurol 1998; 50:318–322, discussion 322

34. Garceau GJ. The filum terminale syndrome (the cord-traction syndrome). J Bone Joint Surg Am 1953;35-A:711–716

35. Vernet O, O'Gorman AM, Farmer JP, McPhillips M, Montes JL. Use of the prone position in the MRI evaluation of spinal cord retethering. Pediatr Neurosurg 1996;25:286–294

36. Breig A. The Lumbar Spine in Adverse Mechanical Tension in the Central Nervous System: An Analysis of Cause and Effect. New York: John Wiley & Sons; 1978:152

37. Taylor TKF, Coolican MJR. Injuries of the conus medullaris. Paraplegia 1988;26:393–400

38. Yamada S, Zinke DE, Sanders D. Pathophysiology of "tethered cord syndrome." J Neurosurg 1981;54: 494–503

39. Barson AJ. The vertebral level of termination of the spinal cord during normal and abnormal development. J Anat 1970;106(Pt 3):489–497

40. Selçuki M, Unlü A, Uğur HC, Soygür T, Arikan N, Selçuki D. Patients with urinary incontinence often benefit from surgical detethering of tight filum terminale. Childs Nerv Syst 2000;16:150–154, discussion 155

41. Tubbs RS, Elton S, Bartolucci AA, Grabb PA, Oakes WJ. The position of the conus medullaris in children with a Chiari I malformation. Pediatr Neurosurg 2000;33: 249–251

42. Nazar GB, Casale AJ, Roberts JG, Linden RD. Occult filum terminale syndrome. Pediatr Neurosurg 1995; 23:228–235

18 Anomalies of Spinal Cord Length and Filum Thickness

Shokei Yamada, Javed Siddiqi, and Shoko M. Yamada

Adults with tethered cord syndrome (TCS) are divided into two groups: group 1 adult TCS patients with spinal dysraphism and group 2 patients without dysraphism who develop signs and symptoms in adulthood.[1–3] A significant number of group 2 patients failed to show an elongated spinal cord and thickened filum terminale that Hoffman et al described in pediatric patients.[4] This chapter reports the statistics derived from the studies on the location of the caudal end of the spinal cord and the thickness of the filum terminale in group 2 adult TCS patients ($N = 104$). Only 35.6% of them were found to have both elongated cord and thickened filum. The data indirectly support that the essential factor for development of TCS is the inelastic filum.

Based on the neurological signs and symptoms localized in the lumbosacral cord and consistent imaging and operative findings, Hoffman et al adopted the term *tethered spinal cord*.[4] They attributed the motor and sensory deficits and incontinence to an increased tension in the elongated spinal cord anchored by a thickened filum terminale. As neurosurgeons' experience continued to increase, however, the concept of tethering-induced disorder broadened to the recognition of an inelastic filum as an essential mechanical factor for development of TCS.[5,6] Earlier in 1993, Warder and Oakes reported that 18% of TCS patients, including both children and adults, had the caudal end of the spinal cord at L1–2 intervertebral space or higher.[7] The authors present the retrospective

analysis of the data on the caudal end of the spinal cord and filum thickness obtained from group 2 TCS in adult and late teenage patients as previously discussed.[8]

■ Materials and Method

One hundred and four patients within the group 2 adult and late teenage TCS, from 17 to 81 years of age, 39 males and 65 females, presented with typical signs and symptoms of TCS (Chapter 15). All the patients lacked spinal dysraphism on imaging studies as well as at operation, except for five patients with bony spina bifida occulta of the S3 through coccygeal vertebrae shown by plain x-ray films. During surgery, the level of the caudal end of the spinal cord was determined by the exit of the lowest coccygeal nerve root, and its location was expressed in relation to the lumbar and sacral vertebral bodies. The filum thickness was measured by the lateral diameter (usually slightly greater than the anteroposterior diameter).

■ Results

The locations of the caudal end of the conus and the diameter of the filum terminale are listed in **Table 18.1**. Only 35.6% of the group 2 TCS patients showed cord elongation and a thickened filum. The caudal end of the spinal cord was found at the L2–3 intervertebral space

Table 18.1   Locations of the Caudal End of the Conus and the Diameter of the Filum Terminale (from total 104 adult cases with TCS)

1. Normal range of caudal end and filum thickness	30 cases (28.8%)
2. Normal range of caudal end and abnormally thick filum	7 cases (6.7%)
3. Low-lying caudal end and normal range filum thickness	30 cases (28.8%)
4. Low-lying caudal end and abnormally thick filum	37 cases (35.6%)

Adding 1. and 2., 37 patients (35.5%) had the caudal end at L2–3 or above, and adding 3. and 4. the diameter of the filum was less than 2 mm in 60 patients (57.7%).

or above in 37 patients (35.6%), and below the L2–3 level in 67 patients (64.4%). The diameter of the filum was less than 2 mm (assumed to be in the normal range) in 60 patients (57.7%) and 2 mm or greater in 44 patients (42.3%).

Of 67 patients with the caudal end below the L2–3, 41 (39.4% of total) had the caudal end opposite to the L3 vertebra, leaving only 26 (25%) with the caudal end below the L3 vertebra. None of the cases with the caudal end at the L3 level was detected by imaging studies as having an elongated spinal cord (Chapter 3).

■ Discussion

Our data clearly demonstrate the variability of the cord length and filum thickness in adults and late teenage patients with TCS, which correspond to the previous report.[8] Warder and Oakes first described no elongation of the spinal cord in adult and pediatric TCS patients.[7] There are also an increasing number of pediatric TCS patients who failed to show these two features (Knierim DS and Won DJ, personal communication, 2007). Other authors diagnosed TCS in small children with a chief complaint of incontinence but without these two anatomical features.[9–11] These facts explain how difficult it is to diagnose TCS by relying on only two features, an elongated cord and a thickened filum. Despite these recent reliable findings, it is still widely believed that an elongated spinal cord and thick filum are the two fundamental features to establish the diagnosis of TCS. Further, this logic extends to such an assumption as the patients without

two features are excluded from TCS or tethered spinal cord, even if they present with typical signs and symptoms of TCS (Chapter 15). The data reported by Yundt et al are noticeable; the normal range of filum thickness was measured as 1.1 to 1.2 mm,[12] whereas the filum thickness in TCS patients ranged from 1.0 to 2.0 mm.[13–15]

We emphasize that the clinical findings[16] are the primary tools for the diagnosis of TCS (Chapter 15), and are assisted by the magnetic resonance imaging (MRI) findings, such as the two features mentioned earlier, fat signal in the filum and syringomyelia.[17] The most consistent MRI finding is the posterior displacement of the conus and filum. This feature is confirmed by intrathecal endoscopy before widely opening the dura and arachnoid membrane, or preoperative percutaneous endoscopy.[6] The further step to prove the lack of elasticity in the filum is the stretch test after exposing the filum. This is the logical approach that utilizes the experimental work on redox changes in cytochrome a,a_3[18] proportionate to cord elongation induced by traction,[18–20] detailed in Chapter 3.

Although fat tissue in the filum has been emphasized for the diagnosis of TCS,[17] fat itself is soft and elastic, and TCS may not develop until fibrous tissue is increased to sufficiently reduce filum elasticity. MRI studies with currently available resolution do not identify the caudal end of the spinal cord, particularly when it is located at the L3 vertebral level. This difficulty can be explained by the inability to locate the exit of the lowest coccygeal nerve root (100 μm in diameter),[2] which is too small to be identified as a landmark of the caudal end of the spinal cord. Commonly, the caudal end at the L3 vertebra is not detected in the group of low-lying cord before surgery.[1–3] It is advisable to consider the conus localization by MRI studies (see Chapter 5, Fig. 5.3). In some cases, fat tissue that extends from the filum into the conus makes the definition of the conus–filum junction impossible by imaging studies. Only at operation, the junction can be determined by the exit of the lowest coccygeal root with microscopic observation (see Chapter 15). The elongation of the spinal cord usually occurs in lumbosacral segments,[13] and the conus diameter is often greater than the normally located conus (S2–4 segments). The relatively large bulk of the conus in these patients may resist traction

forces as much as the lumbar cord segments do, and explain widely spread lumbosacral cord dysfunction in TCS.

■ Conclusion

The length of the spinal cord and the thickness of the filum terminale are of relative importance for the diagnosis of the TCS. Neurological and musculoskeletal abnormalities that indicate or strongly suggest a stretch-induced lumbosacral functional lesion make imaging studies useful. The symptomatic protocol presented in Chapter 15 will assist in the diagnosis for TCS in adults as well as in children.

References

1. Yamada S, Iacono RP, Douglas CD, Lonser RR, Shook JE. Tethered cord syndrome in adults. In: Yamada S, ed. Tethered cord syndrome. Park Ridge, IL: American Association of Neurological Surgeons; 1996:139–165
2. Yamada S, Lonser RR. Adult tethered cord syndrome. J Spinal Disord 2000;13:319–323
3. Yamada S, Won DJ, Kido DK. Adult tethered cord syndrome: new classification correlated with symptomatology, imaging and pathophysiology. Neurosurg Q 2001;11:260–275
4. Hoffman HJ, Hendrick EB, Humphreys RP. The tethered spinal cord: its protean manifestations, diagnosis and surgical correction. Childs Brain 1976;2:145–155
5. Yamada S, Iacono RP, Yamada BS. Pathophysiology of tethered cord syndrome. In: Yamada S, ed. Tethered Cord Syndrome. Park Ridge, IL: American Association of Neurological Surgeons; 1996:29–48
6. Yamada S, Won DJ, Pezeshkpour G, et al. Pathophysiology of tethered cord syndrome and similar complex disorders. Neurosurg Focus 2007;23:1–10
7. Warder DE, Oakes WJ. Tethered cord syndrome and the conus in a normal position. Neurosurgery 1993;33:374–378
8. Yamada S, Won DJ, Yamada SM, Hadden A, Siddiqi J. Adult tethered cord syndrome: relative to spinal cord length and filum thickness. Neurol Res 2004;26:732–734
9. Khoury AE, Hendrick EB, McLorie GA, Kulkarni A, Churchill BM. Occult spinal dysraphism: clinical and urodynamic outcome after division of the filum terminale. J Urol 1990;144(2 Pt 2):426–428, discussion 428–429, 443–444
10. Wehby MC, O'Hollaren PS, Abtin K, Hume JL, Richards BJ. Occult tight filum terminale syndrome: results of surgical untethering. Pediatr Neurosurg 2004;40:51–57, discussion 58
11. Selden NR. Occult tethered cord syndrome: the case for surgery. J Neurosurg 2006;104(5, Suppl):302–304
12. Yundt KD, Park TS, Kaufman BA. Normal diameter of filum terminale in children: in vivo measurement. Pediatr Neurosurg 1997;27:257–259
13. Pang D. Tethered cord syndrome. Adv Pediatr Neurosurg 1986;1:45–79
14. Hochhauser L, Chaung S, Harwood-Nash DS, et al. The tethered cord syndrome revisited [abstract]. AJNR Am J Neuroradiol 1986;7:543
15. Selden NR, Nixon RR, Skoog SR, Lashley DB. Minimal tethered cord syndrome associated with thickening of the terminal filum. J Neurosurg 2006;105(3, Suppl):214–218
16. Yamada S, Siddiqi J, Won DJ, et al. Symptomatic protocols for adult tethered cord syndrome. Neurol Res 2004;26:741–744
17. Yamada S, Zinke DE, Sanders D. Pathophysiology of "tethered cord syndrome." J Neurosurg 1981;54:494–503
18. Yamada S, Won DJ, Yamada SM. Pathophysiology of tethered cord syndrome: correlation with symptomatology. Neurosurg Focus 2004;16:E6
19. Tani S, Yamada S, Knighton RS. Extensibility of the lumbar and sacral cord: pathophysiology of the tethered spinal cord in cats. J Neurosurg 1987;66:116–123
20. Steinbok P, Garton HJ, Gupta N. Occult tethered cord syndrome: a survey of practice patterns. J Neurosurg 2006;104(5, Suppl):309–313

19 Intraoperative Neurophysiological Monitoring of the Lower Sacral Nerve Roots and Spinal Cord

Dachling Pang

Confusing anatomy is often encountered during operations on complex dysraphic lesions in the lumbosacral canal. It is common to see nerve roots embedded in lipoma or scar tissue, or they may not be easily distinguishable from fibrous adhesion bands. Sometimes nerve roots that are bundled tightly by an abnormally thickened arachnoid can look like a thickened filum terminale. Also, the transition between a functional but structurally deformed conus and an intramedullary lipoma is not always visually apparent. Thus some objective means to identify the sacral nerve roots and the conus is necessary to ensure preservation of these neuronal structures. In addition, in some cases of complex transitional lipomas, the tip of the conus is tautly suspended by low sacral roots that are short, stout, and fibrotic. An assessment of their functional integrity is useful for determining whether dividing them, to complete the untethering process, would lead to unacceptable loss of sphincter function.

The first sacral and lower lumbar roots are recognized readily by intraoperative nerve stimulation while palpating for contractions of the respective segmental muscle groups through the surgical drapes. Identification of the lower sacral roots and functional quantification of these roots and their corresponding medullary connections, however, require some objective assessment of perineal sensation and sphincter function.

■ Sensory Monitoring of S2–S4 Segments

The assessment of evoked responses generated by directly stimulating parts of the sex organs, urethra, and anal canal constitutes the mainstay of sensory monitoring of the lower sacral segments. Monitoring of such responses is most useful when the distal conus or dorsal nerve roots are being rather strenuously handled, as in certain difficult resections of large transitional lipomas or during removal of the median fibrous sleeve of a type I split cord malformation. The latency and amplitudes of the waveforms are exquisitely sensitive to structural deformation and ischemic changes to the central sensory pathways. Sensory evoked response monitoring is less useful in the identification of sacral sensory roots because the responses are generated by end organ stimulation. Cortical responses generated by direct dorsal root stimulation give much less predictable waveforms, which are not stable enough for foolproof identification purposes.

Anatomy

The peripheral nerves that supply the bladder, anal canal, and perineal skin, all potentially available for stimulation, are divided into three main groups.

199

1. The pudendal nerve is the primary somatic nerve to this region. The pudendal motor neurons innervating the external sphincter and pelvic floor originate from the Onuf nucleus in the anterior horn of the S2 to S4 cord segments.[1] The sensory fibers come from the corresponding dorsal root ganglia. The mixed fibers course via the S2, S3, and S4 roots to exit the spinal canal through the sacral foramina. Somatosensory impulses travel in this nerve from receptors located in the skin of the genitalia and perineum, pelvic floor, and bulbocavernosus muscles, as well as in the mucosa of the distal urethra and anus.[2,3] Motor fibers in the pudendal nerve innervate the bulbocavernosus muscle, external urethral sphincter, external anal sphincter, and pelvic floor muscles.[4–6] The pudendal nerve is the most easily accessible nerve for evoked response testing.

2. The pelvic splanchnic nerves supply the sacral parasympathetic innervation to the pelvic organs. The motor neurons in this nerve originate in the S2 to S4 cord segments, slightly more caudal than the pudendal motor neurons.[7,8] The fibers are distributed to the pelvic organs via the S2 to S4 nerve roots and inferior epigastric plexus. The pelvic nerve carries sensory afferents from the proximal urethra, bladder wall, prostate, seminal vesicles, and rectum.[9,10] Motor innervation is primarily to the detrusor muscles, the corpus cavernosus, the rectum, and probably the upper smooth-muscle portion of the external urethral sphincter.[10–13] Evoked responses can be elicited on stimulation of the proximal urethra and bladder, presumably due to activation of the pelvic sensory fibers.

3. The hypogastric nerve plexuses carry autonomic (sympathetic) fibers from the intermediolateral cell column of the T11–L2 spinal cord segments.[14] The preganglionic fibers course via the paravertebral sympathetic chain ganglia, inferior mesenteric plexus, superior hypogastric plexus, and finally the inferior hypogastric plexus. The postganglionic fibers are distributed to the smooth muscles of the bladder neck, the smooth-muscled internal urethral sphincter, the parasympathetic intramural ganglia of the detrusor muscles,[15] and probably the intrinsic portion of the external urethral sphincter.[16] The postganglionic fibers also share connections with plexuses around the rectum and anal canal, seminal vesicles, ductus deferens, prostate, and corpus cavernosus in the male, and vagina in the female.[10,11] It is uncertain how much the afferent component of the hypogastric nerves contributes to the evoked response in humans.

Cortical Sensory Evoked Response

Standard recording of the cortical evoked response is made by 5 mm silver or gold-plated cup electrodes or dermal needle electrodes sutured to the scalp. The electrode impedance should be kept below 2000 Ω. The active recording electrode is placed in the midline, ~2 cm behind the Cz electroencephalographic recording site according to the International 10–20 System of Electrode Placement. This has been demonstrated to give maximum cortical response on stimulation of the penile and clitoral skin. The reference electrode can be placed at several sites, although the forehead (F_{Pz}) is convenient and gives a good waveform. Stimuli are delivered at a rate of 3.5 to 5.0 per second, with ~2.5 to 3.0 times the threshold intensity. The recording console consists of high- and low-frequency filters to keep the band pass at 30 to 1000 Hz. The sensitivity of the signal amplifier is usually set at 2 to 10 μV per division.[17] About 250 to 350 responses are averaged to ensure reproducibility of the reading, but weak and unstable signals from severely damaged conuses may require up to 1000 responses to generate an interpretable waveform.[18]

Pudendal Dermatomal Evoked Response

The most commonly used form of pudendal nerve evoked response utilizes stimuli applied to the sensory domain of the dorsal genital nerve. In the male, the dorsal nerve of the penis can be stimulated either bilaterally or unilaterally using 5 mm cup electrodes placed 2 to 3 cm apart at the base of the penis, with the cathode proximal to the anode. Stimuli up to 3.0 or 3.5 times threshold are well tolerated. In the female, the dorsal nerve of the clitoris is stimulated by 5 mm cup electrodes or fine dermal needle electrodes fixed bilaterally to the cleft between the labia major and labia minor. The anodes are placed adjacent to the clitoris bilaterally and the cathode ~2 cm posterior to the anode.[17]

The averaged cortical pudendal evoked response has a similar morphology as the responses obtained from stimulation of the posterior tibial or peroneal nerve. The response has a fairly characteristic "M" pattern, with an initial positive deflection followed by a constant negative, positive, negative, positive waveform.[17] Injury to the S2–4 roots or cord segments is manifested by lengthening of the P1 latency and decreased amplitude of the triphasic waves (**Fig. 19.1**).

Urethral Evoked Response

Cortical evoked responses of very similar morphology and latencies can be obtained using stimulating electrodes embedded in a catheter inserted into the bladder. The catheter has a balloon at its tip, which can be pulled back snugly for anchorage. The location of the urethral electrodes can be kept reasonably constant to eliminate movement artifacts and interference.

Anal Evoked Response

Electrode-bearing catheters can also be inserted into the anal canal for measurement of anal evoked responses. The catheter is anchored by double balloons, the inner one within the anorectal junction and the outer one wedged at the anal verge. The cortical anal responses do not differ from the urethral responses or the pudendal dermatomal responses.[19]

Spinal Evoked Response

Evoked responses can be recorded by electrodes placed on the skin over the spine in humans. They reflect the afferent volley traversing the dorsal columns. The responses progressively increase in latency at more rostral recording locations. Spinal evoked responses are relatively easy to obtain in children, but the amplitudes and waveform definition decrease with age, such that by midteenage years, these responses are more difficult to obtain, as in the case of adults. The response over the mid- to lower lumbar spine consists of an initially positive triphasic potential, representing the volley as it ascends the cauda equina. Over the caudal

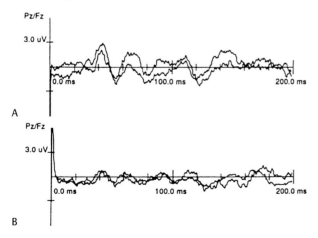

Fig. 19.1 Cortical pudendal nerve evoked responses obtained from a male child with a type I split cord malformation. The neurological deficits are much worse in the left leg. All responses are recorded from P_Z, referenced to F_Z. **(A)** Tracing obtained by stimulating the right dorsal nerve of the penis. **(B)** Tracing obtained by stimulating the left dorsal penile nerve. Note the significant reduction in amplitude in the left responses.

thoracic spine, the response consists of an initially positive, predominantly negative triphasic wave, the negative component of which has several peaks or inflections.[18] The initial portion of this response arises in the intramedullary continuation of the dorsal root fibers, and the subsequent portion reflects synaptic activity concerned with local reflex mechanism rather than the propagation of the response to more rostral cord levels. From the midthoracic to the cervical levels, the response consists of small triphasic potentials that are difficult to follow, presumably arising from multiple ascending pathways including the dorsal and dorsolateral columns.[18]

The only consistent spinal pudendal response has been from stimulation of the dorsal nerve of the penis. The recording electrodes are usually fixed at the T12–L1 interspinous space. The response has a morphology comparable to the spinal response from the posterior tibial and peroneal nerves but with smaller amplitudes and a much shorter latency (**Fig. 19.2**). The spinal pudendal evoked response is sometimes not measurable in overweight individuals, but its presence yields useful information concerning peripheral sensory conduction from the penis since it bypasses the central conduction pathway rostral to the thoracic levels. Because the *cortical* pudendal evoked response has similar latency with the *cortical* posterior tibial response, the central conduction time involved in the pudendal pathways must be considerably longer than that in the posterior tibial pathways.[17,20]

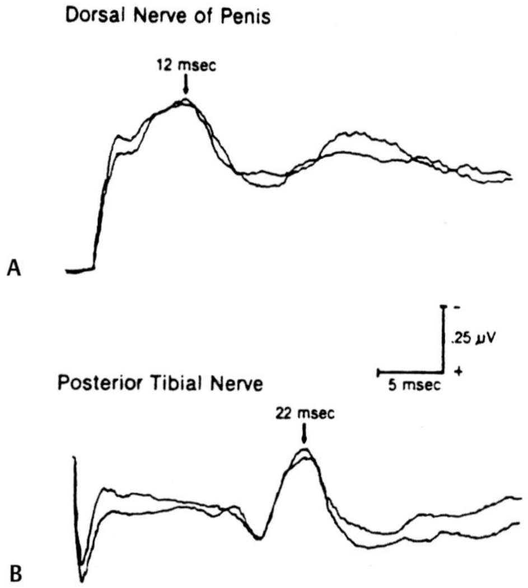

■ Motor Monitoring of the S2–S4 Nerve Roots

Pudendal sensory evoked responses are useful in monitoring intraoperative injury to the conus and lower sacral sensory nerve roots, but they are neither qualitatively nor quantitatively suitable for the identification of the lower sacral roots (especially the motor roots) or conus from nonneural elements. Intraoperative identification requires some way of measuring the one-to-one stimulus-to-response coupling of end organ function when the nerve root in question is being stimulated. For the lower sacral roots, this means the assessment of sphincter function.

Anatomy of the Anal Sphincters

The external anal sphincter consists of a bulky deep part, a fusiform superficial part, and a subcutaneous part decussating behind and in front of the anus.[21] It encloses the lower part of the levator ani, the anorectal junction, and the anal canal in the shape of a funnel. The internal anal sphincter arises from the muscular coats of the rectum and insinuates itself between the rectal mucosa and the upper portion of the funnel.

The external anal sphincter is innervated by the pudendal nerve. This arises from the anterior division of S2 and S3 and both divisions of S4, enters the pudendal (Alcock) canal through the lesser sciatic foramen, and divides into two main branches just proximal to the urogenital diaphragm. The proximal branch, the inferior

Fig. 19.2 Spinal pudendal evoked responses recorded over the T12–L1 interspinous space on stimulation of the **(A)** dorsal nerve of the penis, and spinal responses on stimulation of the **(B)** posterior tibial nerve. Note the much shorter latency of the pudendal response.

hemorrhoidal nerve, supplies the striated muscles of the external anal sphincter; the distal branch, the perineal nerve, supplies the external urethral sphincter. The internal anal sphincter, composed of smooth muscles, is innervated by the hypogastric nerve, derived from the intermediolateral (sympathetic) columns of L1 and L2.[22,23,24] Stimulation of the S2, S3, and S4 roots, therefore, activates only the external and not the internal anal sphincter. Furthermore, unless there is localized disease or trauma to the pudendal branches at the urogenital diaphragm, activity of the external anal sphincter reflects function of the external urethral sphincter.

External Anal Sphincter Electromyography

We are strong advocates of intraoperative electromyographic (EMG) monitoring. During the past decade, as the discriminating capabilities of probe electrodes have become more refined and our dissecting scissors get ever closer to bare spinal cord, intraoperative motor monitoring has risen from being merely helpful to sine qua non.

In truth, we use this technology less as a "monitor" than as an "expositor" because we are more concerned with using EMG for the accurate identification of the motor roots and the detection of functional spinal cord within fibrofatty muddles. For monitoring leg functions, the muscles commonly employed are the sartorius (L1), rectus femoris (L2, L3), anterior tibialis (L4, L5), extensor hallucis longus (L5), and gastrocnemius (S1). Half-inch-long, 25- to 27-gauge needle recording electrodes and input gains of 50 to 80 μV are selected to enable maximum capturing of far-field evoked action potentials of the indexed muscle without undue artifacts[22,25-29] (**Fig. 19.3**).

For monitoring the external anal sphincter, the EMG electrodes are either embedded in an anal plug or anal balloon, which is placed into the anal canal, or are in the form of needles inserted directly into the external anal sphincter transmucosally.[30] The needle electrodes are

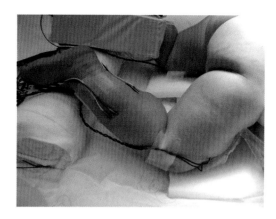

Fig. 19.3 Paired recording needle electrodes in place for the right rectus femoris, anterior tibialis, and gastrocnemius.

more reliable because they are not subject to dislodgment or to having mechanical artifacts during contraction of the sphincter itself. Paired quarter-inch-long 27-gauge needle electrodes are inserted directly through the anal verge on each side to capture activities of the external anal sphincter (S2–4) (**Fig. 19.4**). The needles are securely wedged in place by a soft gauze plug taped to the anal opening, and the electrode wires are further taped to the perianal skin (**Fig. 19.5**). All stimulations and recordings are

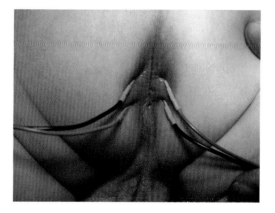

Fig. 19.4 Paired quarter-inch 27-gauge recording needle electrodes in place on each side of the anal verge to capture evoked motor response from both sides of the external anal sphincter.

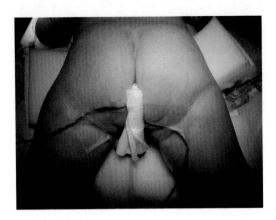

Fig. 19.5 The anal sphincter electrodes are held firmly in place by a soft gauze plug wedged and taped to the anal opening. The electrode wires are also taped firmly to the buttock skin.

done with the Cadwell Cascade Intraoperative Monitoring System (Cadwell Laboratories, Inc., Kennewick, WA) using the Cascade Software Version 2.0.

For nerve root and direct spinal cord stimulation, we used a concentric coaxial bipolar microprobe (Kartush Concentric Bipolar, made by Medtronic Xomed, Inc., www.xomed.com) (**Fig. 19.6**). This microprobe generates extremely focused and confined current spread at its 1.75 mm tip and thus works best at precise

localization of small functioning neuronal–axonal units (**Fig. 19.7**). Larger, double-pronged bipolar electrodes, or worse, monopolar electrodes, which in essence convert the spinal cord into a giant volume conductor, are undesirable because they cause unwanted recruitment of adjacent depolarizable tissues (**Fig. 19.7**).

During nerve stimulation, the cerebrospinal fluid must be continuously suctioned away from the stimulation site to prevent current dispersion. Stimulating currents from 0.5 to 1.5 milliamperes are used depending on target impedance. Supramaximal stimulation of the small sacral roots of infants and young children can usually be accomplished with 0.5 mA (**Figs. 19.8, 19.9**). The larger roots of adults sometimes require higher amperage, as does direct conus stimulation (**Figs. 19.10, 19.11**). The stimulation frequency is usually set at 10 per second. This allows spontaneous random firing due to nerve irritation from surgical manipulation to be distinguishable from the rhythmic evoked contractions.

Sophisticated intraoperative EMG monitoring is extremely helpful in complex lipoma surgery. In resecting transitional and chaotic lipomas, incomplete terminal untethering of the neural placode predictably ends in recurrence of symptoms. Often, with these very large lipomas, the distal neural placode is half obscured

Concentric Coaxial Stimulator

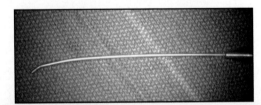

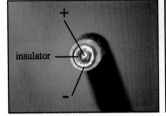

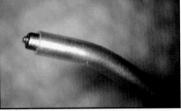

Fig. 19.6 Concentric coaxial bipolar microprobe stimulator, in which the concentric cathode and anode are separated by a coaxial insulator. Tip diameter is ~1.75 mm.

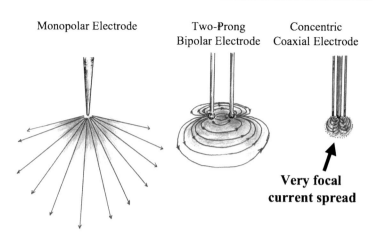

Monopolar Electrode

Two-Prong
Bipolar Electrode

Concentric
Coaxial Electrode

**Very focal
current spread**

Fig. 19.7 Patterns of current spread in three different stimulation electrodes. The concentric coaxial bipolar microprobe has the most focalized current map. The monopolar electrode works by converting the whole body of the patient into a giant volume conductor and has the widest current spread.

by fat and fibrosis so that the extent of "useful" cord cannot be determined visually. This caudal fat–cord–fibrosis jumble can only be sorted out functionally by direct stimulation of the placode and the projecting nerve roots. In other cases, nerve twigs are seen issuing in pairs from the distal placode beyond where it dives into the caudal fat, making it seem impossible to complete the detachment without sacrificing functional cord. This assumption turns out to be spurious. We found that as long as two or three sets of anal sphincter–activating roots, presumably S2 to S4, are identified and preserved on each side of the placode, there should

be no loss of function if the terminal disconnection is made just *caudal* to these roots and everything distal is discarded. The small nerve twigs within the distal stump are probably coccygeal roots and therefore vestigial in humans and have no essential function. No muscle response is seen with stimulating these nerve twigs.

In earlier cases, we also used a pressure-transduced Silastic balloon lodged deep to the anal verge to quantify the anal sphincter contractions,[31] but newer and more sensitive, noise-free recording of anal EMG has since supplanted the balloon.[32]

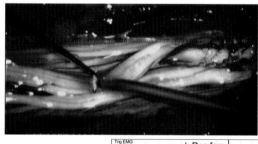

Left L$_4$-L$_5$
Roots
Stimulation

Strong Multiple Left
Leg Muscles, and
Minor Anal Activities

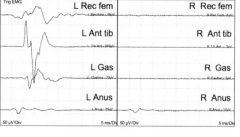

Trig EMG	L Rec fem	R Rec fem
	L Ant tib	R Ant tib
	L Gas	R Gas
	L Anus	R Anus
50 µV/Div	5 ms/Div 50 µV/Div	5 ms/Div

Fig. 19.8 Stimulation of the left L4 and L5 roots (bunched together for demonstration) using the concentric bipolar microprobe stimulator with a current of 1.0 milliampere (mA). Note major evoked electromyographic response from the left anterior tibialis (L Ant Tib), left gastrocnemius (L Gas), and minor response from the left rectus femoris (L Rec Fem) and small twitches from the left anus.

Single Left Small Rootlet
with Bilateral Anal Activation on Stimulation

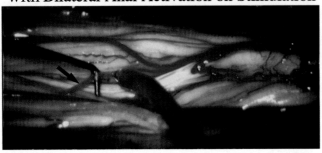

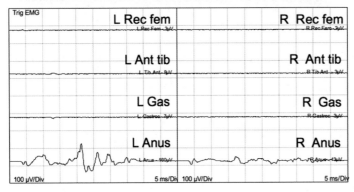

Fig. 19.9 Stimulation of single left S2 rootlet (*arrow*) with a current of 0.5 mA. Note major activities in the left anus and much lower activities in the right anus.

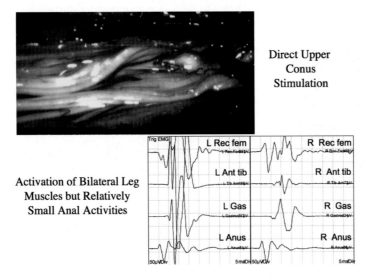

Direct Upper
Conus
Stimulation

Activation of Bilateral Leg
Muscles but Relatively
Small Anal Activities

Fig. 19.10 Direct stimulation of the "upper" conus using the bipolar microprobe stimulator with a current of 2.0 mA. Note: massive bilateral activation of all leg muscles indexed, as well as some anal sphincter activity.

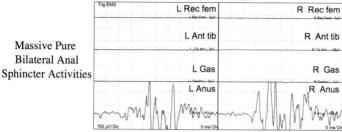

Fig. 19.11 Direct stimulation with current of 1.5 mA of an anomalous "unintegrated secondary neural cord" or isolated lower conus containing only S2–5 roots and no S1 roots. Note massive bilateral activation of the external anal sphincter but complete silence in the leg muscles.

Pelvic Floor Electromyography

Needle recording electrodes can be percutaneously inserted into the "extrinsic" portion of the external urethral sphincter to monitor activity of this sphincter. This technique is routinely used by neurourologists to correlate simultaneous measurements of bladder pressure, urethral pressure, and external urethral sphincter activities. Pelvic floor EMG can thus be used for intraoperative sacral root identification in the same manner as external anal sphincter EMG.

■ Sacral Reflex Monitoring

Two reflexes with centers in the sacral cord can be utilized to assess the integrity of both the sensory and the motor roots as well as their interconnecting intramedullary components.

Bulbocavernosus Reflex

The reflex response of the bulbocavernosus muscle to stimulation of penile nerves can be studied using square wave electrical stimuli applied through ring electrodes on the penis, and recorded either by needle electrodes in the muscle or by surface electrodes fixed to the midline of the perineum between the base of the penis and the anus.[33-35] The averaged response from 50 to 100 stimuli is usually biphasic with an initial negative peak. The latency for most healthy adults is 24 to 42 millisecond[19] but varies with age and maturation in young children. The waveform is also distorted significantly in most cases of myelodysplasia and tends to become "unstable" with very minor manipulations of the conus. The use of this monitoring modality is therefore limited and is feasible only in patients with virtually normal sphincter function preoperatively.

Urethral to Anal Sphincter Reflex

The urethral to anal sphincter reflex can be measured using stimulating electrodes similar to those used in eliciting urethral cortical evoked responses and recording electrodes used in recording external anal sphincter EMG.

The latency is considerably longer (50 to 70 millisecond) than the bulbocavernosus reflex, although their morphologies are similar.[19] The long latency in the urethral–anal sphincter reflex is due partly to the slower conducting velocity of autonomic afferent fibers and partly to a more complex central polysynaptic reflex organization.[17,19]

References

1. Nakagawa S. Onuf's nucleus of the sacral cord in a South American monkey (Saimiri): its location and bilateral cortical input from area 4. Brain Res 1980; 191:337–344

2. Oliver J, Bradley W, Fletcher T. Spinal cord distribution of the somatic innervation of the external urethral sphincter of the cat. J Neurol Sci 1970;10:11–23

3. Todd JK. Afferent impulses in the pudendal nerves of the cat. Q J Exp Physiol Cogn Med Sci 1964;49:258–267

4. Bishop B, Garry RC, Roberts TDM, Todd JK. Control of the external sphincter of the anus in the cat. J Physiol 1956;134:229–240

5. Chantraine A, de Leval J, Onkelinx A. Motor conduction velocity in the internal pudendal nerves. In: Desmedt JE, ed. New Developments in Electromyography and Clinical Neurophysiology. New York: S Karger; 1973: 433–438

6. Mackel R. Segmental and descending control of the external urethral and anal sphincters in the cat. J Physiol 1979;294:105–122

7. Oliver JE Jr, Bradley WE, Fletcher TF. Identification of preganglionic parasympathetic neruons in the sacral spinal cord of the cat. J Comp Neurol 1969;137: 321–328

8. Oliver JE Jr, Bradley WE, Fletcher TF. Spinal cord representation of the micturition reflex. J Comp Neurol 1969;137:329–346

9. Bradley WE, Scott FB. Physiology of the urinary bladder. In: Harrison JH, Gittes RF, Perlmutter AD, et al, eds. Campbell's Urology. 4th ed. Philadelphia: WB Saunders; 1978:87–124

10. Langworthy OR. Innervation of the pelvic organs of the rat. Invest Neural 1965;2:491–511

11. Bouvier M, Gonella J. Nervous control of the internal anal sphincter of the cat. J Physiol 1981;310:457–469

12. McGuire EJ. The innervation and function of the lower urinary tract. J Neurosurg 1986;65:278–285

13. Rockswold GL, Bradley WE, Chou SN. Innervation of the urinary bladder in higher primates. J Comp Neurol 1980;193:509–520

14. Bradley WE, Griffin D, Teague C, Timm G. Sensory innervation of the mammalian urethra. Invest Urol 1973;10:287–289

15. de Groat WC, Ryall RW. Reflexes to sacral parasympathetic neurones concerned with micturition in the cat. J Physiol 1969;200:87–108

16. Elbadawi A. Neuromorphologic basis of vesicourethral function, I: Histochemistry, ultrastructure and function of the intrinsic nerves of the bladder and urethra. Neurourol Urodyn 1982;1:3–50

17. Haldeman S, Bradley WE, Bhatia NN, Johnson BK. Pudendal evoked responses. Arch Neurol 1982;39: 280–283

18. Schweiger M. Method for determining individual contributions of voluntary and involuntary anal sphincters to resting tone. Dis Colon Rectum 1979; 22:415–416

19. Haldeman S, Bradley WE, Bhatia NN. Evoked responses in clinical neuro-urology. Bull Los Angeles Neurol Soc 1982;47:76–90

20. Haldeman S, Bradley WE, Johnson BK. Pudendal somatosensory evoked responses. Neurology 1981; 31:152

21. Lockhart RD, Hamilton GE, Fyfe FW. Anatomy of the Human Body. 3rd ed. Philadelphia: JB Lippincott; 1959:189–193

22. Bailey JA, Powers JJ, Waylonis GW. A clinical evaluation of electromyography of the anal sphincter. Arch Phys Med Rehabil 1970;51:403–408

23. Lawson JON. Structure and function of the internal anal sphincter. Proc R Soc Med 1970;63(Suppl): 84–89

24. Kerremans R. Electrical activity and motility of the internal anal sphincter: an "in vivo" electrophysiological study in man. Acta Gastroenterol Belg 1968; 31:465–482

25. Blank A, Magora A. Electromyographic investigation of the superficial sphincter ani muscle (SSAM) in spinal cord injury. Electromyogr Clin Neurophysiol 1975;15:261–268

26. Lane RH. Clinical application of anorectal physiology. Proc R Soc Med 1975;68:28–30

27. Schnaufer L, Talbert JL, Haller JA, Reid NC, Tobon F, Schuster MM. Differential sphincteric studies in the diagnosis of ano-rectal disorders of childhood. J Pediatr Surg 1967;2:538–543

28. Waylonis GW, Powers JJ. Clinical application of anal sphincter electromyography. Surg Clin North Am 1972;52:807–815

29. Wilson PM. Anorectal closing mechanisms. S Afr Med J 1977;51:802–808

30. James HE, Mulcahy JJ, Walsh JW, Kaplan GW. Use of anal sphincter electromyography during operations on the conus medullaris and sacral nerve roots. Neurosurgery 1979;4:521–523

31. Pang D, Casey K. Use of an anal sphincter pressure monitor during operations on the sacral spinal cord and nerve roots. Neurosurgery 1983;13:562–568

32. Pang D. Intraoperative neurophysiological monitoring of the lower sacral nerve roots and spinal cord. In: Yamada S, ed. Tethered Cord Syndrome. Park Ridge, IL: American Association of Neurological Surgeons Publications Committee; 1996:135–147

33. Dick HC, Bradley WE, Scott FB, Timm GW. Pudendal sexual reflexes: electrophysiologic investigations. Urology 1974;3:376–379

34. Ertekin C, Reel F. Bulbocavernosus reflex in normal men and in patients with neurogenic bladder and/or impotence. J Neurol Sci 1976;28:1–15

35. Siroky MB, Sax DS, Krane RJ. Sacral signal tracing: the electrophysiology of the bulbocavernosus reflex. J Urol 1979;122:661–664

20 Clinical Neurophysiology of Tethered Cord Syndrome and Other Dysraphic Syndromes

Robin L. Gilmore, Sun Ik Lee, and John Walsh

Tethered cord syndrome is a complex developmental malformation, with the underlying pathological anomaly being a dura mater defect or dural schisis. The dural schisis may not be the only developmental defect, but it is probably the most basic one[1] and one that occurs more commonly than is generally recognized.[2,3] Establishing the diagnosis and assessing the extent of functional disability is often difficult but may be aided considerably by the use of several clinical neurophysiological studies, including somatosensory evoked potentials (SSEPs),[4–7] urodynamics with sphincter and pelvic floor electromyography (EMG),[8,9] and anal sphincter EMG and pressure monitoring for intraoperative use.[8,10]

This chapter reviews the contributions of these techniques to the diagnosis and management of patients with tethered cord syndrome. To convey an appreciation for the use of these techniques, the chapter includes a discussion of the relevant developmental anatomy, specifically the development of the neural pathways, assessed by these techniques. In addition to the diagnostic studies, the multimodality monitoring of sensory and motor systems as well as reflex circuits have recently been emphasized as the intraoperative diagnostic tool in many publications.[11–18] These monitoring methods have been shown to reflect not only acute but also chronic insults to the cauda equina or spinal cord. The degree of injury paralleled the degree of electrophysiological changes in an animal study.[19] Thus the spinal cord and cauda equina have been successfully protected by the aid of intraspinal monitoring. The stimulation of the filum has been claimed to be useful when the normal anatomy is distorted by pathological structures.[15,17]

■ Developmental Anatomy of the Spinal Cord

The spinal cord is freer within the vertebral canal than is the brain within the cranium. The spinal dura mater is composed of dense connective tissue with few elastic elements derived from paraxial mesoderm.[20] It is separated from the vertebral internal periosteum by the epidural space, which contains fat cells, blood vessels, and loose connective tissue. The spinal cord needs to be completely free from the vertebral column during development because the rates of growth of the two structures are different. Early in development, the caudal region of the spinal cord undergoes a progressive upward displacement or retrogression relative to the caudal vertebral column.[21] The conus medullaris, which is initially at the coccygeal level in the 30 mm embryo, ascends through the S4 level in the 67 mm embryo, to the L3 level by birth (40 weeks conceptional age),[1] and to the adult L1–2 level by 49 to 50 weeks conceptional age.[22]

The subarachnoid space elongates progressively to accommodate the elongating spinal nerve roots and filum terminale. The filum terminale must also elongate because the cord retains its original coccygeal attachment through this structure. Early dural schisis (below L3) through which the spinal cord comes in direct contact with subcutaneous tissue lends to tethering of the spinal cord to this tissue. Later, subcutaneous adipose tissue penetrates and expands into the intraspinal space.[1] This results in a low conus medullaris and a short, thick filum terminale. It is possible that the adipose tissue is stimulated by its direct contact with neural elements and the abundant arachnoidal vascularity through the dural schisis.

■ Neuroanatomy of Somatosensory Evoked Potentials

Evoked potentials recorded from the body's surface are either near field or far field in nature; that is, the generator source is close or distant to the site of recording. The generators may be in gray matter or white matter. Generators in gray matter produce postsynaptic potentials (PSPs), which may be near field or far field. Near field PSPs are probably responsible for cortical components of SSEPs.

White matter generates compound action potentials (APs), which are propagated through fiber tracts. The latencies of the propagated APs increase proportionately to the distance from the point of stimulation and hence are dependent on the recording electrode position. These are recorded only in close proximation to the fiber tract itself and thus are termed near field potentials (NFPs). Because they are close to the site of origin, the amplitude is relatively large (> 1 μV). Other evoked potentials may be recorded at long distances from the point of propagation and are generated when a traveling impulse (signal) passes through a certain anatomical site or fixed point along the nerve. These are called far field potentials (FFPs). It was previously considered that FFPs reflected the approaching volley recorded beyond the point of termination of an active fiber.[23] More recently, it has been suggested that FFPs are generated because of abrupt changes in the geometry of tissue surrounding

the nerve,[24,25] a change in the medium through which the volley is transmitted, or a change in the direction of the fibers.[26]

In summary, NFPs have a specific distribution (topographic specificity), latencies that vary according to the recording electrode placement, amplitudes > 1 μV, and generally negative polarity. FFPs have a diffuse distribution, fixed latencies, amplitudes < 1 μV, and polarity that probably reflects a volume-conducted positivity.

Potentials are labeled according to polarity and mean latency from a sample of the normal population. As one would expect, latencies change with body growth and nervous system maturation. Hence, labels differ between children and adults.

■ Posterior Tibial Nerve Somatosensory, Motor, and Reflex Evoked Potentials

There are less standard evoked potential component designations for posterior tibial nerve (PTN) SSEPs than for median nerve SSEPs.[25] For the purpose of discussion of generators of SSEP-PTNs, adult terminology is used, with child or infant notation following in parentheses. Following PTN stimulation, electrodes over the popliteal fossa record the electronegative peripheral nerve action potential N8 (N5). Electrodes over the lower spine record two electronegative potentials: the N19 (N11) and the N22 (N14). The N19 (N11) represents the afferent volley in the cauda equina.[27] The N22 (N14) is a stationary potential and probably reflects postsynaptic activity of internuncial neurons in the gray matter of the spinal cord.[27] Electrodes over the cervical spine record another later stationary potential: the N29 (N20). This component may reflect postsynaptic activity in the nucleus gracilis.[28] The P37 (P28) is the first major localized recorded component on the scalp. It reflects the ipsilaterally oriented cortical surface electropositivity, whereas the electronegative end of the dipole may be recorded contralaterally.[29,30] There is a great deal of intersubject variability in the topography of the P37 (P28) in adults[31] and especially in children.[32–34]

This is probably related to the known anatomical difference in the location of the primary sensory area for the leg.[35] When the leg area is located at the superior edge of the interhemispheric fissure, the cortical generator for P37 (P28) is vertically oriented and its amplitude is maximally close to the vertex. When the leg area is located more deeply in the fissure, the cortical generator is more horizontally turned and the P37 (P28) projects ipsilaterally.[30,36]

SSEP is a valuable tool in detecting spinal cord anoxia secondary to inadvertent involvement of supplying vessels around the S1 level. Kothbauer et al[13] used tibial SSEP without any surgical complications. Because the tibial nerve covers predominantly L5 and S1 dermatomes and leaves higher and lower segments relatively uncovered, these authors advocate additional dermatomal SSEP and pudendal monitoring. Monitoring the pudendal nerve activity (S2–S4) had been a promising technique for preventing damage to the sensory roots during the surgery within the cauda equina because it provides additional information at lower sacral levels below S1 that is associated with bowel, bladder, and sexual dysfunction.[37] In 2004, Kothbauer[14] provided an update article in which sensory potentials evoked by tibial or pudendal nerve stimulation were recorded from the dorsal columns via an epidurally inserted electrode and/or from the scalp as cortical responses. Monitoring of the motor system was achieved with motor evoked potentials recorded from limb muscles and the external anal sphincter. Amplitudes and latencies of these responses are then interpreted. The bulbocavernosus reflex, with stimulation of the pudendal nerve and recording of muscle responses in the external anal sphincter, is used for the continuous monitoring of reflex circuitry.[10,13–15]

■ Pathophysiology of Tethered Cord Syndrome

Two decades ago, the usual explanation for the neurological deficit associated with tethered cord syndrome was the effect of traction in preventing the ascent of the spinal cord within the spinal canal during growth. However, Barson[22] pointed out in 1970 that the spinal cord does not ascend significantly after birth. The incongruity in observations is due to the fact that the spine grows most rapidly during embryogenesis and after puberty (during teenage growth spurts), whereas symptoms of tethering are most often observed in early childhood (age 3 to 10 years). James and Lassman reported a clinical case in which, during a postmortem examination, a small bony septum from the midline of the laminae of L3–4 to the underlying vertebral body was found in an aged woman. She had never had any neurological deficits. Had there been significant ascension of the spinal cord after birth, she would have had neurological deficits, so the authors argued.[38] Although this was not necessarily so because issues of the divided cord segments rejoining below the spur and the size of the cleft between cord segments (small or large) were not addressed, the concept that the spinal cord ascended postnatally and produced neurological deficits by traction alone in tethered cord syndrome seemed untenable.

Yamada et al[39] examined the mitochondrial oxidative metabolic changes in the spinal cord before and after subjecting it to stretching. Using reflection spectrophotometry, they monitored in vivo changes in the reduction:oxidation (redox) ratio of cytochrome a,a$_3$ in animal models and in human tethered spinal cords (**Fig. 20.1**). They found a marked metabolic and electrophysiological susceptibility of the lumbosacral cord subjected to hypoxic conditions, especially under traction with hypoxic or electrically stimulating energy stress (**Fig. 20.2**).[39,40] They concluded that symptoms and signs of tethered spinal cord were associated with lumbosacral neuronal dysfunction and that this dysfunction is possibly due to impairment of mitochondrial oxidative metabolism. This is supported by the associated evoked potential changes (see later discussion). Most pediatric neurosurgeons now believe that the chronic stretch on the cord produced by tethering is an essential part of the problem but that

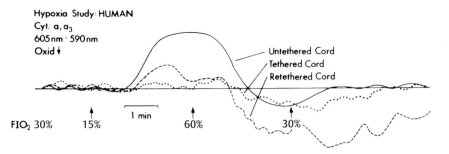

Fig. 20.1 Redox changes during hypoxia in one group of the human tethered cords (type 1). No redox change is seen before untethering (*dotted line*), but a reduction similar to that in normal cat cords is noted after untethering (*solid line*). No reduction occurs while the cord is temporarily retethered (*interrupted line*). FiO₂, fraction of inspired oxygen. (From Yamada S, Zinke DE, Sanders D. Pathophysiology of "tethered cord syndrome." J Neurosurg 1981;54:494-503. Reprinted with permission.)

superimposed insults such as acute flexion episodes or cord hypoxia accentuate symptoms to become more prominent.

Kang et al[41] tethered and untethered the cords of immature kittens and studied the effects of these manipulations on regional spinal cord blood flow, clinical features, and SSEPs. They found that cord tethering caused decreases in regional spinal cord blood flow in the distal spinal cord close to the site of tethering. The decreases in regional spinal cord blood flow (rSCBF) became progressively worse over the weeks following the tethering (**Fig. 20.3**). Untethering of the cord led to an increase in the rSCBF if the untethering occurred by 2 weeks after tethering. Delaying the untethering until 8 weeks caused failure of the rSCBF to recover the normal level. Changes in the evoked potential

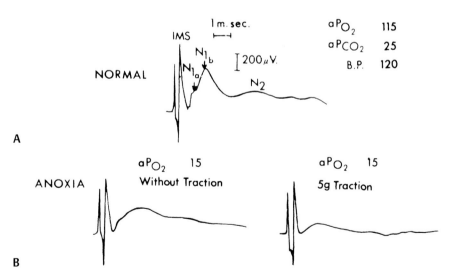

Fig. 20.2 (A) Normal cord potentials in response to dorsal root stimulations. IMS: from the posterior column; N1a: from the afferent terminals; N1b: from the interneurons of the first order; N2: from the interneurons of the second and third orders. **(B)** Marked change in the cord with traction of 5 g. (From Yamada S, Zinke DE, Sanders D. Pathophysiology of "tethered cord syndrome." J Neurosurg 1981;54:494-503. Reprinted with permission.)

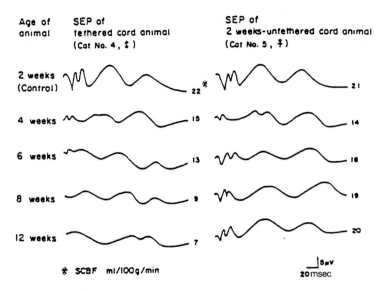

Fig. 20.3 Changes in somatosensory evoked potential (SSEP) were observed if regional spinal cord blood flow (rSCBF) was below 14 mL/100 g/min. Animals untethered after 2 weeks showed normal SSEP, which corresponded with an increase in rSCBF. (From Kang JK, Kim MC, Yim DS, et al. Effects of tethering on regional spinal cord blood flow and sensory-evoked potentials in growing cats. Childs Nerv Syst 1987;3:35–39. Reprinted with permission.)

occurred when rSCBF fell below 14 mL/100 g/min. The decrease in rSCBF had occurred by 2 weeks after tethering.

■ Diagnostic Clinical Neurophysiological Studies

Electrophysiological studies that help with diagnostic formulation include SSEPs after peroneal nerve stimulation (SSEP-PN), after pudendal nerve stimulation (SSEP-PuN), and after posterior tibial nerve stimulation (SSEPPTN), bulbocavernosus reflex (BCR) responses, and urodynamics with sphincter and pelvic floor EMG.

■ Somatosensory Evoked Potentials

It has been a decade since SSEPs were first used to evaluate patients with occult spinal dysraphism. Cracco and Cracco[42] recorded scalp and spinal responses after peroneal stimulation over the cauda equina and rostral spinal cord in adult and child control subjects (**Fig. 20.4**).

These spinal potentials consisted of low-amplitude triphasic waves over the cauda equina and larger potentials over the caudal spinal cord. Scalp potentials had latencies of 30 to 34 millisecond for electropositive components and 40 to 45 millisecond for electronegative components. In patients with sacral lipomas and no or minimal neurological findings, spinal potentials normally recorded over the lower thoracic spine (T9–12) were recorded over the lumbar spine, suggesting caudal displacement of the spinal cord (**Fig. 20.5**). In children with more extensive neurological findings (foot deformities, neurogenic bladders), relatively normal potentials were recorded over the cauda equina, and cerebral potentials were absent.[42] Others have subsequently verified the diagnostic value of SSEPs.[43,44] One group reported a patient who had postoperative SSEP-PN studies that were slightly improved compared with preoperative studies, and the patient had improved clinically.[43]

The authors have systematically studied children and young adults with tethered cord

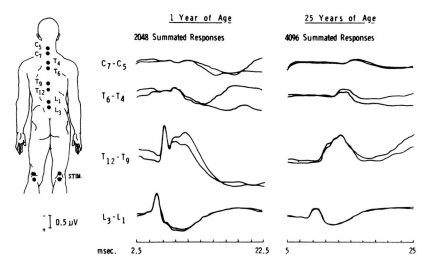

Fig. 20.4 Comparison of bipolar recordings of the spinal response to peroneal nerve stimulation in a 1-year-old infant and in an adult. Over the cauda equina (L3), the response in both the infant and the adult consists of triphasic potentials with poorly defined initial positive phases. In the infant, the response over the caudal spinal cord (T12) consists of a positive negative diphasic potential followed by a broad negative positive diphasic potential; in the adult, it consists of a broad negative potential with two or three inflections. The response over the rostral spinal cord in both the infant and the adult consists of small initially positive triphasic potentials with poorly defined positive phases. (From Cracco JB, Cracco RQ. Spinal somatosensory evoked potentials: maturational and clinical studies. Ann N Y Acad Sci 1982;388:526–537. Reprinted with permission.)

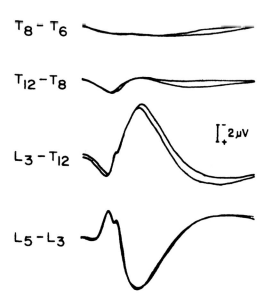

Fig. 20.5 Spinal responses in a 3-year-old child with thoracolumbar myelomeningocele. The large complex response that is recorded over T12 to T9 in normal children is present over L3 in this child, suggesting caudal displacement of the spinal cord. (From Cracco JB, Cracco RQ. Spinal somatosensory evoked potentials: maturational and clinical studies. Ann N Y Acad Sci 1982;388:526–537. Reprinted with permission.)

syndrome using SSEP-PTNs. Because SSEP-PN scalp and spine components are lower in amplitude than those produced by PTN stimulation[45] and because the topography of the scalp component of SSEP-PN is more variable than that of SSEP-PTN, SSEP-PTNs were used rather than SSEP-PNs for evaluation in children suspected of having tethered cord syndrome. Clinical, myelographic, and operative studies were prospectively evaluated in 22 consecutive patients, aged 18 months to 22 years, with symptoms of tethered cord syndrome.[7] Ten had previously undergone repair of lumbosacral meningomyelocele. In 19 patients, the diagnosis was established radiologically and/or intraoperatively. In three patients with clinical symptoms but without radiographically demonstrable lesions, SSEP-PTNs were normal.

Details of SSEP-PTN methodology have been reported elsewhere.[7,33] Briefly, square wave stimuli are delivered to the PTN at the ankle, with an intensity sufficient to cause a twitch of the abductor hallucis muscle or three times the sensory threshold. If the patient were anesthetic to the stimulus, then a sensory threshold three

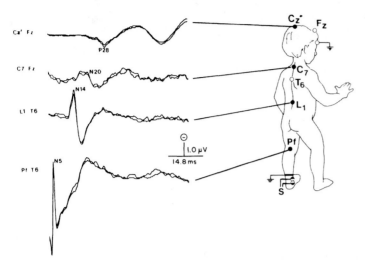

Fig. 20.6 Electrode placement and associated waveforms in somatosensory evoked potentials (SSEPs) after posterior tibial nerve (PTN) stimulation in children. Waveforms shown are from a normal child. The presumed origin of the various peaks is presented in Table 20.2. (From Roy MW, Gilmore R, Walsh JW. Evaluation of children and young adults with tethered spinal cord syndrome: utility of spinal and scalp recorded somatosensory evoked potentials. Surg Neurol 1986;26:241–248. Reprinted with permission.)

times that of a similarly aged control subject was used. The recording montage is presented in **Fig. 20.6**. The bandpass was 30 to 1500 Hz, with 40,000 amplification. Between 1000 and 2000 responses were averaged and replicated. Normative data are largely based on height. Only occasionally will age be used because generally the authors believe height is a better predictor of peak latency[33] (**Fig. 20.7**). Based

upon the absence or presence and the latency of N22 (N14) and P37 (P28), a severity rating scale for SSEP-PTN was developed (**Table 20.1**). The generator of the N22 (N14) is the lumbar spinal cord gray matter (**Table 20.2**). Thus the lumbosacral interneuronal dysfunction reported by Yamada et al[39] might be reflected, especially in abnormalities of the N22 (N14). This is the case.

Table 20.1 Severity Rating Scale for SSEP-PTN*

Severity Score	N22 (N14) Latency	N22 (N14) Amplitude	P37 (P28) Latency
Severity abnormal			
1	absent	absent	absent
2	normal	decreased	absent
3	delayed	normal	absent
4	absent	absent	delayed
Moderately abnormal			
5	absent	absent	normal
5	delayed	normal	normal
6	normal	decreased	delayed
7	normal	normal	delayed
Mildly abnormal			
8	normal	decreased†	normal
9	normal	decreased‡	normal
10	normal	normal	normal

*Notations in parentheses are designations for children (1 to 8 years old).

†P37:N22 amplitude ratio abnormally high

‡P37:N22 amplitude ratio normal (N22 > 0.66 μV in normal children; P37:N22 amplitude ratio = 0.25 to 4.10).

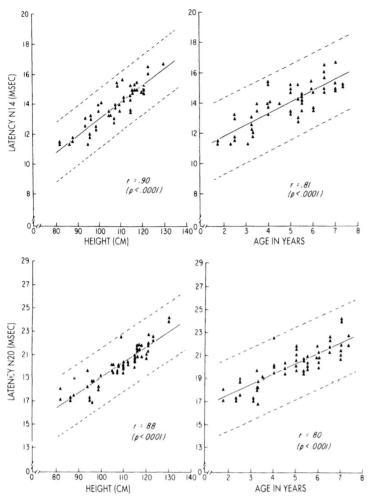

Fig. 20.7 (*Upper left*) Relationship between stature and absolute latency of N14 in children, with height ranging from 82 to 130 cm: x = 1.84 + 0.11 (height), (*Upper right*) Relationship between age and absolute latency of N14 in children aged 1 to 8 years: x = 10.26 ± 0.74 (age). (*Lower left*) Relationship between stature and absolute latency of N20 in children, with height ranging from 82 to 130 cm: x = 4.60 ± 0.14 (height). (*Lower right*) Relationship between age and absolute latency of N20 in children aged 1 to 8 years: x = 15 − 51 ± 0.95 (age). (From Gilmore RL, Bass NH, Wright EA, et al. Developmental assessment of spinal cord and cortical evoked potentials after tibial nerve stimulation: effects of age and stature on normative data during childhood. Electroencephalogr Clin Neurophysiol 1985;62:241–251. Reprinted with permission.)

Table 20.2 Presumed Generators of SSEP-PTN*

Component	Origin
N8 (N5)	Tibial nerve action potential
N19 (N11)	Cauda equina
N22 (N14)	Lumbar cord gray matter
N29 (N20)	Nucleus gracilis
P37 (P28)	Mesial sensory cortex

*Notations in parentheses are designations for children (1 to 8 years old).

The authors developed clinical severity scales using the factors of gait, bowel/bladder continence, motor, sensation, and deep tendon reflexes (**Table 20.3**), and also an operative severity scale based on the presence of lipoma, tension on the filum terminale, and/or extent of adhesions and cord movement after lysis of adhesions (**Table 20.4**). In three patients with clinical symptoms but without radiographically

Table 20.3 Severity Scale for Clinical Assessment of Tethered Cord Syndrome

Gait	*Bowel/Bladder History*
0—unable to walk unassisted	0—total incontinence
1—severe bilateral deficit	1—intermittent incontinence, uncontrolled
2—severe unilateral deficit	2—intermittent incontinence, controlled
3—mild bi- or unilateral deficit	3—increased frequency
4—walks normally	4—total control

Sensation to pinprick
  0—no sensation
  1—diminished sensation
  2—full sensation

Lower limb strength
  Use clinical scale of 0/5 to 5/5 for weakest joint on the limb
  Deep tendon reflexes
  The sum of the ankle and knee score for each lower limb (possible 4+ at each joint)

demonstrable lesions, SSEP-PTNs were normal. In the 19 patients with tethered cord syndrome, the clinical score and SSEP-PTN score correlated significantly ($r = .81$, $p < 0.001$). The location and direction of the tethering structures influenced the SSEP-PTN findings (**Table 20.5**). In patients with involvement primarily of the conus, the N22 (N14) was present but diminished in amplitude. In patients with extensive attachment of the spinal cord, the N22 (N14) was generally absent (**Fig. 20.8**), and frequently the N19 (N11) was also absent. Patients with scalp SSEP-PTN asymmetry tended to have the

Table 20.4 Severity Scale for Operative Findings in Tethered Cord Patients

Lipoma
  0—no lipoma
  1—lipoma not extensively attached
  2—lipoma extensively attached
Filum terminale
  0—flaccid
  1—moderately tight
  2—very tight
Adhesion extent
  0—only filum terminale attachment
  1—loose attachment in addition to filum
  2—extensive, tight adhesions
Cord movement
  Upward movement of the cord after lysis
    of adhesions (cm)

more severe abnormality contralateral to cord deviation or rotation (**Fig. 20.9**).

Postoperative SSEP-PTNs were sometimes improved (**Fig. 20.10** and **Table 20.6**). Findings associated with clinical improvement include an increase in the amplitude of N22 (N14), normalization of the P37 (P28):N22 (N14) amplitude ratio, shortening of the N22 (N14) latency, appearance of previously absent N22 (N14), and a decrease in central conduction time (latency P37 (P28) – latency N22 (N14)).

Some technical points were important: children 8 years old should be tested in the waking state because latency of the scalp component of SSEP-PTN varies with that state.[32–34] The N14 in children (probably generated by structures generating N22 in adults) is considerably higher in amplitude than in adults. Hence, its absence is a more reliable indicator of dysfunction in children.

There is a small but growing literature on evaluating the spinal cord with SSEP-PuN.[12,14,46–48] None of these studies have systematically evaluated the use of SSEP-PuN specifically in patients with tethered cord syndrome, but application to this clinical condition is obvious. The technique consists of stimulating any of several structures innervated by the pudendal nerve. The most accessible structure is the dorsal nerve of the penis, which can be stimulated bilaterally using ring electrodes placed at the

Table 20.5   Clinical and Operative Severity Scores for Patients with Different Degrees of SSEP-PTN Abnormalities

SSEP-PTN Abnormality	No. of Patients	No. of Studies	Clinical Score	Operative Score
Mild	12	20	15.9 ± 1.4	1.3 ± 0.6
Moderate	9	12	9.9 ± 2.0	3.1 ± 1.1
Severe	5	7	8.9 ± 1.3	4.1 ± 1.0

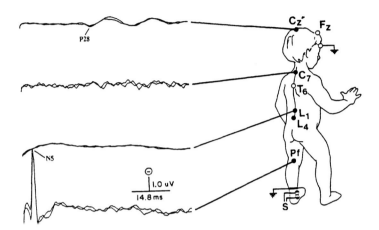

Fig. 20.8 Abnormal somatosensory evoked potential–posterior tibial nerve (SSEP-PTN) with absent N14 (lumbar potential) and N20 (cervical potential) in a child with extensive attachment of the spinal cord.

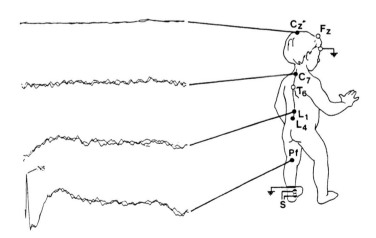

Fig. 20.9 Abnormal somatosensory evoked potential–posterior tibial nerve (SSEP-PTN). This is more abnormal than the study in **Fig. 20.8** in that the lumbar, cervical, and cortical potentials are all absent. The more severe abnormality was contralateral to the spinal cord deviation, with the P28 (cortical potential) absent after left leg stimulation.

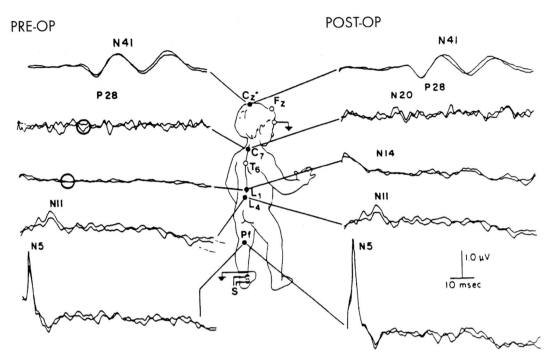

PRE-OP

POST-OP

Fig. 20.10 Preoperative and postoperative somatosensory evoked potential–posterior tibial nerve (SSEP-PTN) in a child who was found at surgery to have extensive tethering and rotation of the sacral spinal cord. Both N14 and N20 (lumbar and cervical spinal cord evoked potentials, respectively) were absent prior to operation (*circles*) and appeared postoperatively. (From Roy MW, Gilmore R, Walsh JW. Evaluation of children and young adults with tethered spinal cord syndrome: utility of spinal and scalp recorded somatosensory evoked potentials. Surg Neurol 1986;26:241–248. Reprinted with permission.)

base of the penis or unilaterally using laterally placed cup electrodes. Stimulation of the urethra[46] or anus[47] is possible using catheter electrodes with tip-inflatable balloons to maintain appropriate stimulus localization (**Fig. 20.11**). Square wave electrical stimuli of 0.3 millisecond applied at 1.7 to 3.1 Hz with an intensity 2.5 times threshold[49] are delivered. Scalp recording electrodes are placed at Cz (2 cm behind Cz, International 10–20 System of Electrode Placement) and Fp_z. Spinal electrodes are placed at the spinous process of T12 or L1 with reference to electrodes at the iliac crest or T6 spinous process. A common bandpass is 10 to 500 Hz. Sampling time ranges from 100 to 200 millisecondsec. Five hundred to 1000 responses are needed for the critical response and 1000 to 2000 responses for the spinal response. Only stimulation of the dorsal nerve of the penis will elicit a spinal response; stimulation of other

Table 20.6 Relationship between Postoperative Clinical Improvement Score and Specific SSEP Changes

	N22 (N14) Appearance	N22 (N14) Increased Amplitude	N22 (N14) – P37 (P28) Latency Decreased
No. of patients	4	3	4
Mean clinical improvement score	2.3	1.3	2

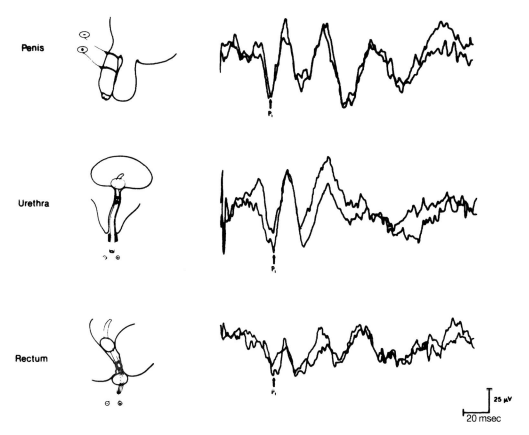

Fig. 20.11 Cortical evoked responses on stimulation of the dorsal nerve of the penis (*upper*), urethra (*middle*), and anal sphincter muscle (*lower*) in the same individual. (From Glick M, Haldeman S. The electrodiagnostic and neurovisceral evaluation of patients with spinal cord injuries. Neurology 1984;34(Suppl 1):209. Reprinted with permission.)

structures innervated by the pudendal nerve will not elicit a spinal response. The mean latencies of the cortical response of the SSEP-PuN is similar to, but slightly longer than, that of the cortical response of the SSEP-PTN: 42.3 + 1.9 millisecond. ~ Amplitude varies depending upon which branch of the PuN is stimulated. The spinal response has a latency of 12.9 + 0.8 millisecond.[50] This latency is much slower than that of the spinal response of the SSEP-PTN, resulting in a long central conduction time (cortical peak latency – spinal peak latency) of ~30 millisecond. This has been attributed to central conduction via smaller fibers than those giving rise to the SSEP-PTN response or to a greater number of synaptic connections in the pathway.[50]

With spinal cord lesions at or above T12, there may be absence or prolongation of the cortical potential. With spinal cord lesions at L1 or below, there will be absence or prolongation of the lumbar potential as well as the cortical potential. In actual practice, the value of this localization is limited because obesity, peripheral neuropathy, or stimulation of the PuN at sites other than the dorsal nerve of the penis will also lead to absence of the spinal potential.

Bulbocavernosus Reflex

The BCR is elicited by squeezing the glans penis or glans clitoridis or pulling on an indwelling Foley catheter. The response, contraction of the external anal sphincter muscle, may be seen or palpated. The absence of a response in a man is highly suggestive of a neurological lesion. Unfortunately, it is absent in up to 20% of normal females.[51]

The corresponding BCR electrophysiological potential is recorded over the perineum using small surface electrodes placed midway between the penis (or vagina) and anus.[52,53] Stimulation electrode placements and parameters are similar to those of SSEP-PuN. Recording parameters are also similar, except that 30 to 100 responses are necessary. With a stimulator, there is often a visible contraction of the pelvic floor. The BCR potentials have a biphasic appearance (**Fig. 20.12**). The latency of the potential is variable: mean = 35.9 millisecond, with a range of 26 to 44 millisecond.[48,49] The BCR potential allows electrophysiological evaluation of cauda equina and conus medullaris function. That is, prolongation of—or, more commonly, absence of—the BCR potential suggests dysfunction of the cauda equina and/or the conus medullaris.[50] Thus both SSEP and BCR studies can indicate function of some of the neural pathways traversing the cauda equina and conus medullaris, two regions frequently involved in tethered cord syndrome.

Pelvic Floor Electromyography

Another means of evaluating the child with tethered cord syndrome is EMG of the perineal floor muscles.[8,54] This technique usually involves placing a concentric needle electrode into the external urethra sphincter muscle. Individual motor unit potentials are examined. Standard criteria for firing rates and other features are used to determine whether the muscles are normal or denervated. Because many pelvic floor muscles are innervated by different sacral roots, careful and thorough EMG examination of several muscles may be necessary to determine the extent of the lesion. Other muscles (in addition to the external urethra sphincter muscle) that can be sampled include the external anal sphincter muscles, the bulbocavernosus muscle, and the ischiocavernosus muscle. This sort of examination is best performed by a physician, usually a urologist, with special

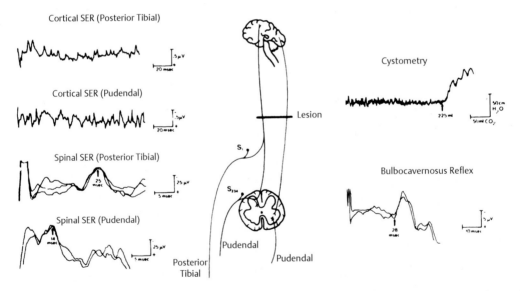

Fig. 20.12 Bulbocavernosus reflex (BCR) responses recorded from different sites in the perineum on stimulation of the dorsal nerve of the penis. SER, sensory evoked response. (From Glick M, Haldeman S. The electrodiagnostic and neurovisceral evaluation of patients with spinal cord injuries. Neurology 1984;34(Suppl 1):209. Reprinted with permission.)

training in the technique. Although EMG can be performed in a patient of any age, it is usually not done in infants or very young children unless there is a critically important diagnostic question regarding the integrity of the S2, S3, and S4 roots.

Intraoperative Electromyographic Monitoring for Tethered Cord Syndrome

The lumbosacral anatomy in patients with tethered cord syndrome is frequently complex. Nerve roots may be embedded in lipoma or may be visually indistinguishable from adhesions or a thickened filum terminale. The S1 and lumbar roots are recognizable by palpation of the contracting muscles after intraoperative electrode stimulation, but identification of the lower sacral roots requires some objective means of measuring sphincteric function.

James et al[9] utilized intraoperative external anal sphincter muscle EMG in 10 patients with spinal dysraphism: four patients with tethered cord syndrome, three with lipomeningocele, and three with other miscellaneous diagnoses. These children ranged in age from 3 weeks to 15 years. Using general anesthesia with the patient in a prone position, an anal plug or catheter containing an electrode or needle electrodes was placed in the anal sphincter muscle for recording purposes.[9] During dissection the conus was stimulated. If contraction of the anal sphincter muscle occurred, meticulous care was undertaken to preserve these structures. No patient deteriorated postoperatively and two noted improvement.

Pang[10] modified this technique by directly recording the "squeeze pressure" using a pressure-sensitive balloon inserted into the anal canal. There is a rationale for using squeeze pressure: it had earlier been noted that there is a direct relationship between anal sphincter muscle integrated EMG and anal canal pressure measurements with an anal balloon.[55] Pang used a double-lumen balloon catheter ordinarily used for intraluminal angioplasty. The balloon does not deform at high pressures so there is a high degree of sensitivity. The stimulation

was done with a disposable monopolar nerve locator stimulator ring and three current intensities: 0.5 (usually sufficient for infants and small children), 1.0, and 2.0 mA. If a sacral root was stimulated and the external anal sphincter muscle contracted, the combined stimulus artifact and spike wave on the pressure tracing was easily recorded. During stimulation, the cerebrospinal fluid had to be continuously suctioned to prevent current dispersion. Pressure responses with unilateral S2, S3, or S4 root stimulation generally generated pressures > 40 to 75 torr, even in plantar flexion of the foot without pressure change. Stimulation of the filum terminale and nonneural tissues always produced stimulus artifact without a pressure wave. Pang found this technique useful in several circumstances: (1) identifying sacral roots embedded in intradural lipoma; (2) identifying the junction between the functional conus and the intramedullary lipoma; (3) differentiating an elongated conus medullaris from a thickened filum terminale; and (4) identifying thickened adhesions (from previous myelomeningocele repair) and sacral roots. The more severely impaired the child or the more complex the disorder, the more the monitoring is needed to prevent nerve root injury, but also the more difficult it is to get satisfactory tracings because the sphincter muscles are paralyzed, and arachnoiditis makes the recording procedures technically much more difficult. In summary, the S2, S3, and S4 roots and the conus can be differentiated from the S1 and lumbar roots, the filum, lipoma, fibrous adhesions, and other nonfunctional fibroneural bands.

In general, motor potential recordings are known to provide immediate and extensive information derived from the motor system function. SSEPs primarily provide direct recording from the sensory tract but also allow for assumption of the motor tract function.[11,12,16,56,57] Shinomiya et al[18] propose the action potential studies of the external anal sphincter, external urethral sphincter, and lower limb muscles, combined with intravesical pressure recordings for safe untethering procedures in patients with lipomas or other anomalous tissue. On the other hand, they doubt that recording from the anal sphincter alone is sufficient to establish the presence of bowel and bladder function, and also SSEP is adequate as an intraoperative monitoring for the reflex arcs in the spinal cord involved in tethered cord syndrome. Even though their opinion is that muscle action potential monitoring is informative of spinal cord and nerve root function as an intraoperative monitoring during the tethered cord release, this study alone has shortcomings due to lack of data to support this method. In addition, muscle relaxants under general anesthesia impair motor action potentials.

Paradiso et al[15] reached a similar conclusion that multimodality intraoperative monitoring reduces the risk of inadvertent injury of neural tissue. They recorded the scalp component of the SSEP after tibial nerve stimulation and free-run EMG of limb muscles supplied by L2–S2 roots, anal and urethral sphincters. SSEP recordings provided almost instant information about the sensory pathway. They pointed out that in tethered cord syndrome, SSEPs are valuable in detecting spinal cord anoxia secondary to inadvertent involvement of supplying vessels above the S1 level and damage to the S1 root,

which carries most of the posterior tibial nerve fibers. They mention that continuous EMG has limitations: (1) presence of EMG activity before manipulation was attempted that was documented in 12 to 16% of cases, and (2) failure to assess nonirritational mechanisms of nerve damage such as ischemia and sharp nerve transection. Evoked EMG was proposed because it assesses the integrity of the nerve fibers between the stimulating site and the muscle. This establishes safe planes and limits of dissection, facilitating maximal detethering at minimal risk of compromising functional neural tissues.[15]

■ Conclusion

Tethered cord syndrome is a stretch-induced functional disorder of the spinal cord. In mechanical insults unlike the vascular injury, both sensory and motor neurons in the spinal cord would be involved due to proximity of each other. A comprehensive preoperative assessment of neurological dysfunction or neurophysiological study of the patients could be helpful in predicting and improving the course of surgical outcome.

References

1. Marin-Padilla M. The tethered cord syndrome: developmental considerations. In: Holtzman RN, Stein BM, eds. The Tethered Spinal Cord. New York: Thieme-Stratton; 1985:3–13
2. Hendrick EB, Hoffman HJ, Humphreys RP. The tethered spinal cord. Clin Neurosurg 1983;30:457–463
3. Hoffman HJ, Hendrick EB, Humphreys RP. The tethered spinal cord: its protean manifestations, diagnosis and surgical correction. Childs Brain 1976;2:145–155
4. Cracco JB, Cracco RQ. Somatosensory spinal and cerebral evoked potentials in children with occult spinal dysraphism [abstract]. Neurology 1979;29:543
5. Cracco J, Cracco RQ, Graziani L. Spinal evoked response in infants with myelodysplasia [abstract]. Neurology 1974;24:359–360
6. Duckworth T, Yamashita T, Franks CI, Brown BH. Somatosensory evoked cortical responses in children

with spina bifida. Dev Med Child Neurol 1976;18:19–24
7. Roy MW, Gilmore R, Walsh JW. Evaluation of children and young adults with tethered spinal cord syndrome: utility of spinal and scalp recorded somatosensory evoked potentials. Surg Neurol 1986;26:241–248
8. Blaivas JG. Urologic abnormalities in the tethered spinal cord. In: Holtzman RN, Stein BM, eds. The Tethered Spinal Cord. New York: Thieme-Stratton; 1985:59–73
9. James HE, Mulcahy JJ, Walsh JW, Kaplan GW. Use of anal sphincter electromyography during operations on the conus medullaris and sacral nerve roots. Neurosurgery 1979;4:521–523
10. Pang D. Use of an anal sphincter pressure monitor for identification of sacral nerve roots and conus. In: Holtzman RN, Stein BM, eds. The Tethered Spinal Cord. New York: Thieme-Stratton; 1985:74–84

11. Albright AL, Pollack IF, Adelson PD, Solot JJ. Outcome data and analysis in pediatric neurosurgery. Neurosurgery 1999;45:101–106

12. Herdmann J, Deletis V, Edmonds HL Jr, Morota N. Spinal cord and nerve root monitoring in spine surgery and related procedures. Spine 1996;21:879–885

13. Kothbauer K, Schmid UD, Seiler RW, Eisner W. Intraoperative motor and sensory monitoring of the cauda equina. Neurosurgery 1994;34:702–707, discussion 707

14. Kothbauer KF, Novak K. Intraoperative monitoring for tethered cord surgery: an update. Neurosurg Focus 2004;16:E8

15. Paradiso G, Lee GY, Sarjeant R, Fehlings MG. Multimodality neurophysiological monitoring during surgery for adult tethered cord syndrome. J Clin Neurosci 2005;12:934–936

16. Phillips LH II, Jane JA. Electrophysiologic monitoring during tethered spinal cord release. In: Clinical Neurosurgery. Vol 43. San Francisco: Williams & Wilkins; 1995:163–202

17. Quiñones-Hinojosa A, Gadkary CA, Gulati M, et al. Neurophysiological monitoring for safe surgical tethered cord syndrome release in adults. Surg Neurol 2004;62:127–133, discussion 133–135

18. Phillips LH 2nd, Jane JA. Electrophysiologic monitoring during tethered cord release. Clin Neurosurg 1996; 43:163–164

19. Kim NH, Yang IH. A study of motor and sensory evoked potentials in chronic cauda equina compression of the dog. Eur Spine J 1996;5:338–344

20. Sensenig EC. The early development of the meninges of the spinal cord in human embryos. Contrib Embryol 1951;34:147–157

21. Streeter GL. Factors involved in the formation of the filum terminale. Am J Anat 1919;25.1–12

22. Barson AJ. The vertebral level of termination of the spinal cord during normal and abnormal development. J Anat 1970;106(Pt 3):489–497

23. Lorente de No R. A study of nerve physiology. Studies Rockefeller Inst. 1947;132:384–477

24. Kimura J, Mitsudome A, Yamada T, Dickins QS. Stationary peaks from a moving source in far-field recording. Electroencephalogr Clin Neurophysiol 1984;58:351–361

25. Lueders H, Lesser R, Hahn J, Little J, Klem G. Subcortical somatosensory evoked potentials to median nerve stimulation. Brain 1983;106(Pt 2):341–372

26. Desmedt JE, Nguyen TH, Carmeliet J. Unexpected latency shifts of the stationary P9 somatosensory evoked potential far field with changes in shoulder position. Electroencephalogr Clin Neurophysiol 1983;56:628–634

27. Seyal M, Gabor AJ. The human posterior tibial somatosensory evoked potential: synapse dependent and synapse independent spinal components. Electroencephalogr Clin Neurophysiol 1985;62:323–331

28. Seyal M, Kraft LW, Gabor AJ. Cervical synapse-dependent somatosensory evoked potential following posterior tibial nerve stimulation. Neurology 1987;37:1417–1421

29. Cruse R, Klem G, Lesser RP, Leuders H. Paradoxical lateralization of cortical potentials evoked by stimulation of posterior tibial nerve. Arch Neurol 1982;39:222–225

30. Seyal M, Emerson RG, Pedley TA. Spinal and early scalp-recorded components of the somatosensory evoked potential following stimulation of the posterior tibial nerve. Electroencephalogr Clin Neurophysiol 1983;55:320–330

31. Emerson RG. Anatomic and physiologic bases of posterior tibial nerve somatosensory evoked potentials. Neurol Clin 1988;6:735–749

32. Gilmore R. The use of somatosensory evoked potentials in infants and children. J Child Neurol 1989;4:3–19

33. Gilmore RL, Bass NH, Wright EA, Greathouse D, Stanback K, Norvell E. Developmental assessment of spinal cord and cortical evoked potentials after tibial nerve stimulation: effects of age and stature on normative data during childhood. Electroencephalogr Clin Neurophysiol 1985;62:241–251

34. Gilmore RL, Hermansen M, Brock J, et al. Effect of sleep on cortical SSEP: age dependency during growth and development. Electroencephalogr Clin Neurophysiol 1986;64:42

35. Penfield W, Rasmussen T. The Cerebral Cortex of Man: A Clinical Study of Localization of Function. New York: Macmillan; 1950

36. Lesser RP, Lüders H, Dinner DS, et al. The source of "paradoxical lateralization' of cortical evoked potentials to posterior tibial nerve stimulation. Neurology 1987;37:82–88

37. Cohen BA, Major MR, Huizenga BA. Pudendal nerve evoked potential monitoring in procedures involving low sacral fixation. Spine 1991;16(8, Suppl):S375–S378

38. James CCM, Lassman LP. Diastematomyelia and the tight filum terminale. J Neurol Sci 1970;10:193–196

39. Yamada S, Zinke DE, Sanders D. Pathophysiology of "tethered cord syndrome." J Neurosurg 1981;54:494–503

40. Yamada S, Knierim D, Yonekura M, Schultz R, Maeda G. Tethered cord syndrome. J Am Paraplegia Soc 1983;6:58–61

41. Kang JK, Kim MC, Kim DS, Song JU. Effects of tethering on regional spinal cord blood flow and sensory-evoked potentials in growing cats. Childs Nerv Syst 1987;3:35–39

42. Cracco JB, Cracco RQ. Spinal somatosensory evoked potentials: maturational and clinical studies. Ann N Y Acad Sci 1982;388:526–537

43. Chehrazi B, Parkinson J, Bucholz R. Evoked somatosensory potentials to common peroneal nerve stimulation in man. J Neurosurg 1981;55:733–741

44. Duckworth T, Yamashita T, Franks CI, Brown BH. Somatosensory evoked cortical responses in children with spina bifida. Dev Med Child Neurol 1976; 18:19–24

45. Chiappa KH. Evoked Potentials in Clinical Medicine. New York: Raven Press; 1983:214

46. Haldeman S, Bradley WE, Bhatia NN. Evoked responses in clinical neuro-urology. Bull Los Angeles Neurol Soc 1982;47:76–90

47. Glick M, Haldeman S. The electrodiagnostic and neurovisceral evaluation of patients with spinal cord injuries. Neurology 1984;34(Suppl 1):209

48. Haldeman S, Bradley WE, Bhatia NN, Johnson BK. Pudendal evoked responses. Arch Neurol 1982;39: 280–283

49. Haldeman S, Bradley WE, Bhatia N. Evoked responses from the pudendal nerve. J Urol 1982;128:974–980

50. Haldeman S. Pudendal nerve evoked spinal, cortical, and bulbocavernosus reflex responses: methods and application. In: Cracco RQ, Bodis-Wollner I, eds. Evoked Potentials. New York: Alan R Liss; 1986:68–75

51. Blaivas JG, Zayed AA, Labib KB. The bulbocavernosus reflex in urology: a prospective study of 299 patients. J Urol 1981;126:197–199

52. Dick HC, Bradley WE, Scott FB, Timm GW. Pudendal sexual reflexes: electrophysiologic investigations. Urology 1974;3:376–379

53. Siroky MB, Sax DS, Krane RJ. Sacral signal tracing: the electrophysiology of the bulbocavernosus reflex. J Urol 1979;122:661–664

54. van Gool JD. Vesico-ureteral reflux in children with spina bifida and detrusor-sphincter dyssynergia. Contrib Nephrol 1984;39:221–237

55. Schweiger M. Method for determining individual contributions of voluntary and involuntary anal sphincters to resting tone. Dis Colon Rectum 1979; 22:415–416

56. Balzer JR, Rose RD, Welch WC, Sclabassi RJ. Simultaneous somatosensory evoked potential and electromyographic recordings during lumbosacral decompression and instrumentation. Neurosurgery 1998;42:1318–1324, discussion 1324–1325

57. Winn H Richard. Editor-in-chief. Youmans Neurological Surgery. 5th ed. Philadelphia: Saunders; 2004

21 Conservative versus Surgical Treatment and Prognostic Evaluation for Tethered Cord Syndrome

Shokei Yamada, George T. Mandybur, Austin R. T. Colohan, and Vivian A. Yamada

This chapter summarizes the previous chapters and reflects on the neurosurgeon's role in the diagnosis and treatment of tethered cord syndrome (TCS). Given that the presentations in the previous chapters clarified the current understandings, the combination of the neurological and musculoskeletal findings and imaging criteria can lead to the diagnosis of TCS.

However, decisions about treatment for TCS are more complicated. Once the diagnosis of TCS is established or when there is an established likelihood that TCS is evolving, the neurosurgeon is required to choose among treatment alternatives that will help patients maintain normal lives while minimizing surgical risks. Additional information about TCS related to various other anomalies and disorders is provided to supplement the previous chapters.

Embryology emphasizes the importance of neurulation and caudal mass regression. The position of the caudal extremity and the development of a normal filum determine the healthy lumbosacral spine and spinal cord. The failure of these two components to develop properly can cause TCS (Chapter 2). The indication and surgical treatment must be definitive in patients with elongated spinal cord attached to inelastic structures, including a fibrous filum, lipoma, or dermoid, and with neurological deficits and musculoskeletal deformities in the lower limbs (Chapter 10).

The pathophysiology of the tethered spinal cord or TCS includes impairment of oxidative metabolism and electrophysiological function (Chapter 3). Mild to moderate metabolic dysfunction caused by low- or medium-grade traction of the experimental cord is reversible. The degree of dysfunction may be related to spinal cord ischemia and corresponds to a mild or moderate form of neurological deficit observed in humans. No histological damage to neurons, glial cells, or vasculature is expected in the spinal cord with such metabolic and electrophysiological dysfunction. However, sudden traction, in addition to steady cord traction, can cause histological damage to neurons. These findings may explain the permanent but partial damage to the lumbosacral cord, particularly to the conus medullaris (Chapter 3).

Neurological and urological examinations must include detailed history taking, specific for the early signs and symptoms of TCS. Neurological signs and symptoms (Chapters 4, 10, and 15) and urological tests (Chapters 7 and 8) must be correlated with lumbosacral lesions above the cord-tethering site. Skin stigmata can be useful when correlated with signs and symptoms and imaging features for diagnosis of TCS (Chapter 10), but older patients often lack these features.

Both autonomic and somatic systems form afferent and efferent reflex arcs, regulate the complex urinary storage and emptying functions, and also participate in the urethral control mechanism. The incontinence in TCS is due to the dysfunction of neurons located within the conus medullaris.[1] A full urodynamic evaluation along with pelvic floor electromyography (EMG) plays an important role in detecting a conus medullaris lesion or sacral neuropathy in patients suspected of having TCS (Chapter 7 and 8). Determination of the postvoid urinary residual for these patients at the clinic is a practical method of detecting early TCS. These methods are valuable in differentiating incontinence due to TCS from psychological incontinence and incontinence due to bladder infection.

Imaging studies have improved the diagnosis of TCS since the advent of computed tomography (CT) and magnetic resonance imaging (MRI). CT or MRI evidence of an elongated cord continuous to a thick filum or a tumor predicts TCS (Chapter 5). For adolescent or adult patients without these MRI features, a posteriorly displaced filum is a useful diagnostic feature for TCS (Chapter 15). To confirm this finding, intraoperative endoscopy confirms the displaced filum posterior to the cauda equina fibers and touching the posterior arachnoid (Chapter 3). In infants with TCS, ultrasonic studies can demonstrate lack of filum and conus movement, which is supposed to be synchronous to cerebrospinal fluid pulsations in normal individuals (Chapter 6).

TCS in the cervical spinal cord (Chapter 9) is clinically manifested like category 2 of the lumbosacral TCS (Chapter 3). The spinal cord lesion is located within a few segments above or below the tethering point because the dentate ligaments hold the cord tightly to prevent stretch-induced cord dysfunction. However, there is experimental evidence that cephalad pulling of a pair of cervical dentate ligaments causes elongation of the cervical cord and extending down to the thoracic cord segments.[2,3] This supports the fact that cervical TCS can really exist. The mechanical causes of tethered cervical spinal cord syndrome include myelomeningoceles (MMCs), lipomyelomeningoceles, and dermoid or postoperative scar formation.

Chapter 14 concentrates on TCS associated with a dermoid or epidermoid tumor. It emphasizes the elimination of the cord tethering effect of a tumor as well as decompression of the cord mass effect. Total resection must be accomplished, although two-staged operations may be required for a large tumor. In addition, an intradural lipoma and dysgenesis of the spinal cord or peripheral nerves must be considered.

Chapter 20 discusses evoked potential studies in conjunction with clinical findings in true TCS [i.e., category 1 cord tethering (Chapter 3)]. The authors found delayed conduction from the spinal cord to the cervical region and cerebral cortex in response to posterior tibial nerve stimulation. This delay is interpreted as impairment of multisynaptic spinal cord conduction, and the postuntethering improvement in evoked potentials is significant. Commonly, straight conduction through the posterior column is not disturbed in TCS patients. Only in category 3 is it likely that the lumbar and cervical somatosensory evoked potentials may be absent, under severe cord tethering or peripheral nerve dysfunction.

■ Severity of Signs and Symptoms and Prognosis

While making treatment decisions, neurosurgeons and other specialists must take into account that the prognosis of TCS patients or those harboring potential cord-tethering disorders depends on several individualized factors. Among these factors are: (1) neurological signs and symptoms must be precisely described (Chapter 4, Chapter 15). (See an example of sensory changes with patchy distribution in **Fig. 21.1.**) (2) The severity of TCS signs and symptoms determines the prognosis; inelastic structures that are immobilizing the spinal cord connected at its caudal end (category 1 patients) are sectioned or resected with better results than category 2 patients. (3) The growth rate of the spinal column in relation to that of the spinal cord influences the spinal cord tension. (4) Forcible cord stretching caused by flexion-extension exercises, a violent impact to the spinal column, or repeated jolting of the spine aggravate signs and symptoms. (5) Impaired oxidative metabolism

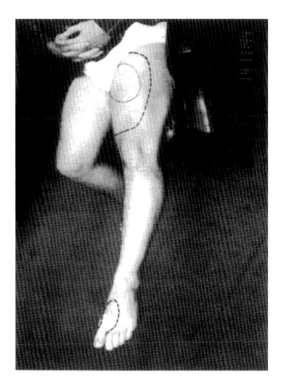

Fig. 21.1 Patchy distribution of sensory deficit (mostly to pain and temperature) is shown in the lower left limb. The dotted line indicates the analgesic area and the dashed lines the hypalgesic area.

associated with TCS is accentuated by any further imposition of hypoxemia, ischemia, or venous stasis, such as that which might be produced during surgical procedures.

The grading system of Hoffman et al[4] for patients with lipomyelomeningoceles (LMMCs) (**Table 21.1**) according to the signs and symptoms is valuable to determine the patient's prognosis (Chapters 3 and 11). This system indicates that the more severe the signs and symptoms, the worse is the outcome. In mild forms of TCS described as type 1 and type 2 (Chapter 3), signs and symptoms often fluctuate. This fluctuation is noted in both adult and young patients. It is not uncommon that after a few days to a few weeks of resting, the patients are often relieved of back and leg pain, and improved in motor, sensory (**Fig. 21.1**), and bladder function. The surgical prognosis of these patients is excellent (Chapter 11). Conservative treatment in these patients is discussed later in this chapter.

Inelastic Filum

The elasticity of the filum determines the degree of cord tethering (Chapters 4, 7, 15, and 20). Fat tissue is soft and elastic but becomes the source of excessive cord tension when the fibrous component increases in fibroadipose tissue. The vulnerability of the spinal cord seems dependent on the volume of each cord segment.[5] The elongated spinal cord (from L1 to S1 segments) is thinner than the normal cord and therefore vulnerable to stretching, whereas the diameter of the conus may be greater than that seen in the normal individual (Chapter 18).

Table 21.1   Grading System for Lipomyelomeningoceles

Grade	Explanation
0	No significant neurological, orthopedic, or urological problem; the patient may have reflex changes and/or sensory deficits
1	Minimal weakness and/or muscle-wasting and/or foot deformity affecting only one leg without significant gait disturbance; normal bladder and sphincter function
2	Neurogenic bladder alone or combined with minimal weakness of one leg, or intact bladder function with minimal weakness affecting both legs
3	Moderate to severe weakness of one leg producing gait disturbance with or without neurogenic bladder, or minimal weakness of both legs combined with neurogenic bladder
4	Severe paraparesis requiring aids for walking, with or without neurogenic bladder
4	Inability to ambulate

Source: Hoffman HJ, Taecholarn C, Hendrick EB, et al. Management of lipomyelomeningoceles: experience at the Hospital for Sick Children, Toronto. J Neurosurg 1985;62:1–8. Reprinted with permission.

Spinal Cord versus Vertebral Column Growth

Although traction effect of an inelastic filum on the lumbosacral cord determines the occurrence of TCS, the growth rate of the vertebral column also influences the severity of the increased tension within the spinal cord that is tethered at its caudal end. From 8 to 9 weeks of gestation, the normal spinal cord begins to ascend in the spinal canal as the growth of the vertebral column is accelerated. The caudal end of the spinal cord is opposite the L3 vertebra by the time of birth[5,6] (Chapters 2 and 15), and it ascends farther to the T12, L1, or L2 vertebral level by 3 years of age[6,7] (Chapters 2 and 10). Because no spinal cord ascension has been recorded thereafter, the overall growth rate of the spinal cord is assumed to be equal to that of the vertebral column after this age (**Fig. 21.2**).[8] A certain degree of tension exists within the normal cord.[2,9] If the spinal cord is anchored by an inelastic filum at or below L3 at the age of 4 years or older, the growth rate of the lumbosacral cord may not match that of the vertebral column[10,11] and is likely to be under excessive tension and further

develop neuronal dysfunction. Both scoliosis and accentuated lordosis allow the spinal cord to take the shortest course in the spinal canal.[12,13] These curvature changes serve as an appropriate means to minimize the tension within the spinal cord. The incidence of a normal (L2–3 interspace or higher) or slightly lower (L3 vertebral level) location of the caudal end of the spinal cord is much higher in adults with TCS (Chapter 15) than in children with TCS[14,15] (Chapter 9) (**Fig. 21.3**). These data can explain the delay of TCS manifestation in adulthood.

Forcible Stretching of the Spinal Cord by Spinal Movement

Performance of flexion-extension exercises or any other strenuous activities associated with spine curvature changes can strain the spinal cord, causing progression of TCS. The fact that the pressure on a large lipoma or LMMC transmits a stretching force to the spinal cord should alert the patients of neurological catastrophe resulting from undue pressure on these anomalies (Chapter 11).

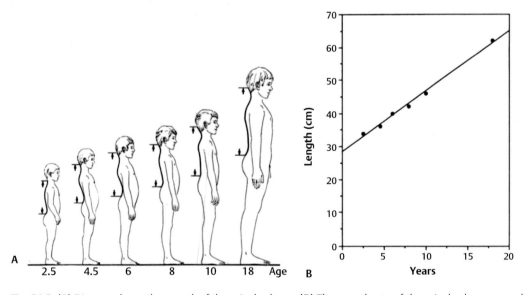

Fig. 21.2 (A) Diagram shows the growth of the spinal column. **(B)** The growth rate of the spinal column was calculated by measuring the distance between the C1 and S2 vertebrae in humans ranging from 2.5 to 18 years of age.

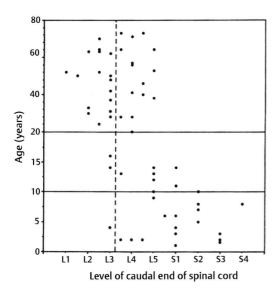

Fig. 21.3 Graph showing the location of the caudal end of the spinal cord relative to the vertebral level. The location of the caudal end is crowded at the L5–S2 vertebral level in TCS patients younger than 20 years of age, and at the L2–4 levels in those 20 years or older.

Oxidative Metabolism

Intraoperative redox studies of cytochrome a,a_3 have indicated that the more functionally impaired the spinal cord function, the more severe are the derangements in oxidative metabolism. This apparent link between neurological and metabolic dysfunction occurred regardless of whether the TCS symptomatology started spontaneously or was initiated by a back injury. Type 1 patients had the best prospects for regaining normal spinal cord function after untethering procedures (Chapter 3). Although the sequence of neurological improvement was slower than in type 1 patients, type 2 patients regained normal or nearly normal motor, sensory, and bladder function. In type 3 patients, recovery from oxidative metabolic impairment was incomplete even though the spinal cord was relaxed after untethering.

Type 1 patients correspond to grades 0 and 1 of the grading system of Hoffman et al.[4] Type 2 patients correspond to grades 2 and 3, and type 3 patients to grade 4 and partly grade 3. These correlations allow for the following conclusions. Type 2 patients should be operated on as soon as the diagnosis is made. The type 1 and type 3 patients need careful evaluation, because neurological signs and symptoms fluctuate; for example, type 1 patients may become almost asymptomatic after 2 weeks of rest, and subtle progression in type 3 patients may be overlooked or undetected. Any degree of symptomatic worsening is an indication for surgical untethering.

■ Treatment

Conservative Treatment

Conservative treatment is desirable for patients with no neurological and musculoskeletal abnormalities despite MRI evidence of an elongated spinal cord attached to a thick filum or a lipoma. Patients with back and leg pain that is accentuated by typical postural changes but with minimal deficit (Chapters 3 and 15) may show only subtle signs of TCS. Surgical untethering protects those patients from progression of neurological deficit and musculoskeletal deformities.

Conservative treatment mainly consists of preventing spinal cord stretching that occurs as a result of straightening the lumbosacral lordosis and consequent elongation of the spinal canal. Patients must be instructed to avoid such postures as (1) sitting legs crossed in a Buddha pose or Yoga sitting, (2) bending over the sink or lavatory[16,17] (see Fig. 15.3 in chapter 15), (3) holding the baby or heavier object at the waist level, (4) holding any weight while standing that causes back and leg pain, (5) sleeping supine in the bed overnight, (6) for woman to lie supine during intercourse, (7) sitting in a slouching position, (8) driving or riding in the car on a bumpy road, until back pain is aggravated, (9) walking, running, or horseback riding long enough to cause back and leg discomfort. (10) deep bending such as athletic practice, toe touching (**Fig. 21.4**), and high leg kicking, although these exercises mainly use flexion of

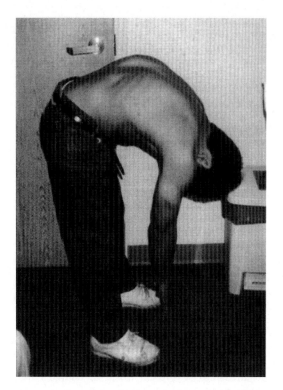

Fig. 21.4 This 16-year-old boy with severe rotational scoliosis began to complain of back and leg pain for several months, interfering with soccer skills. Repeated toe-touch exercises aggravated the pain. Within a few weeks after untethering surgery, he was free of back and leg pain. In 6 months, he underwent corrective spinal fixation surgery and returned to playing soccer.

the hip joints and thoracic spine. These exercises could also straighten the lumbosacral spine and should be avoided. Those patients who show Lhermitte sign should be instructed to avoid hyperflexion of the head and neck.

Because back and leg pain is muscular in nature, muscle relaxants are effective, including (1) medications that control overexcited interneurons in the spinal cord, such as phenobarbital (not as a tranquilizer) and carisoprodol (Soma); (2) muscle relaxants such as valium, methocarbamol (Robaxin); (3) nonsteroidal antiinflammatory agents, such as ibuprofen, celecoxib, (4) steroid for limited period of severe symptomatic exacerbation, (5) opioid derivatives that may be prescribed for only

severe pain that occurs after strenuous physical activities with only intermittent usage, but not longer than a few months to avoid dependency or addiction.

TCS patients should be warned of worsening signs and symptoms by any Valsalva-type maneuver that causes venous congestion and resultant ischemia,[18] and any possibility of tissue hypoxia such as might be produced by strenuous activity, such as skiing at high altitude or diving for a prolonged time. Lying supine on a lipomatous mass during intercourse can result in paraplegia (Hoffman HJ, personal communication,1995).

Surgical Treatment for TCS due to an Inelastic Filum, Sacral MMC, or Caudal MMC

TCS is a syndrome characterized by neurological dysfunction secondary to high tension within the spinal cord, rather than to histological neuronal damage. Intraoperative noninvasive redox studies of cytochrome a,a_3 have demonstrated that a link exists between impairment of oxidative metabolism, regulated by mitochondria in the tethered lumbosacral spinal cord, and neurological dysfunction. Prognosis after surgery appears to be definable by how large the shift toward oxidation of the mitochondrial cytochromes occurs after untethering. Therefore, spinal cord function should return to normal if untethering procedures are performed, as long as the neurons are still metabolically and electrophysiologically at a functional level (Chapters 3, 11, and 15). These scientific results indicate that an untethering procedure should be done as soon as even mild signs and symptoms are noted.

Surgical Treatment for Early Tethered Cord Syndrome

Case 1

The following case is an example of TCS manifestation after repeated strenuous exercises and perfect surgical outcome when treatment was provided in the early stages of TCS. This 22-year-old paramedic trainee presented with difficulty in voiding and intermittent left groin and testicular pain mixed with paresthesia (pins and needles) since 14 years of age. He was toilet trained and walked at 2 years of age. His mother knew that his feet were flat early in childhood, but she, as well as the patient, had noticed an increasingly high arch of both feet and curling of toes (hammertoes) for several years. He recalled that he was not athletic as a child because his body was stiff. The patient underwent intensive physical training and gained flexibility to sit in a yoga position and to touch his toes by his late teens.

On examination, this patient exhibited a slight inversion of the left foot on tiptoe walking (indicating peroneus longus weakness), minimum hypalgesia in the dorsum of both feet, and coccygeal subcutaneous fat and tufts of hair. Ancillary MRI studies showed that there was adipose tissue in the low sacral and coccygeal vertebral canal. Also, testing demonstrated a neurogenic bladder with motor instability of the tonic type and a residual urine volume of 150 mL (via cystometrogram). MRI showed a sacral intraspinal lipoma and posteriorly displaced filum, which was touching the posterior arachnoid membrane (**Fig. 21.5**).

At operation, an inelastic filum was found continuous to a lower sacral and coccygeal fat mass. After cord untethering by sectioning the filum, the patient was relieved of the testicular pain immediately and of incontinence within 1 week. Within 2 months, he noticed that the high arching of the feet and the hammertoes were decreasing. He returned to normal training within 6 weeks.

Case 2

This case represents TCS that developed late in life. This 72-year-old man complained of pain in the back and legs, and weakness and numbness in his distal leg muscles for 9 months. Weakness of the dorsiflexors and plantar flexors of the feet and toes and of the foot everter was found. At operation, the caudal end of the spinal cord was opposite the L5 vertebral level continuous to the fibroadipose filum. The conus ascended 1 cm after

sectioning the filum (**Fig. 21.6**). The patient was relived of pain and improved in motor function. Preoperative spinal cord dysfunction was attributed to the progression of osteoarthritic stenosis that caused restriction of the cord and filum movement and consequently increased cord tension.

Prophylactic Untethering Procedures

The benefits (if any) of prophylactic surgery for potential TCS in patients with cord elongation and filum thickening are still debatable.[19–23] The majority of these patients develop symptomatology early in life, but an increasing number of patients[24–26] develop TCS in adulthood (Chapter 15), as late as 80 years of age in our series. However, it is clear that most of the patients with an MMC or LMMC are anticipated to develop TCS, and its prevention would be repair of these anomalies and cord untethering in category 1[27] and category 2 if possible.

Surgical Treatment for Bladder Control

Chapters 7, 8 and 19 are dedicated to neurourological function in Chapter 13 to sphincter control.

The importance of detecting bladder and rectal control in patients with TCS in its early stage has been recognized. Bladder dysfunction as an early symptom of TCS is reversible but not in the later stage. For this reason, it is imperative for parents to watch diapers of their infant with sacral MMC or LMMC every 15 minutes for 2 hours periodically four times a day. When periodical wetting changes to constant wetting, urgent surgical untethering is mandatory to prevent rapid deterioration of conus function. The following anatomical analysis may explain conus dysfunction: as observed in **Fig. 21.7**; nerve roots of one cord segment take a horizontal course, as do all the nerve roots at 8 to 9 weeks gestation. It is apparent that this cord segment moved neither cephalad nor caudad in relation to the vertebral column during any period of growth. Considering its nerve roots traveling caudad to their dural exits, the cord segment above the horizontal roots is likely to

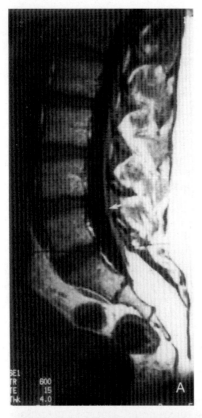

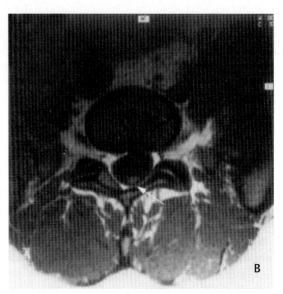

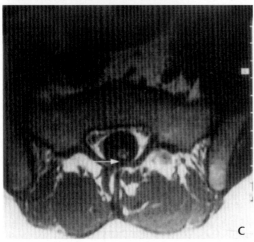

Fig. 21.5 Case 1. **(A)** The spinal cord and filum are displaced posteriorly (*arrow*) and the filum is connected to an intraspinal lipoma. The caudal end of the cord (the lowest coccygeal root) was opposite the S1 vertebral body. **(B)** The spinal cord touches the arachnoid (*arrow*) beneath the L5 lamina. **(C)** The spinal cord segment above the L5 lamina shows some arachnoid space (*arrow*), as does the cord segment below the lamina (not shown).

have stretched or grown cephalad. Likewise, the cord segment below the horizontal roots could have grown caudad, along with the caudad growth of the sacral vertebrae (**Fig. 21.8**). It is postulated that the segments above and below the horizontal nerve roots are under excessive tension as the cause of TCS in this patient.

The growth rate of the dura, within which the tension is higher than within the spinal cord,[9] must be the same as that of the vertebral column because the dural exits of nerve roots

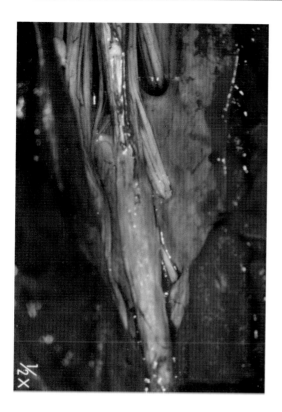

Fig. 21.6 Case 2. This 72-year-old man had a 9-month history of back and leg pain associated with weakness and numbness in the distal legs. A fibroadipose filum was found tethering the spinal cord at the L5 level.

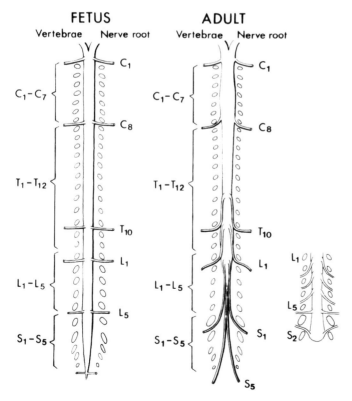

Fig. 21.7 The direction of the nerve roots as they approach the dural exits at 8 to 9 weeks gestation (left), in adulthood (middle), and in tethered spinal cord patients (right).

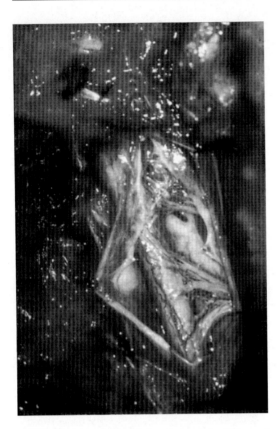

Fig. 21.8 The rootlets of the two consecutive cord segments travel in different directions (cephalad and caudad) and then merge through the same dural exit.

in adults and children remain at the same level as their foramina. The only exception is the sacral sac, which moves from the coccygeal to the S2 vertebral level. It can be concluded that the segments immediately above and below the horizontal nerve roots are under excessively high tension. These are usually the S2, S3, and S4 cord segments. Urinary incontinence was a complaint of these patients.

Surgical Treatment for Tethered Cord Syndrome due to Other Mechanisms

The prognosis of TCS is influenced by the mechanical causes of the syndrome, including diastematomyelia or split spinal cord, scar formation after MMC repair, or dermoid attached

to the cord, and also by other factors such as syringomyelia, neurenteric cyst, and cloacal exstrophy.

Diastematomyelia and Split Spinal Cord

Pang extensively studied the split spinal cord and associated TCS.[28] True diplomyelia is rare and the term *split spinal cord* is preferred[29] From the authors' analysis of various reports,[21,30–33] diastematomyelia provides a unique mechanical cause of cord tethering. In patients with tethered spinal cord[21] or TCS with an inelastic filum[18] the lumbosacral cord is usually stretched between the tethering point and the attachment of the lowest pair of dentate ligaments to the cord. In diastematomyelia, the spinal cord is divided into two lateral halves by a midline bony septum. The following four mechanisms are considered to be responsible for cord stretching: (1) The upper edge of the bony septum incorporated with fibrous tissue, which includes the underlying dura and arachnoid membrane and pia mater, anchors the crotch (bifurcation) of the split cord (**Fig. 21.6**, left and middle). (2) The lower bony edge pushes caudad against the reunited split cords as the spine grows and the cord ascends cephalad rapidly[30] (**Fig. 21.9**, right). (3) The fibrous filum terminale tethers the united spinal cord caudad. The stretching effect on the short cord segment between the inelastic filum (tethering site) and the bony septum (counteracting site) is accentuated with rapid spine growth.[29,31] (4) In some cases, each of the split cords is continuous to a separate filum. Both or one of the half cords, if inelastic, can contribute to TCS development.[34] In addition, congenital dysgenesis of the spinal cord must be considered as a possible cause of neurological deficits. These various factors produce different neurological conditions. The vertebral level of the septum and the location of the elongated cord mainly determine the level of neurological signs. For instance, the bony septum located in the high lumbar (above L2) or thoracic cord causes upper motor neuron lesions. The septum in the caudal portions of an elongated cord causes

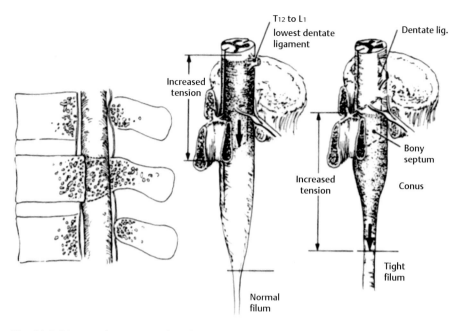

Fig. 21.9 Diagram showing spinal cord stretching in the presence of the diastematomyelic septum.

lower motor neuron lesions. Cord retethering due to scar formation, bony septum regrowth, or vertebral canal narrowing must be considered in cases of neurological recurrence after the surgical repair of the septum and dural scar.

Case 3

The following case is an example of diastematomyelia causing TCS. This 10-year-old boy presented with a 6 month history of numbness and weakness of his left leg, with a tendency to invert the left foot while running. At 2 years of age, he underwent repair of diastematomyelia. The right clubfoot was treated with tendon lengthening and casting at 4 years of age. The patient was able to compete in sports activities until 2 years before admission, when scoliosis was corrected with a Milwaukee brace. Hypalgesia in the left posterior thigh, ankle, and foot, and weakness of the dorsiflexors of the foot and toes and peroneus longus muscle were found. Deep tendon reflexes were hyperactive in his lower limbs except for an areflexic left ankle jerk. Babinski sign was present. Imaging

abnormalities included a wide lumbosacral interpedicular distance, a split spinal cord at the T12 vertebral level, and a thick filum in the lower lumbar and sacral canal.

At operation, subdural and arachnoid scar tissue was found to fill in the gap between two hemicords at the T12 level, extending to the anterior subdural space. The scar tissue was removed and the cord tissue was freed, without finding bony septum or dural reformation between the hemicords. The spinal cord was slightly relaxed. However, the caudal end of the spinal cord was tethered by a thickened fibrous filum (**Fig. 21.10A**). The filum was sectioned and the spinal cord ascended cephalad, forming a 1.5 cm gap between the upper and lower ends of the sectioned filum (**Fig. 21.10B**).

After surgery, the sensory deficit disappeared and motor function improved. The patient could walk faster within 2 months. He returned to school in 6 weeks and regained nearly normal motor function in his lower limbs within 6 months.

Comment. This patient presented with the signs and symptoms of combined upper and

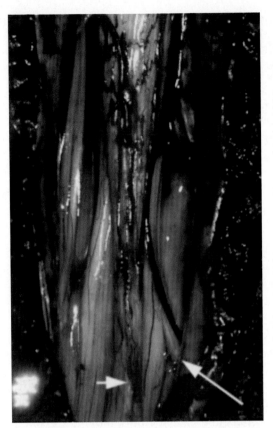

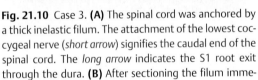

A

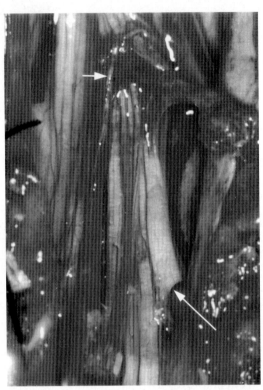

B

Fig. 21.10 Case 3. **(A)** The spinal cord was anchored by a thick inelastic filum. The attachment of the lowest coccygeal nerve (*short arrow*) signifies the caudal end of the spinal cord. The *long arrow* indicates the S1 root exit through the dura. **(B)** After sectioning the filum imme- diately below the attachment of the lowest coccygeal nerve to the cord, the conus ascended and was relaxed. The coccygeal nerve attachment (*short arrow*), which was below the S1 root (*long arrow*) before untethering, is now far above the same root.

lower motor neuron lesions. The former lesion was due to the traction of the cord by the scar-septum, formed after the diastematomyelia operation. The latter lesion was between the caudal end of the spinal cord and the septum. TCS lesions related to diastematomyelia may be produced above or below the septum, as demonstrated in **Fig. 21.9**.

Tethered Cord Syndrome following Myelomeningocele Repair

Scott described untethering procedures for the patients who developed TCS after repair of MMC in detail.[35] The authors describe one of the complicated cases below.

Case 4

The repair of an MMC is known to be followed by the delayed onset or progression of neurolog-ical signs and symptoms similar to TCS (Chapter 11) or true TCS.[33,35] This 22-year-old woman was admitted with complaints of progressive weakness in both distal lower limbs. The history of this patient dated back to less than 24 hours after birth when she underwent MMC repair. Although she never had bladder and bowel con-trol (which required intermittent catheteriza-tion), her motor and sensory function remained normal.

She continued to swim but gave up basketball because jumping and running caused urinary incontinence. About 1 year before admission, the patient began to have numbness and pain in both legs and difficulty running. Neurological signs consisted of weakness of the extensor hallucis longus and brevis muscles bilaterally and the peroneus longus muscle on the left, hypalgesia in the dorsum of both feet and in the perianal area (corresponding to the S3–5 dermatomes), bilateral hyporeflexia of the Achilles tendons, bilateral high-arched feet and right-sided hammertoes, scoliosis, and exaggerated lordosis. A postural pain triad was present (Chapter 15). MRI showed a posteriorly displaced elongated cord.

After L5–S2 laminectomy, the dura and arachnoid were opened in the midline, and the elongated cord was found 0.5 to 1.0 mm underneath the intermediate arachnoid. Scar tissue connecting the arachnoid as well as the intermediate arachnoid (Chapter 11) and the fibroadipose filum was removed and the spinal cord was isolated (**Fig. 21.11**). After complete dissection of the L5, S1, and S2 nerve roots, the caudal spinal cord was moved cephalad, with its tip 2 cm above the tethering level. In relation to the horizontally traveling L5 roots, the L4 roots ran caudad and the S1 roots cephalad to their dural exits, except some of the S1 anterior rootlets traveled caudad.

Postoperatively, the patient regained normal motor and sensory function within 2 weeks, except for the perianal sensory loss that slightly

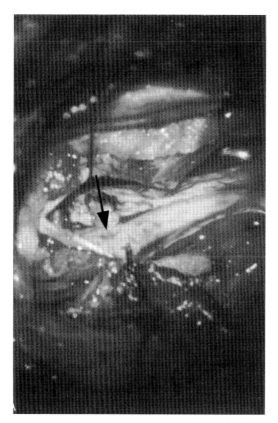
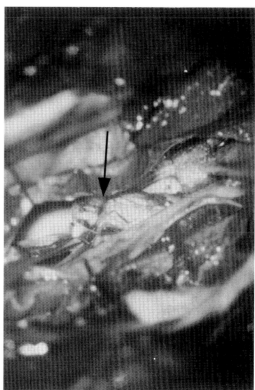

A   **B**

Fig. 21.11 Case 4. **(A)** Intraoperative photograph shows a fibroadipose filum continuous to the cord in the patient who presented with tethered cord syndrome after myelomeningocele repair (*arrow* indicates caudal end of the spinal cord). **(B)** The caudal part of the cord ascended and is slightly buckled (*arrow*) after the filum was removed.

decreased in area. The postural pain triad also disappeared, and she gained bladder sensation for the first time in her life, although she continues intermittent catheterization.

Comment. Motor and sensory dysfunction in the lower limbs was reversible because of its early manifestation. Bladder dysfunction could have been due to one of the following factors: (1) neuronal dysgenesis in the conus, (2) severe cord tethering during fetal growth, or (3) mechanical or circulatory damages to the conus before and after the first MMC repair. Cord tethering due to scar formation after MMC repair cannot be predicted, no matter how meticulously repair is done, particularly after the second or third repair (Chapter 11). During repair, however, it is important to pay special attention to the release of the caudal end of the cord.

Split Spinal Cord and Syringomyelia

Pang described that syringomyelia is often associated with split spinal cord.[28]

Case 5

The following case describes a patient with a combination of TCS and split spinal cord and later development of syringomyelia in the lumbosacral cord subsequent to an untethering procedure. This $3^1/_2$-year-old boy presented with progressive difficulty walking for 6 months. At birth, a lumbar MMC was found and repaired. He was well until 3 years of age, when he began to show weakness in the lower extremities, with inversion of both feet while walking. No bowel or bladder dysfunction was noted. CT showed a split spinal cord attached to the filum terminale. The residual MMC plaque was ~5 × 4 × 3 cm.

At operation, the spinal cord was found to be slightly looped inside the MMC. The spinal cord was split at the cephalic end of the MMC and reunited at its caudal end (**Fig. 21.12**). On sectioning the fibroadipose filum at the L5 level, its cephalic end ascended 7 mm and the spinal cord was relaxed. The arachnoid membrane was closed only at its cephalic and caudal ends with 8–0 nylon sutures, and the dural defect

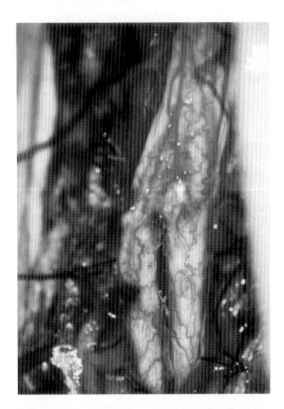

Fig. 21.12 Case 5. Intraoperative photograph shows the attachment of the small myelomeningoceles (*arrows*), which is located at the bifurcation of the split cord. The thick filum was sectioned below the reunion of the hemicords (beyond the photographic field).

was covered by a Silastic sheet graft, which was secured to the surrounding dural edge with 6–0 nylon sutures.

After the untethering procedure, the patient returned to normal activity within a few months. However, at the age of 10 years, he again noted inversion of the feet during walking. MRI demonstrated a swollen cord with an isolated syrinx at the L1–2 vertebral level. At operation, the Silastic sheet, which was surrounded by a thin membrane, was removed and the elongated spinal cord was exposed. The syrinx was found cephalic to the bifurcation of the split cord, and its inner wall was shiny and smooth.

Syringosubarachnoid shunting was performed, and the spinal cord regained its normal contour. The arachnoid membrane was closed

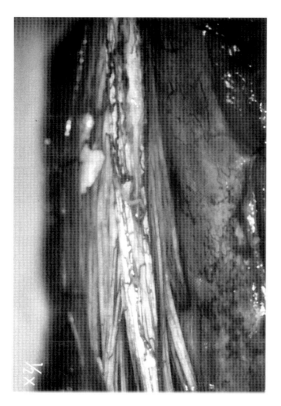

Fig. 21.13 The thickened hemicord (on the right) is continuous to an inelastic filum, whereas the thin hemicord is continuous to an elastic filum, and stretch test (Chapter 3) showed 50% elongation. The inelastic filum was sectioned for cord untethering.

watertight with 6–0 nylon sutures over the tube to secure cerebrospinal circulation before the dura was closed. By the time of discharge, the foot inversion had subsided, and he walked normally within 6 weeks.

Comment. The postoperative syringomyelia may be merely an enlargement of isolated hydromyelia, related to arachnoid adhesions, or stretch-induced central cord degeneration.[36]

There are also cases where only one of the split hemicords is tethered by a thick and inelastic filum (**Fig. 21.13**).

Cloacal Exstrophy

Cloacal exstrophy, a type of caudal agenesis, is a congenital malformation characterized by evagination of the intestines between two bladder halves, an imperforate anus, and an omphalocele. Spinal dysraphism can occur in association with cloacal exstrophy. Some spinal defects have been reported in association with cloacal exstrophy, including MMC,[37] LMMC, double discontinuous LMMC,[38] and lipomeningomyelocystocele.[39] Patients with an imperforate anus may have spinal deformities with varying degrees of neurological deficit.[40,41] In Cohen's study,[42] spinal abnormalities associated with cloacal exstrophy represent a spectrum of occult spinal dysraphism or skin-covered spina bifida. Carey et al described the omphalocele, exstrophy, imperforate anus, spinal defects (OEIS) complex.[43] The VACTER syndrome designates a combination of vertebral, anal, cardiac, tracheoesophageal, renal, and limb abnormalities, whereas VATER lacks the cardiac component.[28] As contrasted with spina bifida cystica (MMC), the skin overlying the back is closed in these syndromes, and there is a lesser degree of dysplasia of the spinal cord and its overlying tissues and no association with hydrocephalus or hindbrain malformation. Chapter 16 describes the clinical aspects of occult spinal dysraphism that has been treated surgically in adult TCS patients. Cloacal exstrophy is now considered a treatable problem with excellent survival rates and even the potential for urinary continence.[37,44–46]

Case 6

This patient was born at 34 to 36 weeks gestational age to a 41-year-old mother. During pregnancy, the mother took prenatal vitamins, Premarin (conjugated estrogen), Flexeril (chlorobenzaprine), and Butazolidin but denied any alcohol or tobacco use. Family history also revealed that the father was an exterminator who frequently used volatile gases and liquid insecticides, including trichlorobenzene, chlordane, pentachlorophenol, and benzene hexachloride. The pregnancy was complicated by premature labor. Upon physical examination of the infant, multiple congenital anomalies were noted: an omphalocele with a vesicle intestinal fissure, cloacal exstrophy, and an imperforate anus. Skeletal anomalies included severe sacral

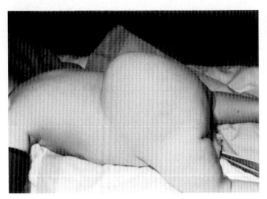

A

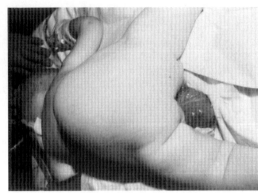

B

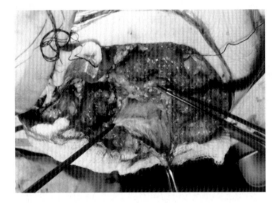

C

Fig. 21.14 Case 6. **(A)** Photograph, dorsal view of a patient with a large meningomyelocystocele. **(B)** Photograph showing an imperforate anus and cloacal exstrophy. **(C)** After opening fibroadipose tissue, the subdural components were exposed and a low-lying spinal cord was found surrounded by a membrane (held by a pair of fine forceps, to upper right) and the dura (held by the two pairs of heavier forceps).

dysgenesis and dysplasia with a left congenital hip dislocation, bilateral talipes equinovarus, and notable arthrogryposis of the knee joints. Abdominal ultrasound demonstrated mild hydronephrosis of the right kidney but no ureteral dilation.

In the lumbar area, there was a large skin-covered mass that was diagnosed as an LMMC (**Fig. 21.14A,B**). Neurologically, mild spastic paraparesis was seen with a sensory deficit at S1 and below. Chromosomal studies showed a normal 46XX pattern with no associated syndromes. A CT scan of the head showed a Chiari malformation associated with a slightly enlarged ventricular system.

The patient underwent surgical repair of the omphalocele and intestinal malformation and casting of both lower extremities for the skeletal deformities. Surgical repair of the lipomeningomyelocystocele and untethering of the spinal cord was performed 9 months

later. Thick adipose tissue surrounded the meningomyelocystocele extending from the L5 vertebral body to the lower sacrum, 15 cm in the vertical dimension and 25 cm in the horizontal dimension. The size of the myelomeningocystocele itself was almost spherical, 8 cm vertically and 10 cm horizontally. The spinal cord extended to the S2 vertebral level and was partly surrounded by the anterior meningocele sac. This portion of the cord was tethered by a fibrous scar that was part of the sac wall (**Fig. 21.14C**). Under the microscope, careful isolation of the spinal cord and nerve roots was performed. Optical studies of redox states of cytochrome a,a_3 were done before and after untethering of the spinal cord. Marked shifts from reduction toward oxidation of the cytochrome redox state after cord untethering were noted in the spinal cord segment 1 cm above the neck of the myelomeningocystocele. The oxidative shifts indicated an improvement in oxidative metabolism. Twelve years after surgery, the patient is ambulating quite well.

Neurenteric Cyst

A neurenteric cyst associated with TCS is also well known (Chapter 2). The signs and symptoms are similar to those due to diastematomyelia.

Scoliosis

There are three types of scoliosis: (1) congenital,[47] (2) idiopathic,[47] and (3) scoliosis associated with spinal dysraphism[11,12,24,32] or tumors.[48] The first and second types are beyond the scope of this book. Scoliosis is very common in the third category.[32] In the authors' observations, all TCS patients have some (mild to severe) degree of scoliosis, which subsides to various extents after untethering procedures. If complicated with congenital deformities due to such conditions as hemivertebrae,[49] facet deformity, unilateral pedicle fusion,[28] or spondylosis,[50] scoliosis worsens even after cord untethering, and corrective surgery of the spine may become necessary.

Case 7

The following case is an example of scoliosis associated with cord tethering. A 16-year-old high school boy, active in soccer, had been exhibiting progressive scoliosis since early childhood. Scoliosis became increasingly rotational (**Figs. 21.4, 21.15**), and for the past 1 or 2 years, he suffered from back and leg pain, especially after playing soccer. No neurological deficit was detected.

At operation, the inelastic filum was sectioned, and the spinal cord ascended and relaxed. Back and leg pain subsided immediately after surgery. A few months later, scoliosis was corrected by instrumentation, and he returned to soccer practice within 6 months.

Ependymomas and Tethered Spinal Cord

The patient harboring an ependymoma at the junction of the conus and the filum may present with TCS. A firm inelastic filum is always

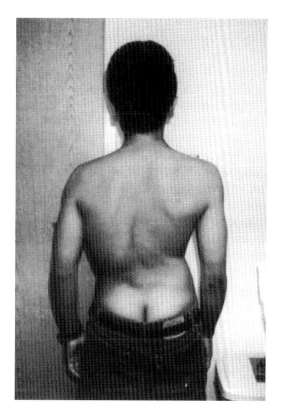

Fig. 21.15 The rotational scoliosis is to the left in the thoracic level and to the right in the lumbosacral level. The spinal cord takes a course in the concave side of the spinal canal to minimize cord tension. The patient was still able to touch his toes before the untethering procedure. The history is described in the text. The lateral view of this patient is seen in **Fig. 21.4**.

the mechanical cause of cord tethering, and the ependymoma is an incidental finding by MRI studies or at operative exposure. It is the authors' practice to expose the caudal end of the conus for filum resection to detect any abnormalities in the area. This can prevent future conus involvement by an enlarging ependymoma. The intraoperative or percutaneous endoscopy can easily identify an ependymoma before opening the dura or before the surgery if MRI studies suggest a small mass. Because the ependymoma may spread extensively into the conus in the future,

Case 8

This is an example of TCS with a coincidental conus ependymoma. This 50-year-old man had a $1^1/_2$-year history of progressive weakness in the left lower extremity along with back and left leg pain. The weakness was first noticed when the patient had difficulty running while playing tennis. This was followed by slapping his left foot while running and by difficulty in tiptoe walking. Pain in the low back and left leg gradually increased. He then began to notice thinning of the muscle bulk below the left knee. He denied difficulty in bladder or rectal control or sexual function. On examination, weakness of the extensor hallucis longus and brevis, tibialis anterior, and peroneus longus muscles, hypalgesia in the dorsum of the left foot, and hyporeflexia of the Achilles tendon were noted. The left foot was inverted on tiptoe walking. MRI indicated an intradural mass at the L1 and L2 vertebral level.

At operation, after L1 and L2 laminectomy and dural opening, a tumor was found underneath the arachnoid, originating from the caudal tip of the conus and upper filum. The soft vascular tumor was totally removed, including a pial capsule and the 0.3 cm long conus tip where two coccygeal nerves were exiting, and a 0.5 cm long portion of the filum. The fibrous inelastic filum was removed another 0.5 cm caudad to secure cord untethering. The cauda equina fibers surrounding the tumor were protected during tumor dissection.

Within 1 week after surgery, the patient regained normal strength of the extensor hallucis longus, and the other muscles have continued to improve. He returned to playing tennis in 6 months. Leg pain subsided over 6 months.

Tail or Dorsal Midline Proboscis

A tail that contains a coccygeal LMMC or meningomyelocystocele is often associated with TCS (Chapter 10). A rare case of dorsal midline proboscis that protruded from the upper lumbar canal is shown in **Fig. 21.16A–C**. A hemilipomyelomeningocele was found in the proboscis, which originated from one of the two compartments separated by a diastematomyelic septum.[51]

■ Conclusion

The following is a suggested selection process for conservative versus surgical treatment of TCS.

Group 1

For the patient who presents with progressive signs and symptoms typical for TCS and characteristic imaging, such as an elongated spinal cord continuous to a thickened, adipose filum or a tumor, or a posteriorly displaced filum, a consensus is that surgical untethering should be performed. Symptomatic patients with diastematomyelia should follow the same rule.

Group 2

Asymptomatic patients with MRI findings as described earlier have a potential TCS and must be followed carefully to detect even the slightest changes in signs and symptoms. For patients with a caudal or small transitional lipoma or LMMC, surgical removal or repair should be performed at an appropriate time around 4 years of age or even earlier (Chapter 11). A dermoid or epidermoid tumor may be treated similarly. A dermal sinus with a connection to the dura and the spinal cord, complicated with frequent recurrences of infection, may be removed earlier than 4 years of age.

Asymptomatic patients with a large caudal or transitional lipoma of LMMC need special consideration for the benefit and risks of surgical procedures. Surgical procedures for cord untethering or decompression are often limited to partial removal or repair of these anomalies. Even after meticulous dissection of fibroadipose tissue away from the spinal cord or nerve roots, circulatory deprivation might result in neurological deficits,[52] including urinary incontinence[39] (Chapters 7, 8, and 11). For this reason, surgical repair may be delayed until the patient

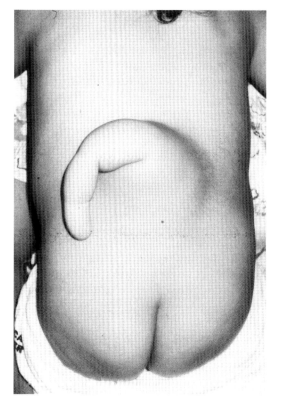

A

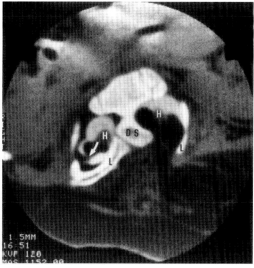

B

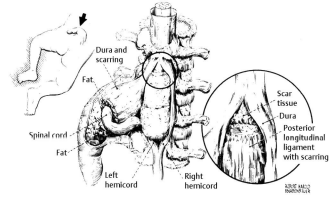

C

Fig. 21.16 (A) A case of lumbar proboscis found in an infant shows a hemispinal cord originated from the hemispinal canal and U-turns in the fingerlike protrusion. **(B)** The entire course of the hemicord is surrounded by a thin layer of meninges continuous to a lipomyelomeningocele by computed tomographic scan. **(C)** A reconstructive drawing shows the relationship of the split cords to the midline diastematomyelic septum.

develops neural tissue maturity and is prepared with homeostatic responses to surgical insult.

Asymptomatic patients with MRI evidence of an elongated cord anchored by a thick filum have a potential to develop TCS later. Prophylactic surgery, however, may not be necessary for patients who compensate by neural plasticity until 80 years of age. The question arises whether surgical treatment is indicated or justified in these patients after evaluating the risks.[19]

Group 3

The patient has mild signs and symptoms such as motor and sensory dysfunction, incontinence, or musculoskeletal deformities suggestive of TCS, but there are no typical imaging findings to indicate cord tethering. It is confusing to patients when various diagnoses have been offered by physicians on trying to explain their symptoms, particularly for those who were diagnosed to have failed back syndrome. Detailed reports on imaging (MRI or CT) studies often describe a lumbar or sacral disk hernia, protrusion, or bulging but often fail to describe neural structure. Differential diagnosis is made with detailed history taking and physical examinations (Chapters 4, 9, and 15), and additional MRI or CT findings such as posteriorly located conus and filum and capacious lumbosacral canal, and associated osteoarthritic changes. Axial MRI is helpful to determine if the conus or filum is touching the posterior arachnoid wall, particularly at the most prominent lordotic level (e.g., the lumbosacral joint, see case 1, **Fig. 21.5**) (Chapter 11). The posteriorly located structures such as osteoarthritic lamina, articular facet, or thickened ligamentum flavum functions like the bridge for violin strings when the patient extends the lumbosacral spine.

Lateral radiographic studies of the adult spine have shown that the canal length between the T10 and S2 vertebrae elongates by 1.5 cm on extreme flexion.[17] From our studies, the same canal elongates in 6-foot-tall men by 2.0 to 2.5 cm when they bend over the sink slightly. The patients with TCS complained of aggravation of back pain immediately in this position.

Group 4

Progressive or fluctuating signs and symptoms (back and leg pain, motor, sensory, or bladder dysfunction, or musculoskeletal deformities suggestive of TCS) are noted in patients who previously had stable neurological deficits with typical imaging characteristics. This patient must be followed closely for detection of any minor progression of neurological deficits, so that early treatment of the patient can be initiated.

References

1. Yamada S, Yamada BS, Won DJ. Tethered cord syndrome. In: Corcos J, Schick E, eds. The Textbook of the Neurogenic Bladder, 2nd ed. London: Informa. 2008:363–372

2. Tubbs RS, Salter G, Grabb PA, Oakes WJ. The denticulate ligament: anatomy and functional significance. J Neurosurg 2001;94(2, Suppl):271–275

3. Turnbull IM, Brieg A, Hassler O. Blood supply of cervical spinal cord in man: a microangiographic cadaver study. J Neurosurg 1966;24:951–965

4. Hoffman HJ, Taecholarn C, Hendrick EB, Humphreys RP. Management of lipomyelomeningoceles: experience at the Hospital for Sick Children, Toronto. J Neurosurg 1985;62:1–8

5. Barson AJ. The vertebral level of termination of the spinal cord during normal and abnormal development. J Anat 1970;106(Pt 3):489–497

6. Hawass ND, el-Badawi MG, Fatani JA, et al. Myelographic study of the spinal cord ascent during fetal development. AJNR Am J Neuroradiol 1987; 8:691–695

7. Reimann AF, Anson BJ. Vertebral level of termination of the spinal cord with report of a case of sacral cord. Anat Rec 1944;88:127–138

8. Vaughan VC III. Developmental pediatrics, growth and development. In: Nelson WE, Vaughan VC III, McKay RJ, eds. Textbook of Pediatrics. 9th ed. Philadelphia: WB Saunders; 1969:15–57

9. Tunituri AR. Elasticity of the spinal cord dura in the dog. J Neurosurg 1977;47:391–396

10. Sarwar M, Virapongse C, Bhimani S. Primary tethered cord syndrome: a new hypothesis of its origin. AJNR Am J Neuroradiol 1984;5:235–242

11. Yamada S, Iacono R. Tethered cord syndrome. In: Pang D, ed. Disorders of the Pediatric Spine. New York: Raven Press; 1995:159–173

12. McLone DG, Herman JM, Gabrieli AP, Dias L. Tethered cord as a cause of scoliosis in children with a myelomeningocele. Pediatr Neurosurg 1990-1991; 16:8–13

13. Yamada S, Schreider S, Ashwal S, et al. Pathophysiological mechanisms in the tethered spinal cord syndrome. In: Holtzman RNN, Stein BM, eds. The Tethered Spinal Cord. New York: Thieme-Stratton; 1985:29–40

14. Yamada S, Won DJ, Yamada SM. Pathophysiology of tethered cord syndrome: correlation with symptomatology. Neurosurg Focus 2004;16:E6

15. Warder DE, Oakes WJ. Tethered cord syndrome and the conus in a normal position. Neurosurgery 1993;33:374–378

16. Yamada S, Lonser RR. Adult tethered cord syndrome. J Spinal Disord 2000;13:319–323

17. Tani S, Yamada S, Fuse T, Nakamura N. [Changes in lumbosacral canal length during flexion and extension—dynamic effect on the elongated spinal cord in the tethered spinal cord]. No To Shinkei 1991;43: 1121–1125

18. Yamada S, Zinke DE, Sanders D. Pathophysiology of "tethered cord syndrome." J Neurosurg 1981;54: 494–503

19. Drake JM. Occult tethered cord syndrome: not an indication for surgery. J Neurosurg 2006;104(5, Suppl):305–308

20. Till K. Occult spinal dysraphism: the value of prophylactic surgical treatment. In: Sano K, Ishii S, LeVay D, eds. Recent Progress in Neurological Surgery (Excerpta Medica). New York: Elsevier; 1973:61–66

21. Hoffman HJ, Hendrick EB, Humphreys RP. The tethered spinal cord: its protean manifestations, diagnosis and surgical correction. Childs Brain 1976;2: 145–155

22. Sutton LN. Lipomyelomeningocele. Neurosurg Clin N Am 1995;6:325–338

23. Till K. Spinal dysraphism: a study of congenital malformations of the lower back. J Bone Joint Surg Br 1969;51:415–422

24. Pang D, Wilberger JE Jr. Tethered cord syndrome in adults. J Neurosurg 1982;57:32–47

25. Scully RE, Mark EJ, McNeely WF, et al. Case records of the Massachusetts General Hospital. Weekly clinicopathological exercises. Case 47-1992. A 25-year-old man with chronic intermittent coccygeal pain and mild bladder dysfunction. N Engl J Med 1992;327: 1581–1588

26. Yamada S, Iacono R, Morgese V, et al. Tethered cord syndrome in adults. In: Menezes A, Sonntag VK, eds. Principles in Spinal Surgery. New York: McGraw-Hill; 1996:433–445

27. Yamada S, Won DJ. What is the true tethered cord syndrome? Childs Nerv Syst 2007;23:371–375

28. Pang D. Split cord malformation. In: Pang D, ed. Disorders of the Pediatric Spine. New York: Raven Press; 1995:203–251

29. Moes CAP, Hendrick EB. Diastematomyelia. J Pediatr 1963;63:238–248

30. Guthkelch AN. Diastematomyelia with median septum. Brain 1974;97:729–742

31. James CCM, Lassman LP. Diastematomyelia and the tight filum terminale. J Neurol Sci 1970;10: 193–196

32. Keim HA, Greene AF. Diastematomyelia and scoliosis. J Bone Joint Surg Am 1973;55:1425–1435

33. McLone DG, Naidich TP. Myelomeningocele: outcome and late complications. In: McLaurin RL, Schut L, Venes JL, et al, eds. Pediatric Neurosurgery. 2nd ed. Philadelphia: WB Saunders; 1989:53–70

34. Yamada S, Yamada SM, Mandybur GT, Yamada BS. Conservative versus surgical treatment and tethered cord syndrome prognosis. In: Yamada S, ed. Tethered Cord Syndrome. Park Ridge, IL: American Association of Neurological Surgeons; 1996: 183–202

35. Scott RM. Delayed deterioration in patients with spinal tethering syndromes. In: Holtzmann RNN, Stein BN, eds. The Tethered Spinal Cord. New York: Thieme-Stratton; 1985:116–120

36. Schlesinger AE, Naidich TP, Quencer RM. Concurrent hydromyelia and diastematomyelia. AJNR Am J Neuroradiol 1986;7:473–477

37. Howell C, Caldamone A, Snyder H, Ziegler M, Duckett J. Optimal management of cloacal exstrophy. J Pediatr Surg 1983;18:365–369

38. Gorey MT, Naidich TP, McLone DG. Double discontinuous lipomyelomeningocele: CT findings. J Comput Assist Tomogr 1985;9:584–591

39. Vade A, Kennard D. Lipomeningomyelocystocele. AJNR Am J Neuroradiol 1987;8:375–377

40. Duhamel B. Embryology of exomphalos and allied malformations. Arch Dis Child 1963;38:142–147

41. Duhamel B. From the mermaid to anal imperforation: the syndrome of caudal regression. Arch Dis Child 1961;36:152–155

42. Cohen AR. The mermaid malformation: cloacal exstrophy and occult spinal dysraphism. Neurosurgery 1991;28:834–843

43. Carey JC, Greenbaum B, Hall BD. The OEIS complex (omphalocele, exstrophy, imperforate anus, spinal defects). Birth Defects Orig Artic Ser 1978;14: 253–263

44. Diamond DA, Jeffs RD. Cloacal exstrophy: a 22-year experience. J Urol 1985;133:779–782

45. Hurwitz RS, Manzoni GAM, Ransley PG, Stephens FD. Cloacal exstrophy: a report of 34 cases. J Urol 1987; 138(4 Pt 2):1060–1064

46. Mee S, Hricak H, Kogan BA, Molnar JJ. An 18-year-old woman born with cloacal exstrophy. J Urol 1986; 135:762–764

47. McGowan DP, Bernhardt M, White AA III. Biomechanics of the juvenile spine. In: Pang D, ed. Disorders of the Pediatric Spine. New York: Raven Press; 1995:27–50

48. Epstein FJ, Constantini S. Spinal cord tumors of childhood. In: Pang D, ed. Disorders of the Pediatric Spine. New York: Raven Press; 1995:371–388

49. Pang D. Tethered cord syndrome. Adv Pediatr Neurosurg 1986;1:45–79

50. Harvell JC Jr, Hanley EN Jr. Spondylolysis and spondylolisthesis. In: Pang D, ed. Disorders of the Pediatric Spine. New York: Raven Press; 1995:561–574

51. Yamada S, Mandybur GT, Thompson JR. Dorsal midline proboscis associated with diastematomyelia and tethered cord syndrome. Case report. J Neurosurg 1996;85:709–712

52. Cochrane DD. Cord untethering for lipomyelomeningocele: expectation after surgery. Neurosurg Focus 2007;23:1–7

Index

Note: Page numbers followed by f and t indicate figures and tables respectively.